Trauma Resuscitation

The team approach

Second Edition

Edited by:

Carl L. Gwinnutt MB BS FRCA
Consultant in Anaesthesia

Peter A. Driscoll BSc MD FFAEM
Consultant in Emergency Medicine
Hope Hospital, Manchester, UK

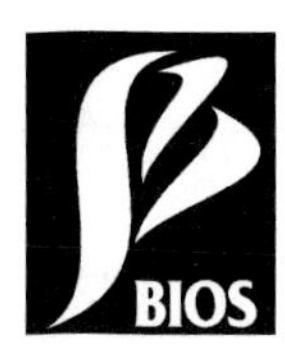

First published © The Macmillian Press Limited 1993
Second Edition © Bios Scientific Publishers Limited 2003

A CIP catalogue record for this book is available from the British Library.

ISBN 1 85996 009 X

BIOS Scientific Publishers Ltd
9 Newtec Place, Magdalen Road, Oxford OX4 1RE, UK
Tel. +44 (0)1865 726286. Fax +44 (0)1865 246823
World Wide Web home page: http://www.bios.co.uk/

Production Editor: Andrew Watts
Typeset by Phoenix Photosetting, Chatham, Kent
Printed by Bell & Bain, Glasgow, Scotland

Contents

Contributors

Professor David Alexander
Aberdeen Centre for Trauma Research
Bennachie
Royal Cornhill Hospital
Aberdeen

Glynne Andrew
Consultant and Honorary Senior Lecturer in Trauma and Orthopaedic Surgery
Hope Hospital
Salford

Damien Bates
Specialist Registrar
Department of Emergency Medicine
Hope Hospital
Salford

Danny Bryden
Consultant in Anaesthesia and Intensive Care Medicine
Royal Hallamshire Hospital
Sheffield

Simon Davies
Trauma Nurse Coordinator
North Staffordshire Hospital
Stoke-on-Trent

Peter Driscoll
Consultant and Honorary Senior Lecturer in Emergency Medicine
Hope Hospital
Salford

Susan Fletcher
Consultant Anaesthetist
Hope Hospital
Salford

Olive Goodall
Lead Nurse
Department of Emergency Medicine
Hope Hospital
Salford

Carl Gwinnutt
Consultant Anaesthetist
Hope Hospital
Salford

Nicola Hewer
Sister
Department of Emergency Medicine
Addenbrooke's Hospital
Cambridge

Chris Johnson
Consultant Anaesthetist
Southmead Hospital
Bristol

Philip Johnson
Charge Nurse
Department of Emergency Medicine
Hope Hospital
Salford

Tim Johnson
Consultant in Pain Management and Anaesthesia
Hope Hospital
Salford

Alan Kay
Consultant Plastic and Reconstructive Surgeon
Frenchay Hospital
Bristol

Peter Kelly
Consultant in Emergency Medicine
The Lister Hospital
Stevenage
Hertfordshire

Roop Kishen
Consultant in Anaesthesia and Intensive Care Medicine
Hope Hospital
Salford

Susan Klein
Thompson Research Fellow in Psychotherapy
Research Coordinator
Aberdeen Centre for Trauma Research
Bennachie
Royal Cornhill Hospital
Aberdeen

Kieran Lennox
Consultant in Anaesthesia and Intensive Care Medicine
North Staffordshire Hospital
Stoke-on-Trent

Lesley Light
Lead Nurse
Department of Trauma and Orthopaedics
Yeoville District Hospital
Somerset

Gabby Lomas
Senior Nurse Practitioner
Department of Emergency Medicine
Hope Hospital
Salford

Anthony McCluskey
Consultant in Anaesthesia and Intensive Care Medicine
Stepping Hill Hospital
Stockport

Peter Oakley
Consultant in Anaesthesia and Trauma
North Staffordshire Hospital
Stoke-on-Trent

David Patton
Consultant and Honorary Senior Lecturer in Maxillofacial Surgery
Morriston Hospital
Swansea

Richard Protheroe
Consultant in Anaesthesia and Intensive Care Medicine
Hope Hospital
Salford

Rory Rickard
Specialist Registrar
Department of Plastic and Reconstructive Surgery
Frenchay Hospital
Bristol

Susan Robinson
Consultant in Emergency Medicine
Addenbrooke's Hospital
Cambridge

Mark Scriven
Consultant General and Vascular Surgeon
Maelor Hospital
Wrexham

Aruni Sen
Consultant in Emergency Medicine
Maelor Hospital
Wrexham

Jasmeet Soar
Consultant in Anaesthesia and Intensive Care Medicine
Southmead Hospital
Bristol

Jill Windle
Lecturer Practitioner
Department of Emergency Medicine
Hope Hospital
Salford

Abbreviations

ABG	Arterial blood gases
ADH	Anti-diuretic hormone
AP	Anterioposterior
APLS	Advanced paediatric life support
ARDS	Acute respiratory distress syndrome
ASA	American Society of Anesthesiologists
ATNC	Advanced Trauma Nursing Course
ATLS	Advanced trauma life support
BAT	Blunt abdominal trauma
CI	Cardiac index
CK	Creatinine kinase
CO	Cardiac output
COX	Cyclo-oxygenase
CPAP	Continuous positive airway pressure
CPP	Cerebral perfusion pressure
CPR	Cardiopulmonary resuscitation
CRPS	Complex regional pain syndrome
CSF	Cerebrospinal fluid
CT	Computerized tomography
CVP	Cerebral venous pressure
DAI	Diffuse axonal injury
DIC	Disseminated intravascular coagulation
DIP	Distal interphalangeal
DPL	Diagnostic peritoneal lavage
DT	Delirium tremens
ECG	Electrocardiography
ED	Emergency Department
EDH	Extradural haematoma
ERCP	Endoscopic retrograde cholangio-pancreatography
FAST	Focused abdominal sonography for trauma
FBC	Full blood count
FDP	Flexor digitorum profundus
FDS	Flexor digitorum superficialis
GCS	Glasgow Coma Scale
GP	General Practitioner
GSW	Gunshot wound
HDU	High dependency unit
HPPF	Human plasma protein fraction
IABP	Intra-aortic balloon pump
ICH	Intracerebral haematoma
ICP	Intracranial pressure

ICU	Intensive care unit
IDH	Intradural haematoma
ISS	Injury severity score
iv	Intravenous
IVP	Intravenous pressure
JVP	jugular venous pressure
KE	Kinetic energy
LMA	Laryngeal mask airway
LSP	Life-saving procedures
LV	Left ventricular
LVEDP	Left ventricular end diastolic pressure
MAP	Mean arterial pressure
MILS	Manual inline stabilization
MODS	Multiple organ dysfunction syndrome
MOF	Multiple organ failure
MRC	Medical research council
MRI	Magnetic resonance imaging
MTOS	Major Trauma Outcome Study
NAI	Non-accidental injury
NSAID	Non-steroidal anti inflammatory drug
OER	Oxygen extraction ratio
PA	Posterioanterior
PAC	Pulmonary artery catheter
PAFC	Pulmonary artery flotation catheter
PAOP	Pulmonary artery occlusion pressure
PAT	Penetrating abdominal trauma
PCA	Patient controlled analgesia
PICU	Paediatric intensive care unit
PIP	Proximal interphalangeal
PTSD	Post traumatic stress disorder
PVR	Pulmonary vascular resistance
ROSPA	Royal Society for the Prevention of Accidents
RSD	Reflex sympathectomy dystrophy
RSI	Rapid sequence induction
RTA	Road traffic accident
RTS	Revised trauma score
RVEDP	Right ventricular end diastolic pressure
SCI	Spinal cord injury
SCIWORA	Spinal cord injury without radiological abnormalities
SDH	Subdural haematoma
SV	Stroke volume
SVR	Systemic vascular resistance
TARN	Trauma Audit Research Network
TNCC	Trauma Nursing Care Course
TOE	Transoesophageal echocardiography
TTE	Transthoracic echocardiography
VAD	Ventricular assistance device
VF	Ventricular failure

Preface

The evolution of trauma care in developed countries around the world has created new and exciting roles for all the personnel involved in the resuscitation and recovery of critically injured patients. The stress on strict roles for the nurse, doctor, paramedic and ancillary staff is now being replaced by a greater emphasis on the 'team approach'. This acknowledges the interactive nature of the procedures undertaken by the trauma team and the need for close cooperation at all stages of the resuscitation. It is an approach at its most successful when based on a formally organized team structure whereby tasks and roles are allocated appropriately. This enables procedures to be undertaken simultaneously, thereby reducing resuscitation times. In addition, it puts each member of the trauma team in the position of being responsible for evaluating the patient and the situation, anticipating the next most appropriate action even as one is being performed, and communicating with each member of the team to provide the best care.

This book has been created with this new vision of the multi-member trauma team in mind. The objective of the authors is to present a comprehensive view of trauma management and its sequelae that relates to both doctors and nurses involved with trauma resuscitation. The general approach to the clinical management of the patient is similar to that espoused by the internationally recognized Advanced Trauma Life Support Course (ATLS), the Advanced Trauma Nursing Course (ATNC) and the Trauma Nursing Core Course (TNCC).

In addressing both doctors and nurses, the book emphasizes the importance of all personnel involved having a good understanding of the pathophysiological changes underlying a trauma resuscitation. This enables greater cooperation between personnel and facilitates the anticipation of the patient's needs. Consideration is therefore given to the relevant mechanisms of injury, the physiological response to injury and a practical system of identifying and addressing life-threatening conditions. Trauma care is reviewed in a systematic way, body system by body system. In addition, in the chapters concerned with areas where injury is commonly life threatening, particular attention is paid to the applied anatomy and physiology of the normal system. Following this, the pathophysiological changes due to trauma and the clinical management of these patients is reviewed.

For further information, the interested reader is referred to the section at the end of each chapter. This lists both medical nursing literature which can be used to follow up on particular aspects of trauma care. We are also aware that protocols evolve in the lifetime of a book as further evidence becomes available. To cope with this a list of key websites are also listed so that topic updates can be easily obtained.

No attempt has been made to highlight either the nurses' or doctors' allocated tasks since the aim of the book is to emphasize the need for an integrated team approach. At certain points in the text however, the nurses' role has been stressed and technical procedures which, in the UK, would be mainly undertaken by doctors, have been highlighted for easy reference. The extent to which nurses and doctors carry out particular tasks will depend on training and local policy. With limitations in medical personnel, as seen in many countries, the trauma nurse could be expected to take over more of the doctor's role. In all situations though, the philosophy of the trauma team should be understood by all members, so that consistent good care can be achieved.

The authors recognize that trauma care is delivered in an expansive variety of settings. It is our desire to equip all personnel, no matter what environment in which he/she practises, with information that can assist them in developing the appropriate decision-making skills required in managing the injured patient. We are confident that *Trauma Resuscitation: The Team Approach* will help all carers to reach their potential as members of the trauma team and, by doing so, improve the patient's chances of returning to a full and active life.

Carl L Gwinnutt
Peter A Driscoll

Trauma websites

All the chapters in this book are referenced with websites that provide further information on the subject. There are millions of websites on the internet and these vary hugely in quality and accuracy. Below are a few simple rules to follow when using websites.

- The easiest way to find information on the web is by using a *search engine* and typing in key words. Different search engines have different ways of finding sites so they will not all give the same results. The main search engine used for this book was Google. At the end of each chapter there is a list of key words that may help you with your search. Some search engines are listed below:

  www.google.com
  www.yahoo.com
  www.altavista.com
  www.ask.co.uk

- Some websites act as *portals* to other sites. They have usually chosen a list of useful links to websites covering particular topics. Hopefully these sites have been vetted for quality and accuracy.
- *Accuracy.* Much of the information on the web has not been peer reviewed and may have been put on the web several years ago. A degree of judgement is usually required when looking at the site. Questions to ask include who wrote the site and is the site dated? Many sites are produced by professional associations and universities and tend to be of good quality; others are put together by individual enthusiasts and quality can vary immensely. Some sites are updated regularly while many languish in the past.
- *Ease of use.* Some complex sites may take a long time to download depending on the type of connection you use. Large images may also be slow to download. All the sites recommended are relatively straightforward to download from the web.
- *Journals.* Many journals are now available online. Whilst some are free, most require a subscriptions. The library in your hospital or university may have electronic subscriptions to journals. Your librarian should be able to assist you in obtaining access to journals online, by providing you with passwords for those journals the library has a subscription for.

Each chapter is followed by a list of sites that are specific to that subject. The sites listed below are general websites that cover a number of trauma topics. All the sites we have listed are free.

www.trauma.org

This is an excellent trauma website which includes interactive moulages.

http://www.swsahs.nsw.gov.au/livtrauma/default.asp

This is the trauma website of the Liverpool Hospital, Sydney, Australia. It has some useful sections on all aspects of trauma.

www.bestbets.org

Provides evidence-based answers to common clinical questions, using a systematic approach to reviewing the literature.

www.cdc.gov/ncipc/default.htm

US national injury prevention homepage: full of useful facts and figures and prevention issues.

www.update-software.com/ccweb/cochrane/revabstr/mainindex.htm

This site provides abstracts to the Cochrane database of evidence-based reviews.

http://freemedicaljournals.com/

This site gives a list of the journals that are currently freely available on the internet. This includes many trauma journals.

www.ncbi.nlm.nih.gov/entrez/query.fcgi

PubMed, a service of the National Library of Medicine, provides access to over 11 million MEDLINE citations back to the mid-1960s and additional life science journals. PubMed includes links to many sites providing full text articles and other related resources.

http://www.who.int/violence_injury_prevention/surveillance.htm

This is the WHO website containing international data on cause of death including trauma statistics.

www.cdc.gov/ncipc/default.htm

US national injury prevention homepage: full of useful facts and figures and prevention issues.

Jas Soar

Introduction

P.A. Driscoll

What is the size and extent of the problem?

The world is currently waging a war on its streets, in the work place and at home. At the start of this millennium the number of trauma deaths exceeded 3.2 million worldwide. In the UK alone, the annual number of deaths from trauma is 14.5 – 18,000, but the USA can boast a figure approximately ten times greater. Each day 3 thousand die and 30 thousand are seriously injured on the world's roads. Developing countries are reporting similar findings as road traffic crashes begin to exceed deaths due to infectious diseases. 85% of the deaths and 90% of the disability adjusted life years lost from road traffic crashes are in the low and middle-income countries. As in all wars, it is the youth of the country that takes the heaviest losses. It remains the most common cause of death in industrialized nations, in people under 35. However by 2020 it is anticipated that trauma will be the second or third leading cause of death in all countries.

Disability from trauma far exceeds the number of fatalities. For example 31 people in Portugal sustain some disability for every vehicular death and in the USA there are 19.4 million non-fatal injuries per annum (i.e. one every 2 seconds). Overall, casualties from this 'trauma war' occupy more hospital beds and cause the loss of more working days, than cancer and cardiac patients combined. For the British taxpayer, the cost of this slaughter is high – £2.22 billion per annum, i.e., around 1% of the gross national product (WHO estimation). In the USA, the figure is put at $400 billion. The final cost is even higher because there is a loss of national talent and tax revenue, in addition to the emotional and material consequences suffered by each family affected. The cumulative effect of trauma patients who survive, but in a crippled state, adds to the financial pressure.

What areas of the body are being injured?

Trauma is usually caused by a blunt mechanism in the developed world. This leads to multiple injuries, with usually one system severely affected and one-to-two others areas damaged to a lesser degree. Overall, the incidence of life threatening injuries in different systems is: head 30–70%, chest 20–35%, abdomen 10–35% and spine 5%. In excess of 40% of the trauma victims also have orthopaedic injuries but these are not usually life threatening.

When is death following trauma occurring?

In 1983, Trunkey's group at San Francisco General hospital reviewed 862 trauma deaths over a 2-year period. They concluded the fatalities occurred in one of three phases. The first peak is at, or shortly after, the time of injury. These patients die of major neurological or vascular injury and most are unsalvageable with present day technology but 40% could be avoided by various prevention programmes. UK data would support this conclusion.

In the US data, the second peak occurred several hours after the injury. These patients commonly die from airway, breathing or circulatory problems. The majority of these cases are potentially treatable. This period has become known as the 'golden hour' to emphasize the time following injury when resuscitation and stabilization are critical. UK data does not show a specific peak in this time frame. In England and Wales there is a steady fall off in the death rate over time. In contrast in Scotland there are very few deaths until the "third peak" described below.

This final peak in the US data occurs days or weeks after the injury. These victims are dying from multiple organ failure, acute respiratory disease syndrome or overwhelming infection. It is now known that inadequate resuscitation in the immediate or early post injury period leads to an increased mortality rate during this phase.

Is trauma care getting better in the UK?

In 1988, a Royal College of Surgeons' investigation on 11 health districts in England and Wales found that a third of the trauma deaths, occurring after arrival in hospital, were preventable. These deaths resulted from missed diagnosis, hypoxia, continuing haemorrhage and lack of timely surgery.

Lecky *et al* summarised the progress made by 2001. They found there had been a 3% reduction in the overall severity adjusted odds of death in England and Wales. Of interest was that most of this improvement occurred before 1994 and appeared to correspond to the increase in consultant presence in the initial management of severely injured patients (i.e., ISS over 15) (25% in 1989 to 40% in 1994). There was also a rapid spread of the advanced trauma courses (e.g., ATLS, TNCC, ATNC). After 1994, the mortality rate has remained steady with the best 10% of hospitals having a standardised mortality rate difference of 85 compared to the bottom 10%.

It is not clear why progress has stopped. One possibility is that the UK never took on board the development of whole trauma systems as advocated in North America. Consequently they go to the nearest hospital rather than the most appropriate. Furthermore, within the receiving hospital itself the organised trauma care found in many resuscitation rooms may not continue once the patient goes to theatre or the ward.

Are there problems with the current system of managing the trauma victims in the UK?

Prevention

There are few cases that are true 'accidents', i.e., "an event without apparent cause". For example, the man who crashes his car after drinking alcohol has **not** had an accident. All traumatic events are an interaction between host, agent, social culture and the legal system. The Transport and Road Research Laboratory (UK) estimates that 65% of road traffic "accidents" were due to human error. 80% of the pedestrians injured were themselves at fault, with children and the elderly being the worst offenders.

The link between alcohol abuse and many types of injury has been well documented. In the UK it is a factor in at least 28% of all fatal car crashes, and in the USA, 40–50%

of the people dying following trauma have a blood alcohol level greater than 100 mg%. Alcohol can also influence the clinical course of the patient by affecting the diagnostic signs and physiological and immunological response to trauma. Compared to alcohol, other drugs cause fewer road traffic crashes. Nevertheless the incidence of prescription and illegal substances being found in road users is increasing.

Prevention by legislation has been used effectively in various countries over the past years, with laws on smoke alarms, flame resistant clothing, drink/driving, seat belts, child car seats, car design and motorcycle helmets being introduced. Education has also been used to some effect. Unfortunately, trauma, like all diseases, is more common in the socially deprived and would be improved by material changes in the social conditions.

Prehospital care

The standard of care in the pre-hospital phase varies significantly between countries as well as between districts inside the same country. Studies from the UK have shown an increase in pre-hospital time over the years. This is likely to be due to the increase in the use of advanced skills by paramedics. Unfortunately this increase in expertise is not matched by an increase in survivors. Indeed there is evidence to show that using advanced skills in the critically ill patient increases their chance of dying. It would appear these patients need to rapidly transported to an appropriate facility where anaesthetic or surgical intervention can be carried out quickly. In contrast patients who are haemodynamically stable do benefit from advanced care at the scene of the incident and go onto have lower disability scores once they leave hospital. What is required therefore are trained paramedics who can judge when to intervene and when to move. Unfortunately the current UK paramedic receives little audit and feedback on their management of the patients and so there is no accumulation of knowledge and experience. This situation is perpetuated by there being little medical input into the service and the very limited communications between the hospital and the on site team. The result is a profession that is not utilizing its post training learning experiences.

On Admission

In Briton, trauma victims frequently arrive late at night when inexperienced junior doctors staff the Emergency departments. This can lead to delays in getting senior help once the clinician realizes there is a problem. There are also difficulties in carrying out necessary investigations and prioritising patients' injuries. Delays in carrying out the life saving procedures (LSP) have to be prevented as this has a strong (negative) correlation with physiological changes in the patient in the resuscitation room. The time for the LSP also affects the overall survival of the trauma patient.

Trauma teams are not exclusive to Trauma Centres. Indeed many District General hospitals (or their equivalent in Europe and the USA) have such teams. This has the theoretical advantage of bringing together a group of people with the appropriate expertise to manage the multiply injured patient. In the UK, the teams usually comprise junior doctors with limited experience in handling the complex problem of trauma management. The organization of the teams is informal with members arriving at different times and carrying out procedures in an ad hoc manner. There is no overall co-ordination and no allocation of duties to the team members. There is also no national guidance on the organization of the ideal trauma team, its structure and who should be in charge.

Once resuscitation starts the next problem encountered is the poor knowledge base for the management of the pathophysiological changes after trauma. Reliance is put on clinical skills and inadequate monitoring devices recording variables such as blood pressure and heart rate. This leads to lesser degrees of hypoxia and hypovolaemia not being recognized, resulting in too little oxygen and fluid being given too late. It is therefore not surprising that hypoxia and hypovolaemia are the chief causes of preventable death in industrialized nations.

The role of the team in trauma care

It can be seen from the previous discussion that there is considerable scope for improvement in all aspects of trauma care. A fully integrated team of trained nurses and doctors needs to be present to deal with the trauma victim when he arrives at the hospital. An efficient, organized resuscitation needs to be commenced which leads to initial stabilization, diagnosis and definitive management.

It has been shown that the most efficient team organization is achieved by having each team member carrying out individual tasks simultaneously. This process is known as 'horizontal organization'. The least efficient technique in which each task is carried out sequentially, is known as 'vertical organization. If tasks are to be performed simultaneously, precise allocation of tasks to team members is essential, or there is chaos. Each procedure is divided into manageable units and allocated to individual team members by a designated nursing and medical team leader. These tasks must be divided evenly among the team to prevent overloading of any particular member.

When these organizational changes are introduced significant reductions in resuscitation times can be achieved. In particular, the time to carry out the life saving procedures is shortened and this is known to correlate with the short and long term survival of the patient.

The initial management of the trauma victim can be a difficult and stressful time, which could easily become overwhelming without prior planning. The allocation of staff to specific roles within the team, relieves the stress and ensures that the department functions safely, whilst the injured patient receives immediate assessment and life saving intervention.

To enable these organizational changes to be introduced, the team members have to have the skills to carry out the particular tasks. A key way of achieving this is by having all the staff dealing with trauma victims, complete an Advanced Trauma course. To this should be added specific training in team work and leadership so that the group functions as a unit rather than collection of individuals with no common aim. This certainly should be the aim for the future. Until this is achieved however, the necessary organizational changes required for the team approach can still be made with appropriate departmental or hospital training. The following chapters provide information on which these changes can be based. For those who have already completed the above courses, the following chapters will act to reinforce the knowledge and skills acquired and hopefully act as a spurt to encourage others to undertake similar training.

References and further reading

Anderson I, Woodford M, De Dombal F et al. Retrospective analysis of 1000 deaths from injury in England and Wales. *BMJ* 1988; **296:** 1305–8.
Anderson I, Woodford M, Irving M. Preventability of death from penetrating injury in England and Wales. *Injury* 1989; **20:** 69–71.
ATLS for doctors, Course manual. 6th Edition. The American College of Surgeons Committee on Trauma, The American College of Surgeons, 1997, Chicago.
Boyd C, Tolson M. Evaluating trauma care: the TRISS method. *J Trauma* 1987; **27:** 370–378.
Committee on trauma. Hospital and prehospital resources for optimal care of the injured patient. Am C Surgeons Bull 1986; 71.
Driscoll P, Vincent C. Variation in trauma resuscitation and its effects on outcome. *Injury* 1992; **23:** 111–115.
Driscoll P, Vincent C. Organizing an efficient trauma team. *Injury* 1992; **23:** 107–110.
Driscoll P. Trauma: today's problems, tomorrows answer. *Injury* 1992; **23:** 151–158.
Lecky F, Woodford M, Bouamra O, Yates D. Lack of change in trauma care in England and Wales since 1994. *EMJ* 2002; **19:** 520–23.
Lecky F, Woodford M, Yates D. Trends in trauma care in England and Wales 1989–97. *Lancet* 2000; **355:** 1771–5.
Nantulya V, Reich M. The neglected epidemic: road traffic injuries in developing countries. *BMJ* 2002; **324:** 1139–41.
Nicholl J, Hughes S, Dixon S, Yates D. The costs and benefits of paramedic skills in pre-hospital trauma care. HMSO 1998, London.
Roberts I, Abbasi K. War on the roads. *BMJ* 2002; **324:** 1107–8
Royal College of Surgeons Report. The management of patients with major injuries. Report of a Working Party 1988; Royal College of Surgeons, London.
TNCC Course manual (second edition). Emergency Nurses Association 1988, Award Printing Corporation, Chicago, Illinois.
Trunkey D. Trauma. Scientific America 1983; **249:** 28–35
West J, Trunkey D. Systems of trauma care: a study of two counties. *Arch Surg* 1979; **114:** 455–460.
Wyatt J, Beard D, Gray A, Busuttil A, Robertson C. The time of death after trauma. *BMJ* 1995; **310:** 1502.

1 Resuscitation and stabilization of the severely injured patient

P Driscoll, D Bates, G Lomas

Objectives

The objectives of this chapter are:

- to understand the structure and function of a trauma team;
- gain an overview of the whole of the management of the patient in the resuscitation room.

Many of the points mentioned will be reinforced and described in greater detail in the ensuing chapters. The reader may find it useful, therefore, to concentrate initially on the team structure and function. After studying Chapters 2, 3 and 4, this chapter should then be re-read so that the clinical issues described can be considered.

1.1 Introduction

The efficient management of the severely injured patient is dependent on a team approach and a predetermined system to guide the personnel through the initial assessment and life-saving procedures. These two essential elements will enable each member to carry out their allotted task simultaneously. In so doing, the time to resuscitate the patient is reduced, and his chances of surviving increased.

It is important, therefore, that each member of the team is familiar with both their own role and that of their colleagues. Accordingly, a comprehensive view of the medical and nursing management of the trauma patient is given so that members of the team can:

- see where their role fits into the overall organization;
- appreciate the importance of their role;
- anticipate what may be required as the resuscitation progresses;
- extend their role in an emergency.

1.2 Pre-hospital information and communication

The Emergency Department (ED) usually receives some warning, via ambulance control, that a severely injured patient is about to arrive. This time is best spent marshalling, briefing and preparing the trauma team. The increasing use of telemedicine systems also allows direct contact between the paramedic crew and the receiving hospital, thus the paramedical staff can receive advice while providing hospital staff with essential information (Box 1.1).

BOX 1.1	Essential pre-hospital information
	- Nature of the incident - Number, age and sex of the casualties - The patients' complaints, priorities and injuries - Airway, ventilatory and circulatory status - The conscious level - The management plan and its effect - Estimated time of arrival

Detail of the mechanism of the injury is crucial as it gives valuable information about the forces the patient was subjected to, particularly the direction of impact. Further help comes from a description of the damage to vehicles or the weapon used (*Figure 1.1*) which will often be provided by the pre-hospital team.

1.3 The trauma team

The group of nurses and doctors who make up the trauma team need to be summoned once the pre-hospital information is received, and should all be in place when the patient arrives. The personnel must be immediately available and pre-organized to ensure that any delays are avoided.

1.3.1 Team members

The trauma team should comprise the following nursing, medical and radiological staff:

Nursing staff

- A nursing team leader.
- An 'airway nurse'.

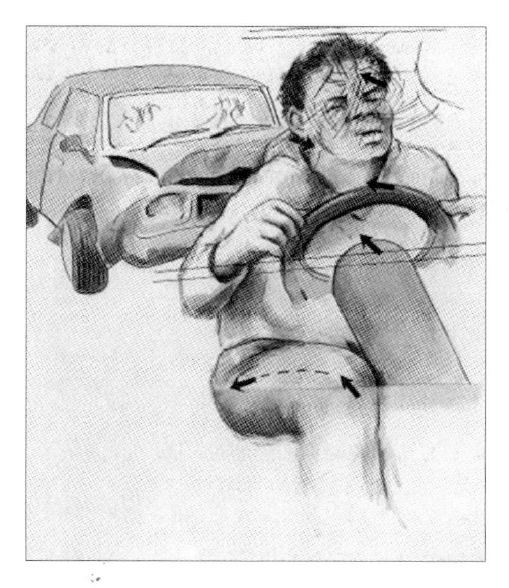

Figure 1.1 Diagram of a frontal road traffic accident. Arrows indicate areas of potential injury.

- Two 'circulation nurses'*.
- A recording nurse.
- A 'relatives' nurse.

Medical staff

- A medical team leader.
- An 'airway doctor'.
- Two 'circulation' doctors*.

Radiographer*

In all cases, the nursing and medical personnel chosen for the respective roles must be appropriately trained. Seniority per se is no guarantee of competence!

1.3.2 Objectives of the trauma team

- To identify and treat life threatening injuries.
- To identify other problems and arrange appropriate investigation and treatment.
- To arrange and transfer to definitive care.

On first sight it appears that many personnel will be taken away from the department for a long time. However, the aim is to achieve an efficient and rapid correction of all the immediately life-threatening conditions. Once this has been completed, only the core personnel need to remain and those marked with an asterisk can return to their normal duties.

1.3.3 The roles of the team members

Each member has to be thoroughly familiar with his/her respective duties so that tasks can be performed simultaneously for the maximum benefit of the patient in the shortest possible time. It is also essential that problems are anticipated rather than reacted to once they develop. When nurses and doctors pair up to tackle the various tasks, the efficiency of the team improves. However, assignments may vary between units depending on the resources available and the skill of the personnel.

Team leaders

Nursing team leader

- Coordinates the nursing team.
- Prepares sterile packs for procedures.
- Assists the circulation nurses and brings extra equipment as necessary.

Medical team leader

- Coordinates the specific tasks of the individual team members.

- Examines the patient.
- Assimilates and records the clinical findings from other members of the team.
- Arranges investigations in order of priority.
- Liaises with specialists who have been called.
- Question the ambulance personnel to ascertain the mechanism of injury, the pre-hospital findings and the treatment given so far.
- Depending on the skills of the rest of the team, carries out particular procedures, such as diagnostic peritoneal lavage (DPL) or chest drain insertion.

Airway personnel

Airway nurse

- Assists in securing the airway and stabilizing the cervical spine.
- Establishes a rapport with the patient giving psychological support throughout his ordeal in the resuscitation room. Ideally all information should be fed through her to the patient.

Airway doctor

- Clears and secures the airway whilst taking appropriate cervical spine precautions.
- Ensures adequate ventilation with a high concentration of oxygen.

Circulation personnel

Circulation nurses

- Assists with the removal of the patient's clothing.
- Assists with insertion of iv infusions, chest drain and urinary catheterization.
- Connects the patient to the monitors and measures the vital signs.
- Monitors the fluid balance.
- Assists in special procedures, for example a thoracotomy.
- Commences chest compressions if cardiopulmonary resuscitation is required.

Circulation doctors

- Assists in the removal of the patient's clothes.
- Establishes peripheral intravenous infusions and takes blood for investigations.
- Carries out certain procedures, for example chest drain insertion, urinary catheterization.
- Carries out other procedures depending on their skill level.

Recording nurse

- Keeps contemporaneous records of the patient's vital signs, fluid infusions and drug administration.
- Notes times of interventions and arrival of other specialities.
- Helps with filling in request cards and liasing with laboratories.

Relatives nurse

- Cares for the patient's relatives when they arrive.
- Liases with the trauma team to provide the relatives with appropriate information and support.
- Accompanies the relatives if they wish to be present in the resuscitation room.

Radiographer

- Takes two standard x-rays of the chest and pelvis on all patients subjected to blunt trauma. A more selective approach is used with victims of penetrating trauma.

To avoid chaos and disorganization, there should be no more than six people physically touching the patient. The other team members must keep well back.

1.4 Preparation

It is the nurses' responsibility at the beginning of every shift to ensure that the resuscitation room is fully stocked and the equipment in working order and ready for use. Therefore only minimum preparation should be necessary immediately prior to the arrival of the patient. Before the patient arrives, the trauma team should assemble in the resuscitation room and ideally each member should undertake universal precautions. However, if these are not available, rubber gloves, plastic aprons and glasses must be worn, as all blood and body fluids should be assumed to carry HIV and hepatitis viruses. Whilst protective clothing is being put on, the team leaders should brief the personnel, ensuring that each member knows the task for which they are responsible. A final check of the equipment, by the appropriate team members can then be made.

Trauma victims often have sharp objects such as glass and other debris in their clothing, hair and on their skin. Ordinary surgical gloves give no protection against these, consequently the personnel undressing the patient must initially wear robust gloves.

1.5 Reception and transfer

On arrival the patient should be triaged using a recognized system and, when appropriate, transferred to the resuscitation room. Once there, the nursing team leader needs to start a stop clock or note the time accurately, so that the times of events can be recorded.

Most trauma patients will arrive immobilized on a long spinal board that facilitates the transfer from the stretcher to the ED trolley. Nevertheless, this manoeuvre must be coordinated to avoid rotation of the spinal column and exacerbation of pre-existing injuries (*Figure 1.2*). Team members should also check that lines and leads are free so that they do not become disconnected or snagged. If the victim is not on any lifting device, six people are required for transfer. The team must be well drilled in this technique and coordinated by a team leader experienced in the safe transfer of patients with possible spinal trauma. One of the airway personnel should stabilize the head and neck, as four lift the patient from the side and a sixth removes the ambulance trolley.

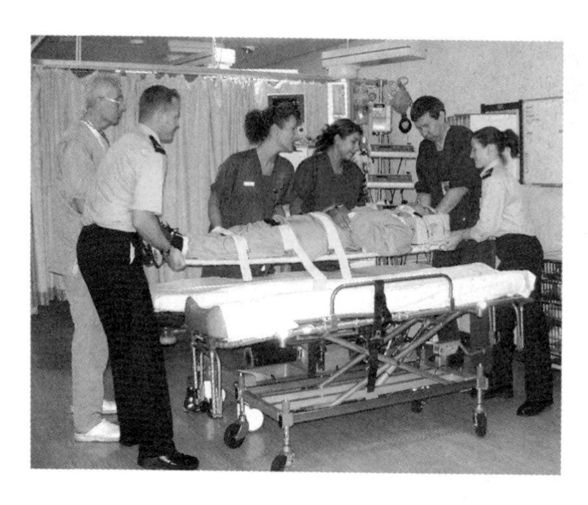

Figure 1.2 Patient being lifted onto a trolley on a back board

1.6 Assessment and management

Management now consists of a three-phase approach followed in all patients, consisting of:

(i) primary survey and resuscitation;

(ii) secondary survey;

(iii) definitive care.

1.6.1 Primary survey and resuscitation

The objective of this phase in the resuscitation is to identify and treat any immediately life-threatening conditions. While every patient is nursed as an individual, the team must follow a strict routine in order to perform efficiently. Five parameters are dealt with in the order in which, if untreated, they would lead to the death of the casualty:

A: Airway and cervical spine control

B: Breathing

C: Circulation

D: Dysfunction of the CNS

E: Exposure and environment

Although the tasks are described sequentially they should be carried out simultaneously, whilst at the same time, information is obtained from the ambulance personnel (see later).

Airway and cervical spine control

Although ensuring a patent airway is of paramount importance, the airway personnel must initially assume the presence of a cervical spine injury, particularly if the patient is a victim of blunt trauma or if the mechanism of injury indicates this region may have been damaged (see Section 7.3). Consequently, none of the activities used to clear and secure the airway must result in movement of the head or neck (*Figure 1.3*).

While the airway nurse manually immobilizes the cervical spine, the airway doctor talks to the patient. This not only establishes supportive contact, but also can be used

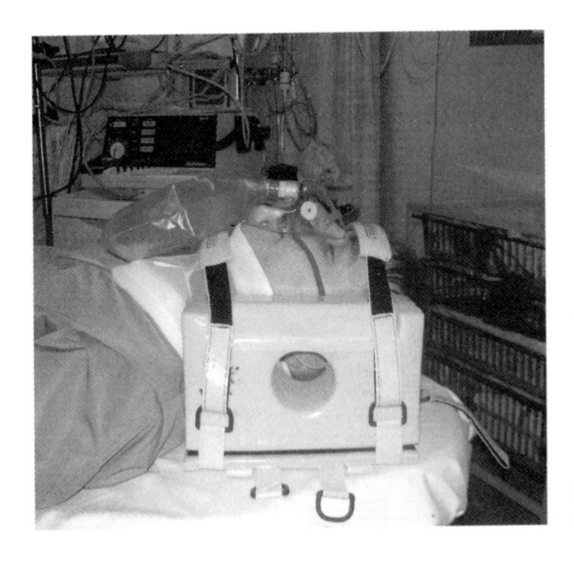

Figure 1.3 Neck stabilization with semirigid collar, blocks and tape

to assess the airway. If the patient replies with a normal voice, giving a logical answer, then the airway can be assumed to be patent and the brain adequately perfused with oxygenated blood. An impaired or absent reply indicates that the airway could be obstructed, the most common cause of which is the tongue. This must be pulled forward using either the chin lift or jaw thrust techniques (see Section 2.4). In the unconscious patient, the airway can initially be maintained by the insertion of an oropharyngeal (Guedel) airway, or if the mouth cannot be opened, a nasopharyngeal airway. Relative contraindications to the use of this device are facial injuries or possible base of skull fracture. If this does not improve the situation the airway must be checked for obstruction. Vomit or other liquid debris is best removed with a rigid sucker; pliable suckers are more likely to kink and obstruct. If passed nasally, they can also enter the cranial vault in the presence of a fractured cribriform plate (see Section 2.4.1). If the patient has a pharyngeal (gag) reflex, he is capable of maintaining his own airway and no attempt must be made to insert an oral airway as this may precipitate vomiting, cervical movement and a rise in intracranial pressure (ICP). Again a nasopharyngeal airway may be tried in these situations because it is less likely to stimulate a gag reflex.

Trauma victims rarely have empty stomachs. In combination with chest and abdominal injuries and alcohol ingestion there is a high risk of vomiting and aspiration of gastric contents. Therefore in the absence of a gag reflex early endotracheal intubation is required to minimize this risk. This needs to be carried out by medical members of the team with adequate anaesthetic training and experience, using the procedures described in Section 2.6.

If the patient starts to vomit while still immobilized on a spinal board, they can be turned on their side. If not on a board, the trolley should be tipped head down and the vomit sucked away as it appears in the mouth. It is impractical to nurse the patient on their side, so until airway protection is achieved constant supervision is necessary.

Once the airway has been cleared and secured, 100% oxygen should be administered. In the spontaneously breathing patient this is via a nonrebreathing mask with a reservoir, attached to a high flow (12–15 l/min) oxygen source. If intubated, he should be ventilated with an appropriate breathing system.

Once the airway has been secured, the neck is inspected quickly for:

- swellings and wounds, which can indicate there is local injury or damaged blood vessels;
- subcutaneous emphysema from a pulmonary, pharyngeal or oesophageal injury;
- tracheal deviation resulting from a tension pneumothorax (see below);
- distended neck veins indicate there is a rise in the central venous pressure. This can result from a tension pneumothorax, cardiac tamponade or damage to the great vessels (see Section 3.4);
- laryngeal crepitus indicating laryngeal trauma.

To enable the airway nurse now safely to release the patient's head and neck, the cervical spine needs to be secured using a semirigid collar and head blocks. The only exception to this rule is the restless patient who will not keep still. In this case, immobilizing the head and neck whilst allowing the rest of the patient's body to keep moving can damage the cervical spine. A suboptimal level of immobilization is therefore accepted, consisting of only a semirigid collar.

Breathing

There are five immediately life-threatening thoracic conditions which must be searched for, and if found treated (Box 1.2).

The earliest clues as to whether any of these conditions exist are the respiratory rate and effort. These need to be monitored at frequent intervals by one of the circulation nurses, as they are very sensitive indicators of underlying lung pathology. At the same time, the medical team leader should inspect both sides of the chest, assessing the patient's respiratory effort, colour and for signs of trauma. Any obvious injury, the use of accessory muscles of respiration or paradoxical chest movement must be noted. This is followed by auscultation and percussion in the axillae, to assess ventilation of the periphery of the lungs. Listening over the anterior chest mainly detects air movement in the large airways, which can give a false impression of the adequacy of ventilation. Consequently, differences between the two sides of the chest can be missed, especially if the patient is being artificially ventilated.

If there is a difference in air entry and percussion note between the right and left sides of the patient's chest, there is usually a local thoracic problem. This may be the result of either a pneumo- or haemothorax. If a pneumothorax is suspected, it is vital to determine if it is under tension. A build-up of pressure in the pleural cavity can rapidly compromise the lungs and circulation with fatal consequences (see Section 3.4.1). If the findings support this diagnosis, a wide bore cannula connected to a syringe should be inserted into the second intercostal space in the midclavicular line on the affected side. The aim is to release the positive pressure in the chest. If there is sudden release of air, the diagnosis is confirmed and a chest drain can subsequently be inserted

BOX 1.2 Immediately life-threatening thoracic conditions

- Tension pneumothorax
- Cardiac tamponade
- Open chest wound
- Massive haemothorax
- Flail chest

on that side. Alternatively, if there is no rapid decompression of the pleural cavity, then an urgent chest x-ray must be taken before a chest drain is placed.

In the primary survey, only a massive haemothorax, over 1.5 l in volume is likely to be detected. Initial treatment consists of a chest drain, however there is usually enough time to confirm the clinical suspicion with a chest x-ray before this procedure is carried out.

If there is no air entry to both lungs, then there is either a complete obstruction of the upper airway, or an incomplete seal between face and mask. The maintenance of an effective seal is by no means simple and the airway personnel need to be skilled in the use of a bag and facemask. Ideally a two-person technique should be used, with one holding the mask on and pulling the patient's chin forward with both hands, whilst the other person squeezes the bag. Care must always be taken to maintain cervical immobilization. If this still fails then the airway doctor and nurse should prepare for urgent tracheal intubation.

Open chest wounds need to be covered initially with an Ashermann seal dressing and early insertion of a chest drain to prevent the development of a tension pneumothorax will also be required.

The immediate treatment of a flail segment of chest wall depends on the extent of the underlying pulmonary contusion. If the arterial partial pressure of oxygen is low, or if the patient is becoming exhausted, then he will require intubation and positive pressure ventilation (see Section 2.6).

Any penetrating injury that enters the area indicated in *Figure 3.6* may involve the heart. This can lead to a pericardial tamponade as blood collects in the pericardial sac. If it is suspected, the medical team leader, and one of the circulation nurses, should aspirate the blood using the sub xiphoid percutaneous approach (see Section 3.4.1).

Circulation

Any overt bleeding must be controlled by direct pressure using absorbent sterile dressings and covered with a compression bandage. Tourniquets are not used as they do not completely prevent bleeding and increase tissue damage.

One of the circulation nurses should measure the blood pressure and note the rate, volume and regularity of the pulse. An automated blood pressure recorder and electrocardiography (ECG) monitor must also be connected to the patient. At the same time, the medical team leader should determine if the patient demonstrates any clinical evidence of shock (see Section 4.6). Skin colour, clamminess, capillary refill time, heart rate, blood pressure, pulse pressure and conscious level must all be assessed. Intravenous access should be established using two wide bore peripheral cannulae. If this is not possible then cannulation of a central vein should be performed; in these circumstances, cannulation of the femoral vein can be useful as it avoids the risk of iatrogenic chest injury.

Once the first cannula is in position, blood is drawn for grouping, typing, or full cross-matching, full blood count, analysis of the urea and electrolytes, pregnancy test in women of childbearing age and a bedside blood glucose estimation should be performed. The cannula should not be jeopardized if it is difficult to aspirate blood. Instead, the intravenous (IV) infusion should be started and the required blood sample can then be taken from the femoral vein or artery. An arterial sample also needs to be obtained for blood gas and pH analysis, but can wait until the end of the primary survey.

The initial fluid for infusion can be either crystalloid or colloid; the debate over the type used continues without definitive evidence either way. The volume administered should be guided by: the site of bleeding, the volume lost and the patient's response. Early blood administration will be required in the haemodynamically unstable patient (see Section 4.7.1). To reduce the incidence of hypothermia, all fluids must be warmed before use.

1.6.1.4 Dysfunction

A rapid and gross assessment of the conscious level is made by asking the patient to put his tongue out, to wiggle his toes and to squeeze the clinician's fingers. The patient may respond spontaneously, following verbal command, to pain or not at all. This is known as the AVPU system (Box 1.3). Pupil size and reactivity must also be assessed. These tests will need to be augmented with a more detailed examination during the secondary survey.

It is important to remember that there a number of causes of a reduced level of consciousness apart from head injury (Box 1.4).

BOX 1.3 The AVPU system

- A – Alert
- V – Only responding to verbal stimulus
- P – Only responding to pain
- U – Unresponsive to any stimulus

BOX 1.4 Causes of an altered level of consciousness

- T – trauma to the brain
- I – insulin/diabetes
- P – poisons
- P – psychiatric
- S – shock
- A – alcohol
- E – epilepsy
- I – infection
- O – opiates
- U – urea/metabolic

Exposure and environment

While the patient's dignity must be respected, it is essential that all clothing be removed so that the entire patient can be examined. The presence of injuries, particularly to the spine, prohibits normal removal of clothes. In trauma patients garments must be cut along seams using large bandage scissors, to facilitate their removal with minimal patient movement. If the patient is conscious an explanation can be given and permission sought. Exposed trauma patients can lose body heat rapidly no matter what the season, leading to a fall in the core temperature, particularly if they have a spinal injury. Studies have also shown that if hypothermia is allowed to develop, morbidity and mortality are increased. The resuscitation room should therefore be kept warm and overhead or warm air heaters used.

The rapid removal of tight clothing in gross hypovolaemia can precipitate sudden hypotension due to the loss of the tamponade effect. Therefore these garments should only be removed at the team leader's discretion and only after the establishment of adequate fluid resuscitation.

In order to prevent further discomfort and the risk of developing pressure sores haemodynamically stable patients can be log rolled at this stage and the spinal board removed. Head restraints should be maintained until the cervical spine has been cleared of potential injury.

The well-practised trauma team should complete the objectives of the primary survey and resuscitation phase within 7 min (Box 1.5). Prearrangement with the laboratory for rapid processing and reporting will facilitate the team leaders' evaluation of the patient's state.

BOX 1.5 Objectives of the primary survey and resuscitation phase

- Assessment and stabilization of the airway
- Stabilization of the cervical spine
- Assessment and correction of any ventilatory problems
- Control of any overt haemorrhage
- Assessment of the patient's haemodynamic state
- Insertion of two, large bore, peripheral cannulae
- Blood samples taken and sent to the laboratory
- Assessment of the patient's conscious level
- Establishment of supportive contact
- Removal of the patient's clothes
- Keep the patient warm
- Initial vital signs recorded and monitors connected
- Insertion of a gastric tube if appropriate

The heart rate, blood pressure, respiratory rate, pulse oximetry and ECG should be monitored and recorded at regular intervals to identify any change in the patient's condition. An important question to ask repeatedly is, 'Is the patient getting better or worse'? This helps to determine if the team needs to move rapidly to definitive care. For example, the patient should be taken directly to theatre to gain control of a source of bleeding if there is no response to appropriate intravenous resuscitation.

At this point provision of analgesia should be considered. Usually morphine titrated intravenously is used but there are other methods and agents which can be used depending upon the situation (see Section 16.3).

Only when all the airway, ventilatory and hypovolaemic problems have been corrected can the team continue the more detailed secondary survey

During the primary survey the relative's nurse should greet any of the patient's relatives or friends who arrive, take them to a private room, which has all necessary facilities, and remain with them to provide support and information. Periodically, she will have to go to the resuscitation room to exchange information with both team leaders. If the family wish to be present in the resuscitation room the relatives' nurse should accompany them.

Once the primary survey has been completed, the leaders can disband the non-essential members of the team so that they can return to their normal activities in the department.

1.6.2 Secondary survey

The objectives of this phase are to:

- examine the patient from head to toe and front to back to determine the full extent of his injuries;
- take a complete medical history;
- assimilate all clinical, laboratory and radiological information;
- formulate a management plan for the patient.

Should the patient deteriorate at any stage, the team leader must abandon the secondary survey and reassess the trauma victim's airway, breathing and circulatory state in the manner described in the primary survey

As with the primary survey, a well-coordinated team effort is required. Procedures by individual team members are followed according to a precise protocol and tasks are performed simultaneously rather than sequentially. The common error of being distracted before the whole body has been inspected must be avoided as potentially serious injuries can be missed, especially in the unconscious patient.

During the secondary survey the airway nurse maintains verbal contact with the patient while the recording nurse continues to measure the vital signs regularly and monitors fluid balance.

Unless already obtained in the primary survey, all blunt trauma victims should now have a chest, pelvis and lateral cervical spine x-ray performed. Providing all seven cervical vertebrae as well as the C7–T1 junction can be seen on the x-ray, up to 85% of cervical spine abnormalities will be shown. The easiest way of ensuring an adequate film is obtained on the first attempt is for one of the team members to pull the patient's arms towards their feet as the radiograph is taken (*Figure 1.4*) to remove the shoulders

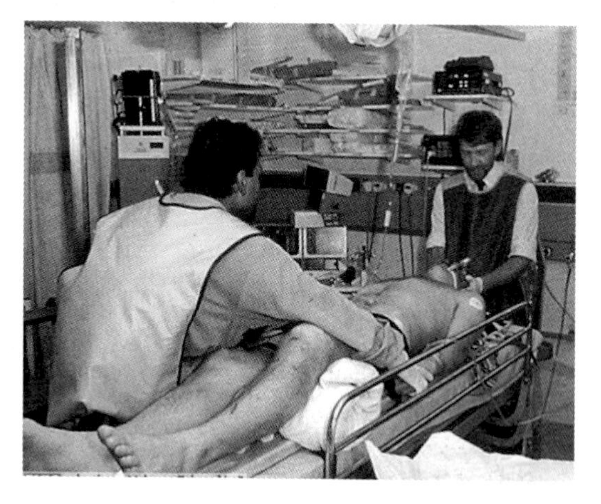

Figure 1.4 **Pulling the arms down for a cervical radiograph**

from the x-ray field. Alternative views (e.g. oblique and 'Swimmer's' view) or investigations (e.g. computerized tomography (CT)) can be used if this fails to give an adequate view. Further cervical spine views will be required before all injuries to the cervical spine can be excluded.

Neurological state

This comprises of an assessment of the conscious level using the Glasgow Coma Scale (GCS), the pupillary response and the presence of any lateralizing signs (see Section 6.5.3). One of the circulation nurses should then continue to monitor these parameters. If there is any deterioration, hypoxia or hypovolaemia must be ruled out before an intracranial injury is considered.

Examination of the peripheral nervous system should be performed. Abnormalities of motor and sensory function can help indicate the level and extent of spinal injury. In male patients the presence of priapism may be the first indication of spinal injury.

If the spinal cord has been transected at or above the mid-thoracic level, there is loss of sympathetic outflow, a reduction in vasomotor tone and peripheral vasodilatation causing hypotension. The degree of vasodilatation depends on how much vasomotor tone is lost. Transection of the spinal cord in the cervical region removes all vasomotor tone and causes profound hypotension. This will not be associated with a tachycardia because the sympathetic innervation of the heart (T1–T4) has also been lost, a condition referred to as 'neurogenic shock' (see Section 7.3.2).

Scalp

This must be examined for lacerations, swellings or depressions. Its entire surface needs to be inspected but the occiput will have to wait until the patient is turned or the cervical spine 'cleared' both clinically and radiologically. Visual inspection may discover fractures in the base of the lacerations. Wounds should not be blindly probed as further damage to underlying structures can result. If there is major bleeding from the scalp, digital pressure or a self-retaining retractor should be used. Although not common, scalp lacerations can bleed sufficiently to cause hypovolaemia; consequently haemostasis is crucial.

Base of skull

Fractures to this structure will produce signs along a diagonal line demonstrated in *Figure 1.5*. Bruising over the mastoid process (Battle's sign) usually takes 12–36 h to

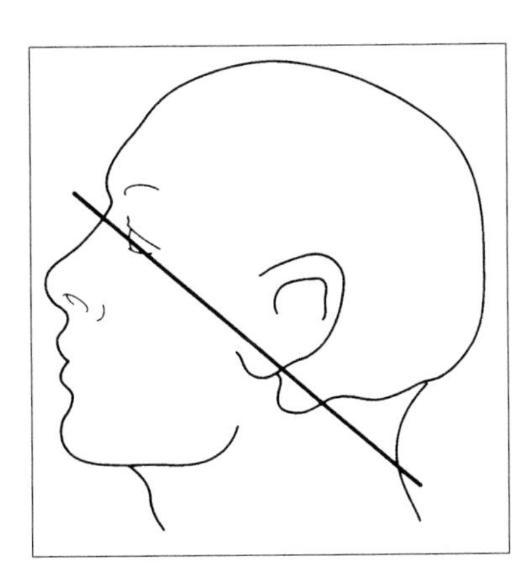

Figure 1.5 Diagonal line demonstrating the level of the base of the skull

appear, it is therefore of limited use in the resuscitation room. A cerebrospinal fluid (CSF) leak via the ears or nose may be missed as it is invariably mixed with blood. Fortunately its presence in this bloody discharge can be detected by noting the delay in clotting of the blood and the double ring pattern when it is dropped onto an absorbent sheet. In this situation nothing, including an auroscope, should be inserted into the external auditory canal because of the risk of introducing infection and hence causing meningitis. As there is a small chance of a nasogastric tube passing into the cranium through an anterior base of skull fracture, these tubes should be passed orally when this type of injury is suspected.

Eyes

The eyes should be inspected before significant orbital swelling makes examination too difficult. Look for haemorrhages, both inside and outside the globe, for foreign bodies under the lids (including contact lenses) and penetrating injuries. Pupil size and response to light, directly and consensually, should be recorded. If the patient is conscious, having them read a name badge or fluid label can be used as a simple test of visual acuity. If the patient is unconscious the corneal reflexes should be tested.

Face

This should be palpated symmetrically for deformities and tenderness. Check for loose, lost or damaged teeth and stability of the maxilla (the mid third of the face), by pulling the latter forward (see Section 8.3). Middle third fractures can be associated with both airway obstruction and base of skull fractures. Only injuries causing airway obstruction need to be treated immediately. Mandibular fractures can also cause airway obstruction because of the loss of stability of the tongue.

Neck

The immobilization devices must be removed for the team leader to examine the neck, therefore the airway nurse will need to reapply manual inline stabilization. The neck should be inspected for any deformity (rare), bruising and lacerations. The spinous processes of the cervical vertebrae can then be palpated for tenderness or a 'step off' deformity. The posterior cervical muscles should also be palpated for tenderness or spasm. The conscious patient can assist by indicating if there is pain or tenderness in the neck and locating the site.

A laceration should only be inspected and *never* probed with metal instruments or fingers. If a laceration penetrates platysma, definitive radiological or surgical management will be needed. The choice depends on the clinical state of the patient (see Section 8.3.1).

Thorax

The priority at this stage is to identify those thoracic conditions which are potentially life threatening, along with any other chest injuries (see Section 3.4). The chest wall must be re-inspected for bruising, signs of obstruction, asymmetry of movement and wounds. Acceleration and deceleration forces invariably leave marks on the chest wall, which should lead the team to consider particular types of injury. Good pre-hospital information is vital to determine the mechanism of injury.

The assessor should then palpate the sternum and along each rib, starting in the axillae and proceeding caudally and anteriorly. The presence of any crepitus, tenderness or subcutaneous emphysema must be noted. Auscultation and percussion of the whole chest can then be carried out to determine if there is any asymmetry between the right and left sides of the chest.

Potentially life-threatening injuries that need to be excluded include:

- pulmonary and cardiac contusions – particularly after blunt trauma;
- a ruptured diaphragm or perforated oesophagus – can follow both blunt and penetrating trauma;
- tear of the thoracic aorta – after a rapid deceleration;
- a simple pneumothorax or haemothorax.

Penetrating chest wounds can injure any of the structures within the thorax. Wounds that appear to cross the mediastinum pose a high risk of damaging the heart, bronchial tree or upper gastrointestinal tract. A high index of suspicion must be maintained and immediate surgical consultation is mandatory.

Abdomen

In the secondary survey, the aim is simply to determine if the patient requires a laparotomy – a precise diagnosis of which particular viscus has been injured is both time consuming and of little relevance. A thorough examination of the whole abdomen is required, including both the perineum and stability of the pelvis. All bruising, abnormal movement and wounds must be noted and lacerations should be inspected but not probed blindly as further damage can result. Any exposed bowel should be covered with warm saline-soaked swabs. If underlying muscle has been penetrated, it is not possible to determine the actual depth of the wound; consequently these cases will require further investigations (see Section 5.4.4).

The abdomen needs to be palpated in a systematic manner so that areas of tenderness can be detected. An intra-abdominal bleed should be suspected if the ribs overlying the liver and spleen (5–11) are fractured, the patient is haemodynamically unstable or if there are seat belt marks, tyre marks or bruises over the abdominal surface. Further investigation of possible abdominal injury can be achieved with ultrasound, CT scanning or DPL, according to local protocols. This should not delay the treatment of the haemodynamically unstable patient who should proceed directly to theatre. Early liaison with the general surgeons is vital.

The detection of abdominal tenderness is unreliable if there is a sensory defect due to neurological damage or drugs, or if there are fractures of the lower ribs or pelvis

Marked gastric distension is frequently found in crying children, adults with head or abdominal injuries and patients who have been ventilated with a bag and mask technique. The insertion of a gastric tube facilitates the abdominal examination of these patients and reduces the risks of aspiration.

A rectal examination should always be carried out. This provides five pieces of information:

- sphincter tone – this can be lost after spinal injuries;
- direct anal or rectal trauma;

- pelvic fractures;
- prostatic position – this can be disrupted after posterior urethral injury;
- blood in the lower alimentary canal.

The rate of urine output is an important indicator in assessing the shocked patient (see Section 4.6). Therefore it should be measured in all trauma patients and in most cases this will require catheterization. If there is no evidence of urethral injury, the catheter is passed transurethrally. If urethral trauma is suspected (Box 1.6), and the patient is unable to urinate, a suprapubic catheter may be necessary. The urine that is voided initially should be tested for blood and a sample saved for microscopy and subsequent possible drug analysis.

BOX 1.6 Signs of urethral injury in a male patient

- Bruising around the scrotum
- Blood at the end of the urethral meatus
- High riding prostate
- Fractured pubic rami
- Inability to pass urine

Extremities

The limbs are examined by inspection, palpation and movement. All the long bones must also be rotated and, if the patient is conscious, he should be asked actively to move each limb.

Any wounds associated with open fractures must be swabbed and covered with a nonadherent dressing. As different surgeons will need to examine the limb, a digital photograph of the wound before it is covered will reduce the number of times the dressings have to be removed.

All limb fractures should be splinted to reduce fracture movement, pain, bleeding, formation of fat emboli and secondary soft tissue swelling and damage.

A detailed inspection of the whole of the patient is needed to determine the number and extent of any soft tissue injuries. Each breach in the skin needs to be inspected to determine its site, depth and the presence of any underlying structural damage that will subsequently require surgical repair. Superficial wounds can be cleaned, thoroughly irrigated and dressed in patients who are clinically stable.

Upon completion of the examination, the presence of any bruising, wounds and deformities must be noted along with any crepitus, instability, neurovascular abnormalities or soft tissue damage. As time delays can result in tissue loss, gross limb deformities need to be corrected and the pulses and sensation rechecked before any radiographs are taken (see Section 9.3).

Back

If a spinal injury is suspected the patient should only be moved by a well-coordinated log rolling technique (*Figure 1.6*). The patient is turned away from the examiner who takes this opportunity to clear away all the debris from under the patient. The whole of the back is assessed, from occiput to heels, looking for bruising and open wounds. The back of the chest must be auscultated, the area between the buttocks inspected and the vertebral column palpated for bogginess, malalignment and deformities in contour. The examination finishes with palpation of the longitudinal spinal muscles for spasm

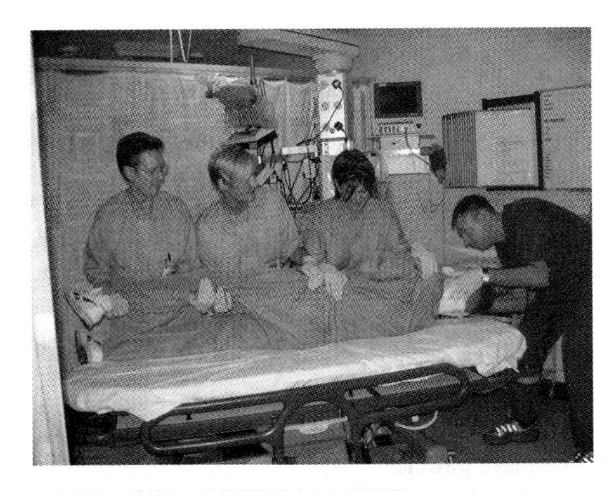

Figure 1.6 **Patient being 'log rolled'**

and tenderness. The patient is then log rolled back into the supine position, after the long spine board has been removed.

At the same time, the nursing team leader will need to make an initial assessment of the risk of pressure sores developing using a scoring system (*Box 1.7*). Meticulous attention to prevention must be made from the outset, particularly for patients with spinal injuries and the elderly because they have a high risk of developing decubitus

BOX 1.7 Pressure sore risk assessment

Age/Sex		**Medications**		**Build**		**Appetite**	
14–49	1	Cytotoxics	4	Average	0	Good	0
50–64	2	Steroids	4	Above average	1	Fair	1
65–74	3	NSAIDs	4	Obese	2	Poor	2
75–80	4			Below average	3	Refusing food	3
>80	5						
Male	1					NBM with ivi	1
Female	2					NBM no ivi	2
Mobility		**Activity in bed**		**Continence**		**Skin condition**	
Independent	0	Independent	0	Continent/catheter	0	Healthy	0
Zimmer/crutches	1	Minimal assist.	1	Occ. incont. urine	1	Rashes/abrasions	1
Assistance	2	Full assist to		Incontinent of urine	2	Dehydrated	1
Few steps only	3	move/sit up	2	Incontinent of faeces	3	Tissue paper	1
Bedfast/traction	4	Immobile,		Doubly incontinent	4	Clammy	1
Transfer/chairfast	5	logrolling	3			Oedematous	1
						Red/discoloured	2
						Broken/sore	3
Conscious level		**Surgery**		**Special risks**		**Neuro deficit**	
Alert	0	< 2 hours	1	Terminal cachexia	8	Diabetes	4–6
Lethargic	1	> 2 hours	2	Cardiac failure	5	MS	4–6
Confused	1	Below waist	2	Perip. Vasc. Disease	5	CVA	4–6
Sedated:		Spinal anaesth	2	Unstable spinal fract	5	Paraplegia	4–6
Sedation score 1	1	Post op epidural	2	Head injury/ skull			
Sedation score 2	2			fracture	5		
Sedation score 3	3			Hb < 100g/l	2		
				Smoker	1		

The sum of the scores for each category is calculated to predict risk, eg 0–8 low risk, 15–18 high risk. This is then used in conjunction with the patient's weight to identify type of mattress required.

ulcers. Remember the patient may have already spent a considerable time in one position before being rescued and, if he requires surgery, he may have to remain in the same position for several more hours. Lying on a hard spinal board can exacerbate these problems. It is therefore important to note how long the trauma victim remains in one position and to move whatever can be moved, every 30 min using hip lifts for example. The spinal board should be removed at the earliest opportunity. This needs to be taken into consideration when compiling the nursing plans.

Medical history

By the end of the secondary survey, the medical team leader must have assembled the patient's medical history. Some information will have already been acquired from the ambulance personnel or relatives. Further sources of information are the patient's general practitioner (GP) and hospital records. A comprehensive medical history may help clarify clinical findings that do not appear to relate to the history of the incident, which led to the victim's condition. The important elements of the medical history can be remembered by the mnemonic AMPLE:

- A – Allergies
- M – Medicines
- P – Past medical history
- L – Last meal
- E – Events leading to the incident

1.6.3 Assimilation of information

As the condition of the patient can change quickly, repeated examinations and constant monitoring of the vital signs is essential. The recording nurse, responsible for recording the latter at 5-min intervals, must be vigilant and bring any deterioration in the respiratory rate, pulse, blood pressure, conscious level and urine output to the immediate attention of the team leaders.

By the end of the secondary survey, the answers to the following questions must be known:

Is the patient's respiratory function satisfactory?

If it is not adequate then the cause must be sought and corrected as a priority.

Is the patient's circulatory status satisfactory?

With less than 20% of the blood volume lost, vital signs usually return to normal after less than 2 l of fluid. If they then remain stable then it implies that the patient is not actively bleeding. Patients whose vital signs initially improve but then decline are either actively bleeding or recommenced bleeding during the resuscitation. They have usually lost over 30% of their blood volume and require an infusion with typed blood and invariably require surgery. The total lack of response to a fluid challenge suggests two possibilities. Either the patient has lost over 40% of their blood volume and is bleeding faster than the rate of the fluid infusion or shock is not due to hypovolaemia. In the case of major haemorrhage, an operation is urgently required, the latter will need invasive techniques to monitor the central venous and pulmonary artery pressures to help guide resuscitation.

Are any further radiological investigations required?

Any hypoxic or haemodynamically problems must be addressed first. Once his condition stabilizes, radiographs can be performed of particular sites of injury or those areas suggested by the mechanism of injury, along with any other specialized investigations. It is an important part of the team leaders' responsibilities to determine the priorities of these investigations.

What is the extent and priorities of the injuries?

The ABC system is used to categorizes injuries so that the most dangerous is treated first. For example, problems with the airway (A) must be corrected before those of the circulation (C).

Have any injuries being overlooked?

The mechanism of injury and the injury pattern must be considered to avoid overlooking sites of damage. Trauma rarely 'skips' areas, for example if an injury has been found in the thorax and femur, but not in the abdomen, then it probably has been missed.

Is tetanus toxoid, human antitetanus immunoglobulin (Humotet) or antibiotics required?

This will depend on both local and national policies that should be known by the team leaders.

Is analgesia required?

Severely injured patients need analgesia. Entonox can be given until the baseline observations are recorded unless there are any contraindications (i.e. pneumothorax and head and abdominal injuries). Intravenous morphine can then be titrated against the patient's pain level.

1.6.4 Definitive care

This can only start once the patient has been adequately assessed and resuscitated. In many cases this will require transfer to either the operating theatre and/or intensive care. It is therefore very important that the transfer from the resuscitation room to these areas is done as smoothly as possible.

While the move is being planned, the medical team leader must complete the medical notes. At the same time the charts, vital signs, fluid balance, drug administration and preliminary nursing care documentation need to be collated. A purpose designed single trauma sheet can facilitate this process (*Figure 1.7*). The relative's nurse can then brief the team leaders about the condition of any relatives or friends who are in the department on the patient's behalf. The medical team leader should accompany her back to the relative's room, to talk to them. If this doctor has had to accompany the patient another clinician, fully versed with the situation, should speak with the relatives.

If the patient is unconscious, his clothing and belongings may provide essential information to help establish his identity. Whether the patient's name is known or not, some system of identification is required, in order that drugs and blood can be administered safely. This becomes more important when there are several patients in the

Name _ _ _ _ _ _ _ Age/D.O.B._ _ _ _ _
Address _ _ _ _ _ _ _ _ _ _ _ _ _ _ _ _
_ _ _ _ _ _ _ _ _ _ _ _ _ _ _ _ _ _ _ _
_ _ _ _ _ _ _ _ _ _ A/E No: _ _ _ _ _ _

Date _ _ _ _ _ Time of arrival _ _ _ _ _
Drugs _ _ _ _ _ Allergies _ _ _ _ _ _
PMH _ _ _ _ _ _ _ _ _ _ _ _ _ _ _ _ _
_ _ _ _ _ _ _ _ _ Last ate _ _ _ _ _ _ _

BLOODS	RESULTS	BLOODS	RESULTS
☐ Hb		☐ WCC	
☐ Hct		☐ PLTS	
☐ Na		☐ BS	
☐ K		☐ Urea	
☐ BM	Time / % O_2		
☐ ABG	pO^2		
	pCO^2		
	pH		
	BE		
☐ Other			

PRIMARY SURVEY

	ASSESSMENT	RESUSCITATION
☐ AIRWAY	☐ Normal Gag Y/N ☐ Unconscious ☐ Facial fractures	☐ Spontaneous *Mask/mask + airway* _ _ _ %O^2 ☐ Ventilated ☐ ETT - *size* _ _ _ ☐ N-G tube
	CERVICAL SPINE ☐ Normal ☐ Suspect injury ☐ Firm collar ☐ In line traction	
☐ BREATHING	*RR ON ARRIVAL................../min* ☐ Trauma (blunt/penetrating) ☐ Pneumothorax (open / closed / tension) ☐ Haemothorax ☐ Flail segment	☐ Chest drain Left Right *Size* _ _ _ *Size* _ _ _
☐ CIRCULATION	*SYSTOLIC BP ON ARRIVAL ....mmHg* ☐ Haemorrhage ☐ External ☐ Internal ☐ Chest ☐ Abdomen ☐ Pelvis	IV (1)-*site* _ _ _ _ *Size* _ _ _ _ _ IV (2)-*site* _ _ _ _ *Size* _ _ _ _ _ Blood ordered ☐ 0 Neg Time _ _ hrs ☐ Grouped ☐ X-match ☐ G + S ☐ Pressure dressings ☐ Arterial blood gases ☐ ECG monitor
☐ DYSFUNCTION	*GCS ON ARRIVAL...................* ☐ Alert ☐ Responds to verbal commands ☐ Responds to pain ☐ Unresponsive Pupils equal : Y / N	☐ In line stabilisation of whole spine

X-RAYS	Findings
☐ C-spine	
☐ CXR	
☐ Pelvis	
☐ SXR	
☐ Long bones	
☐ Spine	
☐ C.T. scan	

DRUGS	Dr. sig.	Sig. given
☐ Tet. tox. 0.5 ml		
☐ Humo. Tet. 250 units		
☐ Analgesics		
☐ Antibiotic		
☐ Anaesthetic drugs		

SECONDARY SURVEY Tick pulses present
Summary of Injuries

PERITONEAL LAVAGE
RBC _ _ _ _ /mm³ WBC _ _ _ /mm³
Bacteria _ _ _ Y/N Food _ _ _ Y/N
Performed by _ _ _ _ Time _ _ _ _ _
USS abdo _ _ _ _ _ _ _ _ _ _ _ _

URINE (Cath / MSU / Other)
Blood _ _ _ _ _ Ketones _ _ _ _
Sugar _ _ _ _ _ Protein _ _ _ _

REFERRALS

	Grade	Time: Called	Time: Arrived
☐ Anaesthetist			
☐ Gen.surgeons			
☐ Orthopaedic			
☐ Neurosurg.			
☐ Thoracic			
☐ Plastic			
☐ Max. fac.			
☐ Other			

DISPOSAL TIME
Ward _ _ _ _ _ _ _ _ _ hrs
ITU _ _ _ _ _ _ _ _ _ hrs
Theatre _ _ _ _ _ _ _ _ hrs
CT scan _ _ _ _ _ _ _ _ hrs
Died _ _ _ _ _ _ _ _ _ hrs
Transfer _ _ _ _ _ _ _ _ hrs

Resuscitation led by :
Initially : _ _ _ _ _ _ _ _ _ _ _ _ _
Finally : _ _ _ _ _ _ _ _ _ _ _ _ _
Chart compiled by :
Name _ _ _ _ _ Signature _ _ _ _

Figure 1.7 Trauma sheet

INCIDENT DETAILS : Time

- Mechanism
- Pre-hospital care

Vital signs at scene :

BP [ ] Pulse [ ] RR [ ] GCS [ ]

NURSING DETAILS

Relatives Name ____________ Phone no. ______

Address ______________________

______________________ Contacted Y/N

Other details

VITAL SIGNS

Hour

Minute

Blood pressure ↕

Pulse ●

180
160
140
120
100
80
60
40
20
0

Respiratory rate

Temperature °C

Arterial oxygen saturation (%)

James Driscoll McCabe 1991

Pupil scale (mm)

1
2
3
4
5
6
7
8

ACTIONS / EVENTS

Hour

Minute

PUPILS

+ Reacts
- No reaction
C Closed by swelling

R Size
Reaction

L Size
Reaction

HAEMACCEL

	G.C.S.	
VERBAL	Orientated	5
	Confused	4
	Inappropriate words	3
	Incomprehensible sounds	2
	None	1
MOTOR	Obeys commands	6
	Localises pain	5
	Flexion to pain	4
	Decorticate movement	3
	Extension to pain	2
	None	1
EYE	Spontaneous	4
	To speech	3
	To pain	2
	None	1
	G.C.S. Total Score	

I.V. Site 1				I.V. Site 2			
Time	Fluid	Vol.	Given	Time	Fluid	Vol.	Given

Total input IV site 1= [ml] Total input IV site 2 = [ml]

TOTAL IV INPUT [= ml]

URINE OUTPUT		OTHER LOSSES	
Catheter / voided		Specify :______	
Time	Vol.	Time	Vol.

TOTAL URINE OUTPUT [= ml]

TOTAL OTHER LOSSES [= ml]

Department of Medical Illustration, S.H.A. H91071270

resuscitation room. If identity bracelets are impractical, then indelible markers can be used to write a number on the patient's skin. The rescue personnel must hand over any possessions brought in with the patient to the nursing staff. These must be kept safely, along with the patient's clothing and property. At the end of the secondary survey, or during it if there are hands to spare, all these articles must be searched. A check is needed for any medical alert card or disc, a suicide note and any medicine bottles or tablets.

No patient must be allowed to leave the department without identification

Jewellery, and when appropriate dentures, need to be removed with permission if conscious and stored in a labelled valuables bag or envelope. As soft tissue can swell, constrictive jewellery must be removed and if this is not possible, it should be cut off. At an appropriate moment, the patient's property is collected, preferably by nurses outside the trauma team, checked, recorded, signed for and locked away. Whatever the outcome of the resuscitation, relatives take a dim view of items of property being misplaced. Nurses are legally responsible for this property and prolonged problems can result from disregarding the patient's seemingly unimportant effects in the heat of the moment. If a criminal case is suspected, all clothing, possessions, loose debris, bullets and shrapnel are required for forensic examination. These, too, must be collected, labelled, placed in individual bags and signed for prior to releasing them to the appropriate authorities according to established procedures.

If a delay in transfer is anticipated, the patient can be given a gentle, preliminary wash to remove any blood, mud or other contaminating material.

Preparation for transfer of the patient

The safe transfer of patients is vital, whether intra- or interhospital. Details are to be found in Chapter 17.

1.7 Preparation of the resuscitation room

As the transfer is under way, the remaining staff can begin preparing the area for arrival of the next trauma victim. Throughout the resuscitation the team should have kept the area as tidy and organized as possible with sharps, open packs and instruments being disposed of as they are used. This is essential for both safety and efficiency. Wet, greasy floors need to be wiped or covered immediately after spillage to avoid accidents to staff. Once the patient has been transferred and the resuscitation area restocked, checked and made ready, the team can get together for a preliminary or definitive debriefing session.

1.8 Summary

To enable the patient to receive the most efficient resuscitation, a group of appropriately trained personnel must be ready to meet him when he arrives at the ED. These people must be coordinated by nursing and medical team leaders so that they are all aware of the tasks they have to perform, and that they are carried out simultaneously.

The first priority is to detect and treat the immediately life-threatening conditions. Following this, a detailed head to toe assessment can be completed. The team leaders can then list the patient's injuries and their priorities for both further investigations and definitive treatment.

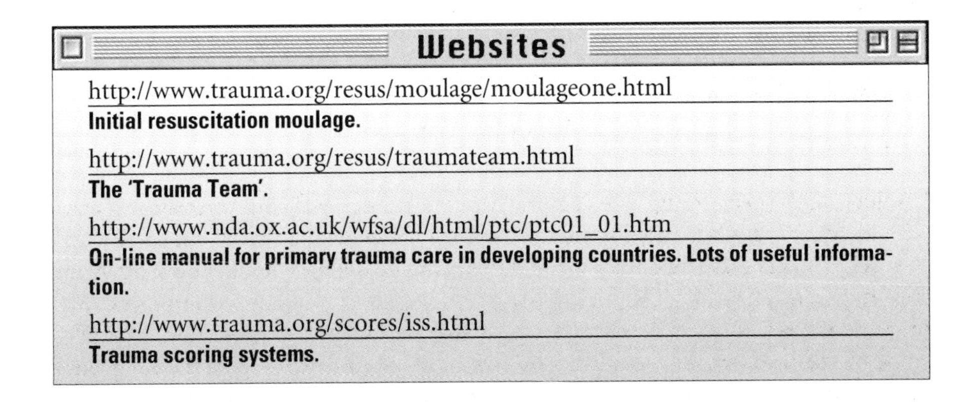

Websites

http://www.trauma.org/resus/moulage/moulageone.html
Initial resuscitation moulage.

http://www.trauma.org/resus/traumateam.html
The 'Trauma Team'.

http://www.nda.ox.ac.uk/wfsa/dl/html/ptc/ptc01_01.htm
On-line manual for primary trauma care in developing countries. Lots of useful information.

http://www.trauma.org/scores/iss.html
Trauma scoring systems.

Further reading

1. **American College of Surgeons Committee on Trauma** (1997) *Advanced Trauma Life Support Course for Doctors.* American College of Surgeons, Chicago, IL.
2. **Driscoll P & Vincent C.** (1992) Variation in trauma resuscitation and its effects on outcome. *Injury* 23: 11.
3. **Driscoll P & Vincent C.** (1992) Organizing an efficient trauma team. *Injury* 23: 107.
4. **Sheehy S, Marvin J & Jimmerson C. (eds)** (1992) *Emergency Nursing, Principles and Practice,* 3rd Edn. CV Mosby, St Louis.

2 The management of the airway and cervical spine control

C Gwinnutt, O Goodall

Objectives

The objectives of this chapter are to teach the team members allocated to manage the trauma patient's airway:

- how to assess and secure the airway;
- basic airway management;
- the use of simple airway adjuncts;
- artificial ventilation;
- advanced airway management;
- the role of drugs to aid intubation;
- the use of surgical airways in the resuscitation room.

2.1 Introduction

Establishing and maintaining a clear airway are essential prerequisites for successful resuscitation and are therefore the first medical interventions in the trauma patient. If the cervical spine is injured, the spinal cord may be jeopardized if any airway intervention is not performed in a controlled manner. This chapter will describe how the airway can be assessed, cleared and secured, at the same time minimizing the risk to the spinal cord.

2.2 Anatomy

Figure 2.1 demonstrates the important surface landmarks of the upper airway.

2.3 Standby preparation and transfer

Although all equipment must be checked on a regular basis, the doctor and nurse responsible for managing the airway and cervical spine must complete a final check of equipment whilst awaiting the arrival of the patient.

On arrival at hospital, the trauma victim's airway must be assessed immediately, even before he is moved from the ambulance to the resuscitation room. If there is evidence of compromise, it should initially be cleared and secured using a simple device (see below). Simultaneously the neck should be secured either with a rigid cervical

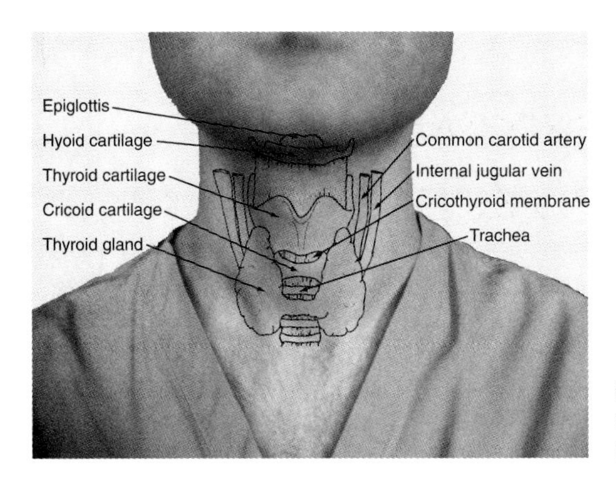

Figure 2.1 Surface markings of anatomy of airway structures in the neck

collar, sand bags and tape or the application of manual inline stabilization (MILS) (*Figure 2.2*). During transfer to, or within the resuscitation room, the doctor and nurse responsible for the airway must ensure that there is no uncontrolled movement of the spine and that any airway device is not displaced.

2.4 Assessing and securing the airway

The quickest way of evaluating the airway is to ask the patient 'Are you alright?' A lucid reply suggests: the airway is clear, the patient has a reasonable vital capacity breath, and cerebral perfusion is sufficient to maintain consciousness.

An impaired response may be due to any of the causes in the following table.

Sign		Cause
Stridor	Noisy breathing, usually on inspiration	Partial obstruction at larynx
Tachypnoea	Increased respiratory rate (> 29/min)	Airway obstruction Intrathoracic injuries Hypovolaemia Hypoxia Hypercarbia Pre-existing medical problem
Agitation	Combative, sweating, tachycardia	Hypercarbia Hypoxia
Impaired ventilation	Reduced rate, depth	Reduced conscious level Airway obstruction

All of the above may be associated with use of the accessory muscles of ventilation (e.g. sternomastoid and scalene muscles) and indrawing of the intercostal, supraclavicular and suprasternal spaces. Whatever the initial cause, if unresolved, this will lead to hypercarbia and further reduction in conscious level.

If there is no attempt at a reply, the patient is usually unconscious. This may be due to a number of causes other than a head injury (Box 1.4).

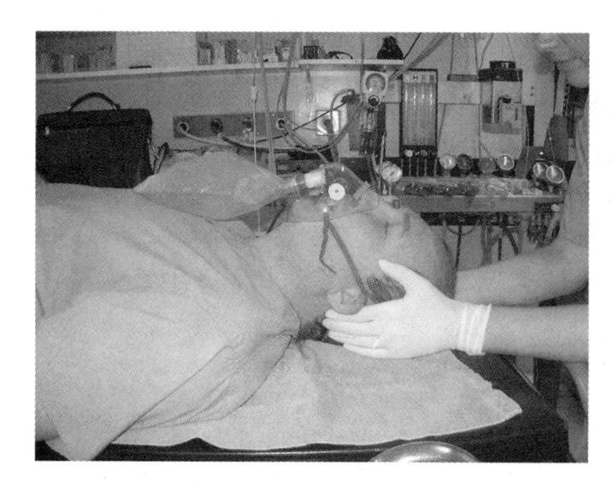

Figure 2.2 Nurse stabilizing the cervical spine

Profound hypoxia or hypovolaemia, alone or in combination, are potent causes of unconsciousness

If the victim is unresponsive and airway personnel suspect that the victim is unconscious, the airway and ventilation must be assessed rapidly by:

- LOOKING – to see if the chest is rising and falling, i.e. is there any respiratory effort?
- LISTENING – close to the patient's mouth for abnormal sounds, that is, is the airway partially obstructed?
- FEELING – with the side of one's face for expired air, that is, is ventilation adequate or absent?

If the airway is inadequate or patient is not breathing (apnoeic), then the commonest cause is the tongue. Loss of submandibular muscle tone allows the tongue to slide back and occlude the oropharynx, while at the same time the epiglottis may obstruct the larynx. Other causes of obstruction are unstable fractures of the maxilla or mandible, haemorrhage in the mouth obstructing the oropharynx, and direct obstruction of the larynx by foreign bodies or swelling. Initial manoeuvres to relieve obstruction of the airway include: chin lift (*Figure 2.3*), jaw thrust (*Figure 2.4*), removal of foreign material (a rigid, Yankauer, sucker for liquid, Magill's forceps for loose, solid debris), gravity by placing the patient semiprone to allow drainage of liquids. It is important that the effectiveness of all of these manoeuvres is assessed using the 'look, listen and feel' method.

2.4.1 Simple airway devices

In the unconscious patient, pulling the tongue forward may be all that is required to obtain a clear airway, but once the jaw is released the obstruction will recur. To overcome this the following devices can be used.

Oropharyngeal (Guedel) airway

- Available in different sizes, an approximate guide is given by the vertical distance from the incisors to the angle of the jaw.

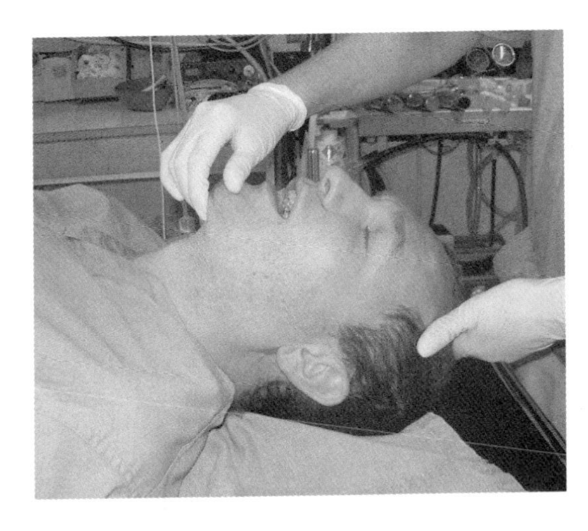

Figure 2.3 **Chin lift. The index and middle finger pull the mandible forward as the thumb assists and pushes down the lower lip and jaw.**

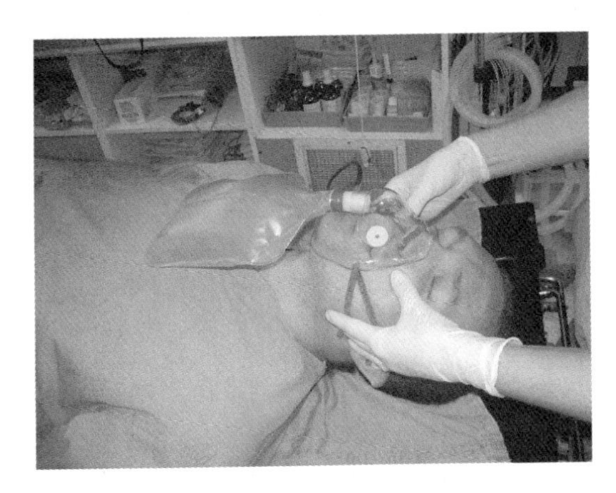

Figure 2.4 **Jaw thrust. The fingers of both hands are placed behind the angles of the jaw with the thumbs placed over the malar prominences. Downward pressure is exerted on the thumbs as the fingers lift the mandible forward.**

- Inserted 'upside down', as far back as the hard palate, then rotated through 180°.
- Fully inserted until the flange lies in front of the upper and lower incisors.
- Only tolerated when pharyngeal reflexes are depressed.

Nasopharyngeal airway

- Size relates to the internal diameter in mm, approximately 7–8 mm for an adult male, 6–7 mm for an adult female.
- Lubricate well, inserted through the nostril (usually the right, unless obviously blocked).
- Advanced along the floor of the nose, parallel to the hard palate using a slight rotational action.
- If resistance is encountered, do not use excessive force, as this can precipitate haemorrhage, try the other nostril.

- Once in place, secure to prevent it being inhaled by inserting a safety pin through the expanded end.
- Used with extreme caution if a basal skull fracture is suspected.
- Better tolerated than the oropharyngeal airway.

After insertion of either device, reassess the airway, repeating the look, listen and feel manoeuvres, auscultate the chest to confirm bilateral ventilation, administer oxygen (see below) immobilize the cervical spine appropriately (*Figure 1.3*).

BOX 2.1 Complications from airway insertion

- Trauma to all structures encountered, provoking bleeding
- Partial or complete airway obstruction
- Laryngeal spasm because the device is too long
- Vomiting because the patient has a gag reflex

2.5 Breathing

In all trauma patients, the aim should be to achieve an inspired oxygen concentration of 100%. The concentration of oxygen delivered is often referred to as the FiO_2 (fractional inspired oxygen concentration) and expressed as a decimal rather than a percentage, e.g. 21% = FiO_2 0.21.

2.5.1 Spontaneous ventilation

If the actions described above result in a patent airway and resumption of breathing, a close fitting mask with a reservoir should be placed over the patient's nose and mouth and connected to oxygen at a flow rate of 15 l/min. This type of mask meets the patient's peak inspiratory flow rate and reduces entrainment of air and results in an $FiO_2 = 0.85$ (85%) (*Figure 2.2*).

2.5.2 Artificial ventilation

If the patient is apnoeic or breathing inadequately:

- Ventilate using a bag-valve-face mask, preferably a 'two-man' technique, at a rate of 10–12 breaths per min (*Figure 2.5*).
- Attach oxygen at 15 l/min, to increase the FiO_2 to 0.5.
- Adding a reservoir bag increases the FiO_2 to approximately 0.9.
- Watch for bilateral chest movement, auscultate bilaterally to ensure ventilation of both lungs.

Note:

1. The use of the reservoir ensures that the bag refills with a greater proportion of oxygen than room air. With a tight-fitting mask this method allows an FiO_2 of up to 0.9.
2. The one-way valve prevents expired gas entering the self-inflating bag.
3. Inadequate ventilation may occur due either to a leak between the patient's face and mask, or gas being forced down the oesophagus as the bag is squeezed. The latter

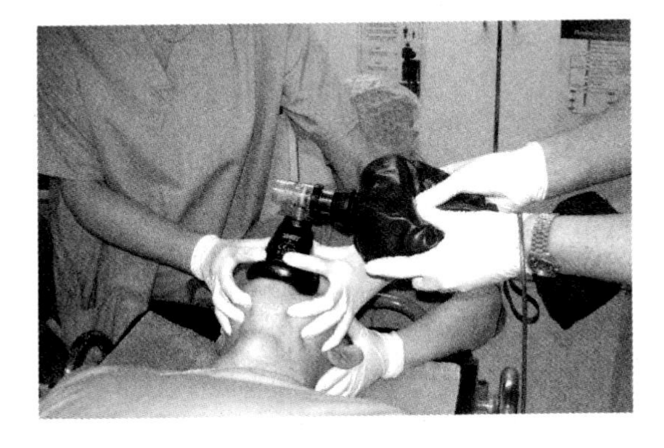

Figure 2.5 Two person bag-valve-mask ventilation with reservoir bag and oxygen source

will cause gastric distension, further impairing ventilation and predispose to regurgitation.

Cricoid pressure

This procedure is usually reserved for use during intubation. However, it can minimize gastric distension during ventilation with a facemask and thereby reduce the chance of aspiration (see Section 2.6.6).

2.6 Advanced airway control

If it is inappropriate or impossible to maintain a patent airway and achieve adequate ventilation using basic techniques (Box 2.2), one of the following advanced techniques should be used:

- tracheal intubation;
- laryngeal mask airway (LMA) or Combitube;
- surgical airway.

The preferred method is tracheal intubation as it has several advantages: it facilitates ventilation and allows a high concentration of oxygen to be delivered, isolates the airway and reduces the risk of aspiration of gastric contents or blood from maxillofacial injuries, and the airway can be suctioned to remove secretions or inhaled debris. However, in many trauma patients intubation will require the administration of drugs to overcome the laryngeal reflexes.

BOX 2.2 Indications for advanced airway techniques

- Unconscious with loss of protective reflexes
- Poor airway with basic techniques, e.g. severe facial trauma
- Specific need for ventilation, e.g. head injury
- Compromise of normal respiratory mechanism, e.g. chest injury
- Anticipation of airway obstruction, e.g. inhalation injury to the upper airway

2.6.1 Endotracheal intubation

Preparation

- Check all equipment required is present and functioning (*Figure 2.6*).
- Draw up and label all drugs required.
- Ensure adequate and secure intravenous access.
- Start pre-oxygenating the patient.

The procedure

Because most trauma patients will not have an empty stomach, they are at risk of regurgitation and aspiration of gastric contents; therefore cricoid pressure should be applied during laryngoscopy and intubation. The optimal position for intubation is with the patient's neck flexed and the head extended at the atlanto-occipital joint (often likened to 'sniffing the morning air'). *This should only be performed in trauma patients where there is no actual or possible injury to the cervical spine.*

Standard intubation technique

- The laryngoscope is held in the *left* hand.
- The mouth opened using the index and thumb of the right hand in a scissor action.
- The blade of the laryngoscope is inserted along the right side of the tongue, displacing it to the left.
- The tip of the laryngoscope is advanced into the gap between the base of the tongue and the epiglottis (vallecula).
- Force is applied in the direction the handle is pointing (*Figure 2.7*), thereby lifting the tongue and epiglottis to expose the larynx.
- There should be *no* wrist movement, all the force comes from the upper arm.
- The tube is advanced from the right hand corner of the mouth through the cords.
- The laryngoscope is withdrawn taking care not to dislodge the tube.
- The cuff is inflated and ventilation commenced.
- The position of the tube is confirmed (see below) and it is secured in place.

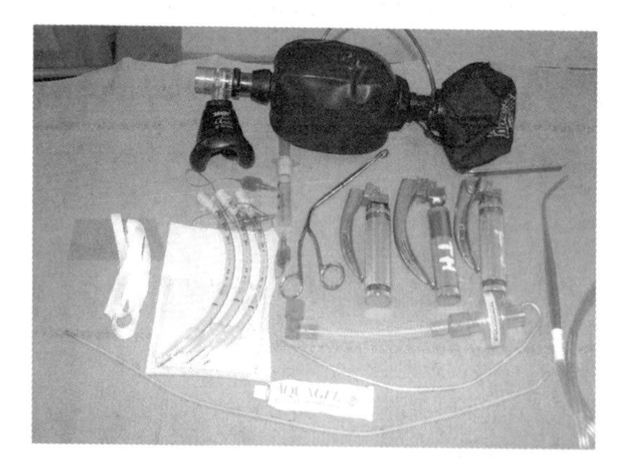

Figure 2.6 Equipment required for endotracheal intubation

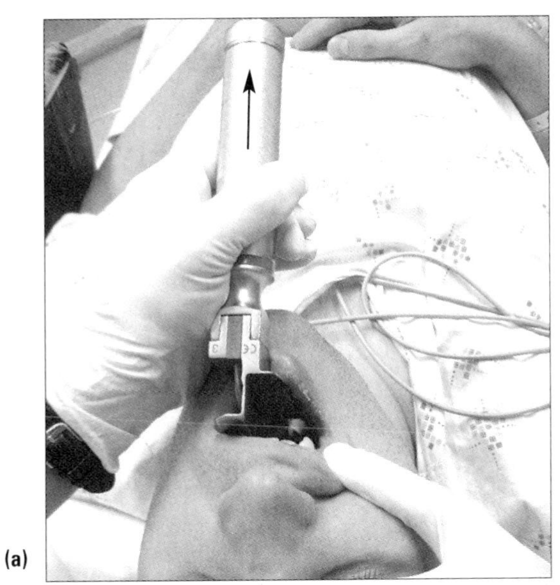

(a)

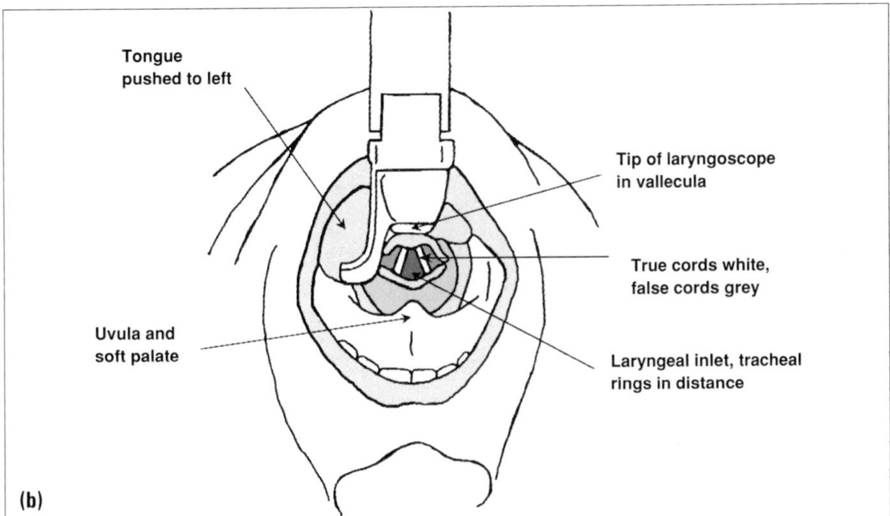

(b)

Figure 2.7 (a) Direct laryngoscopy. Arrow shows direction of force. Epiglottis just visible. (b) Diagramatic representation of view of laryngoscopy.

Where there is known or suspected injury to the cervical spine the head and neck must be maintained in neutral alignment during intubation. When the collar, blocks and tapes are in position, mouth opening and laryngoscopy are compromised, the view of the larynx is impaired and intubation becomes very difficult. The following technique is recommended:

- the collar is removed and replaced by MILS to allow increased mouth opening;
- the laryngoscope is inserted in the manner described above into the vallecula;
- if the view of the larynx is impaired, a gum elastic bougie is used as an introducer;
- keeping the laryngoscope in place, the bougie is passed behind the epiglottis, its tip pointing anteriorly so that it passes into larynx;

- a tracheal tube (usually 1–2 mm smaller in diameter than normal, e.g. 7 mm) is slid over the bougie into the larynx;
- the tube is then held in place and the bougie withdrawn;
- the cuff is inflated, ventilation commenced and the position of the tube is confirmed (see below).

McCoy laryngoscope

A very useful alternative laryngoscope for difficult intubations. The tip of this laryngoscope is hinged and can be elevated using the lever on the handle. The device is inserted in the normal way into the vallecula and when the tip is elevated, it 'lifts' the epiglottis anteriorly and may reveal the larynx, allowing intubation in the manner described above (*Figure 2.8*).

Confirming correct tube placement

- Detection of carbon dioxide in expired gas (end tidal CO_2).
- Look for symmetrical movement of the chest wall with ventilation.
- Listen in both axillae for breath sounds and over the stomach for absence of sounds.
- Oesophageal detector device.

When the tube is in the correct place and secured, cricoid pressure should only be released on the instruction of the person carrying out the intubation.

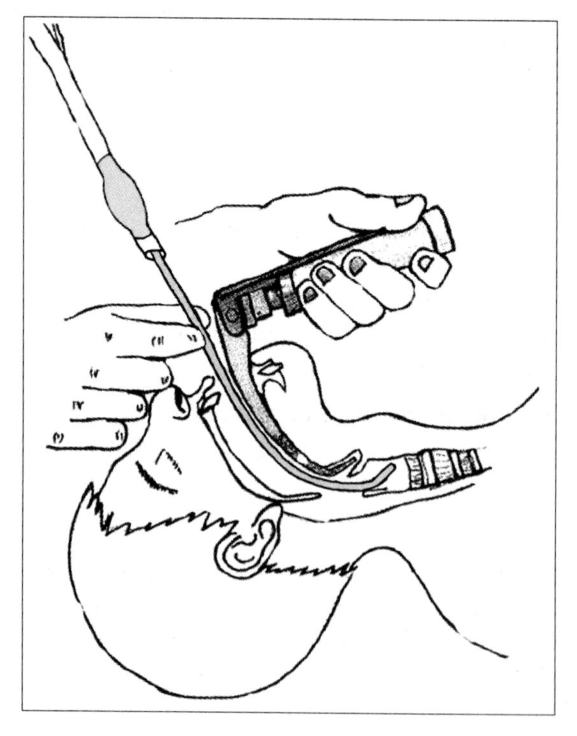

Figure 2.8 Direct laryngoscopy using McCoy and bougie

Notes:

(i) Difficult intubation. Do not persist without intermittently oxygenating the patient. A tip is to take a deep breath when picking up the laryngoscope and once you feel the need to breathe again, so will the patient.

(ii) Oesophageal intubation. If suspected (no CO_2 in expired gas), deflate the cuff and withdraw tube completely. Reattempt intubation after oxygenation.

(iii) The oesophageal detector device. If the tube is in the trachea, it is possible to aspirate air rapidly into a 50-ml syringe attached to the tube, without resistance. If the tube is in the oesophagus, on aspiration, the oesophageal mucosa will obstruct the end of the tube and air cannot be aspirated.

(iv) Endobronchial intubation (usually the right). This will produce poor ventilation, decreased chest movement and reduced breath sounds on the unventilated side. Deflate cuff, withdraw tube 1–2 cm, reinflate cuff and recheck position. Do not confuse with a developing pneumothorax when unilateral breath sounds are heard (see Section 3.7.2).

(v) Any patient arriving intubated must have the position of the tube confirmed as described above. Do not assume that intubation has been carried out correctly or that the tube is still in the trachea.

Complications

Endotracheal intubation does have well recognized complications (see Box 2.3).

BOX 2.3 Complications following endotracheal intubation

1. Trauma – lips, teeth, tongue, jaw, pharynx, larynx, cervical spine
2. Hypoxia – prolonged attempt, unrecognized oesophageal intubation, intubation of the right main bronchus, failed intubation
3. Vomiting – degree of unconsciousness misjudged

Breathing

Following successful intubation, the patient must be ventilated with a high concentration of oxygen.

(i) Use a self-inflating bag with a reservoir and oxygen attached at 15 l/min. Ventilate so that the chest is seen to rise and at a rate of 12–15 breaths/min.

(ii) Use a mechanical ventilator if trained in its function;

 (a) set a tidal volume of 7–10 ml/kg at a rate of 12 breaths/min;

 (b) set the pressure limit initially to 25 mmHg (3 kPa, 30 cmH_2O);

 (c) set the FiO_2 to 1.0 (100%, no air mix);

 (d) attach to the patient and switch on.

The final determinant of the adequacy of ventilation is analysis of an arterial blood sample. A chest x-ray will also be required to allow identification of chest injuries and demonstrate the position of the tracheal tube. A large bore gastric tube should also be inserted to deflate and empty the stomach. A nasal approach for this tube is contraindicated if a base of skull fracture is suspected.

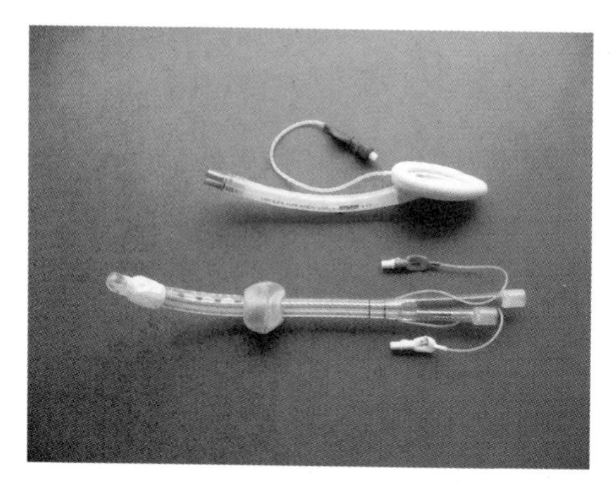

Figure 2.9 **LMA and Combitube**

Suction

If the airway is soiled by blood or vomit, tracheobronchial suction can be carried out preceded by a period of pre-oxygenation. A flexible, sterile catheter, less than half the diameter of the tracheal tube, is threaded down the tracheal tube. Once in place, suction is commenced in an intermittent fashion as the tube is withdrawn with a rotatory motion. The patient should not be deprived of oxygen for longer than 30 s and on no account must the suction be connected directly to the tracheal tube. Once the suction catheter has been removed, the patient must be ventilated for at least 1 min before the procedure is repeated. The patient's ECG and oxygen saturation must be monitored throughout this procedure.

Suction may cause:

- hypoxia from a decrease in lung volume, particularly if suction is prolonged;
- arrhythmias from sympathetic and vagal stimulation;
- hypertension and a rise in intracranial pressure.

Tracheal intubation may not always be possible for a number of reasons and there are two alternative airway management devices currently in use (*Figure 2.9*):

- laryngeal mask airway or LMA;
- Combitube.

2.6.2 Laryngeal mask airway

The LMA is inserted blindly, without the need for laryngoscopy. Once in place, the tip sits in the upper oesophagus and an inflatable cuff forms a low-pressure seal around the glottis. Although designed for use in spontaneously breathing patients, it can be used in conjunction with artificial ventilation provided care is taken not to generate high pressure in the airway (> 25 cmH_2O). Although made in a variety of sizes, those most commonly used in adults are 3 or 4 in females, 4 or 5 in males.

Advantages of the LMA

- It can be inserted with the neck maintained in a neutral position with a collar, etc., but it is easier if replaced with MILS.

- Artificial ventilation via the LMA is better than via a face mask.
- It is easier to insert than a tracheal tube, and the skill is learnt faster than intubation.
- There is considerable but not absolute protection against aspiration, particularly from above, that is, the nasopharynx.
- Insertion is often successful when tracheal intubation would be predicted to be difficult.
- Reflexes need to be suppressed to the same degree as for insertion of an oropharyngeal airway; muscle relaxants are not required.

Preparation for insertion is as described above for intubation.

The procedure (Figure 2.10)

- The cuff is deflated and the back of the mask is lubricated.
- The LMA is held in the dominant hand using the index finger as a 'splint'.
- The patient's mouth is opened and the LMA advanced behind the upper incisors and along the hard palate, with the open side facing but not touching the tongue.
- The mask is further inserted towards the pharynx, using the index finger to provide support.
- When the index finger is fully inserted the mask is held with the opposite hand and the finger removed.
- The mask is finally advanced until resistance is felt.
- The cuff is then inflated via the pilot tube.

The patient can then be allowed to breathe a high concentration of oxygen spontaneously or ventilated, with appropriate checks made.

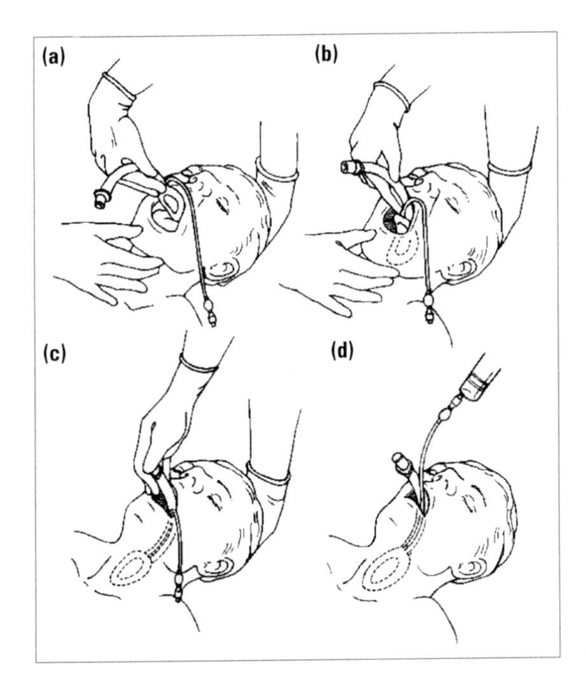

Figure 2.10 Insertion of LMA. Reproduced from Gwinnutt CL, *Clinical Anaesthesia* (1996), with permission from Blackwell Science.

Limitations of the LMA

- Difficult or impossible insertion if mouth opening is less than 1.5 cm, for example trismus, seizures, pre-existing disease of the temporomandibular joints.
- Poor ventilation if high airway pressures are required, e.g. pulmonary contusions, oedema.
- Inadequate in the presence of glottic or subglottic pathology, e.g. burns, foreign bodies.
- Difficult to insert if cricoid pressure is being applied.

Recently, an LMA with a modified cuff the 'Proseal LMA' has been introduced. This is claimed to have a higher seal pressure and therefore is more suited for use when ventilation is required. It also allows a gastric tube to be passed via a second lumen.

2.6.3 The Combitube

This is a double lumen tube that is inserted blindly and designed to allow artificial ventilation whether it enters the oesophagus or trachea. Once inserted, the two cuffs are inflated and ventilation of the patient is attempted assuming oesophageal placement (most commonly, > 90% of insertions). If this is unsuccessful ventilation is attempted via the tracheal lumen. At present the Combitube is not recommended for patients breathing spontaneously. The Combitube is available in two sizes, 37FG (small adult) and 41FG.

Advantages of the Combitube

- It can be inserted with the neck maintained in a neutral position.
- Ventilation is as effective as via a tracheal tube.
- It prevents aspiration of gastric contents whether in the oesophagus or trachea.
- It protects from soiling from above the larynx.
- The Combitube functions effectively in the presence of a cervical collar.
- It allows generation of relatively higher airway pressures compared to a standard LMA.
- It has been successfully used in a variety of difficult trauma scenarios.

Insertion

- The cuffs are fully deflated and the distal part of the Combitube is lubricated.
- Bending the device into a 'hockey-stick' shape aids insertion.
- The patients head and neck are maintained in a neutral position, the mouth opened and the jaw lifted.
- The device is inserted taking care to remain in the midline and advanced until the two black lines reach the teeth or gums.
- The large (No. 1) or pharyngeal cuff is inflated with air (approximately 1 ml/kg), and the small (No. 2) cuff with 10–15 ml air.
- As oesophageal placement almost always occurs, ventilation commences via the longer or No. 1 lumen and appropriate checks made to confirm ventilation (*Figure 2.11a*).

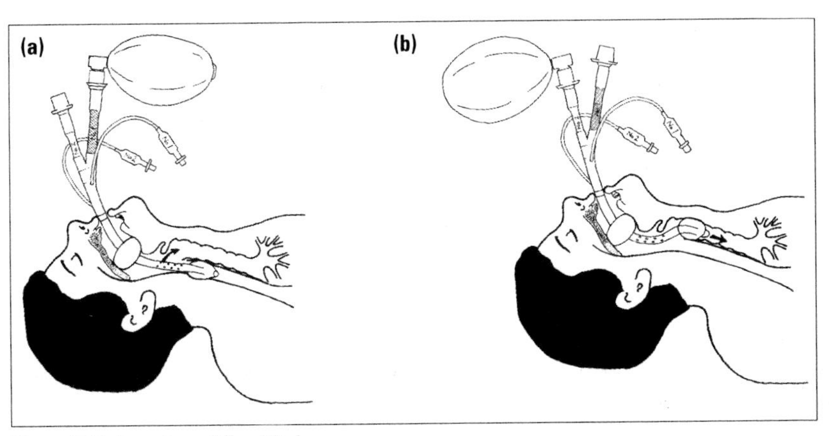

Figure 2.11 Insertion of Combitube

- If the lungs are not ventilated, ventilation is attempted via the shorter (No. 2) lumen and appropriate checks made (*Figure 2.11b*).
- Once correctly inserted and ventilation is confirmed, fixation is not essential.

Limitations of the Combitube

- Difficulty in acquiring training in insertion as it is not in daily use.
- Difficult insertion where there is restricted mouth opening.
- Risk of oesophageal perforation in the presence of known or suspected oesophageal pathology.
- Pharyngeal or laryngeal trauma on insertion, usually due to incorrect technique or overinflation of the pharyngeal balloon.
- Inability to ventilate via either lumen, usually because inserted too far and pharyngeal cuff occludes the larynx.
- Limited number of sizes and single use only.

Despite the potential problems identified above, both the LMA and Combitube are useful devices in airway management and have recently been included in the American Society of Anesthesiologists (ASA) difficult airway management algorithm.

Occasionally it may not be possible to intubate the trachea or achieve adequate oxygenation using the above devices. In such circumstances the airway nurse and doctor must be able to perform a surgical airway (see below).

2.6.4 Drugs used to facilitate advance airway management

The reflexes in the larynx must be abolished to facilitate intubation. Occasionally, this occurs as a result of the severity of injuries sustained, and the trachea can be intubated. However, such patients have a high mortality rate. More often, drugs are used to abolish the reflexes, usually a combination of an anaesthetic agent to ensure unconsciousness followed by a neuromuscular blocking drug ('muscle relaxant'). Further doses or infusions are then administered to maintain unconsciousness and prevent the patient becoming distressed and allow artificial ventilation. The LMA (and Combitube on the vast majority of occasions) do not pass through the larynx; administration of an anaesthetic agent alone is sufficient to allow insertion. The other most commonly used drugs are analgesics, usually opioids. Anaesthetic drugs may also be administered to modify the cardiovascular response to airway management, for example in the head injured when such responses may increase intracranial pressure (ICP) as a result of an increase in cerebral blood flow (see Section 6.3).

The decision to use these drugs will depend upon several factors:

- the type of device to be used;
- the presence of airway obstruction;
- any predicted difficulties with intubation;
- the presence of specific injuries.

The use of these agents must be restricted to those with anaesthetic training because of the potential problems associated with their use

Patients requiring intubation who have no evidence of airway obstruction, where there is no reason to expect difficulty with intubation, or they can already be adequately ventilated with a bag-valve-mask device, then it is appropriate to administer an intravenous anaesthetic agent followed by a muscle relaxant, to provide optimal conditions for intubation (see below).

In a patient where there is any predicted difficulty with intubation (see Box 2.4), the airway is compromised or ventilation impaired (e.g. severe facial trauma, laryngeal oedema), anaesthetic drugs will render the patient apnoeic and totally dependent on the airway nurse and doctor to secure the airway and maintain ventilation. If difficult or impossible ('can't intubate, can't ventilate'), hypoxia will be exacerbated and force the airway doctor to create a surgical airway under poor and hurried conditions. Under these circumstances, the alternatives are as follows, but all require considerable skill in airway management.

1. Inhalation induction of anaesthesia. The patient breathes an increasing concentration of an inhalational agent (e.g. sevoflurane in oxygen), until unconscious and the pharyngeal reflexes depressed. Direct laryngoscopy is then performed; if the larynx can be seen, either a tracheal tube can be passed (which may provoke coughing) or a muscle relaxant can be administered, knowing that intubation will be possible. This technique requires a clear airway and normal respiratory effort to ensure delivery of an adequate concentration of anaesthetic agent to the lungs. There will

BOX 2.4 Typical conditions predisposing to difficult intubation

Pre-existing conditions	Anatomical abnormalities	Obvious trauma
Pregnancy	Obesity	Faciomaxillary
Rheumatoid arthritis	Bull neck	Neck and cervical spine
Ankylosing spondylitis	Prominent dentition	Larynx
Acromegaly	Poor dentition	Airway obstruction

be a significant period between loss of consciousness and securing the airway during which the patient is at risk of aspiration.

2. Fibreoptic bronchoscopy. The airway is anaesthetized using topical (local) anaesthesia. The bronchoscope is advanced under direct vision, via either the nose or mouth into the trachea, while spontaneous ventilation is maintained. The tracheal tube is advanced over the bronchoscope into the larynx. This requires a cooperative patient if conscious and a relatively bloodless field to allow visualization of the anatomy through the bronchoscope.
3. In the conscious patient, with severe compromise of the airway and predicted difficulty with intubation or ventilation, the safest option is to perform a needle cricothyroidotomy under local anaesthesia. An anaesthetic agent and muscle relaxant can then be administered to optimize the conditions for intubation, knowing that if it fails, the patient can be oxygenated.

Pharmacology

Induction agents used to induce loss of consciousness in patients are generally short acting anaesthetic agents. Strictly speaking, only a muscle relaxant is needed to facilitate intubation, however paralysis alone would be extremely unpleasant and associated with potentially harmful reflexes (e.g. hypertension, tachycardia, increase in ICP).

Intravenous anaesthetic agents depress myocardial contractility and cause vasodilatation or both, resulting in hypotension. In those trauma patients who are already hypovolaemic, this effect is exaggerated. Ketamine has the least adverse effects unless the patient is profoundly hypovolaemic when its actions are similar to all other drugs.

Etomidate

- Presentation: 10 ml ampoules, 2 mg/ml, ready for use (eliminates the risk of dilution errors).
- Dose: 0.15–0.3 mg/kg intravenously.
- Loss of consciousness within 30–45 s, duration of 6–10 min.
- Associated with a relatively greater degree of cardiovascular stability, helping maintain vital organ perfusion.
- Reduces oxygen demand by the brain, cerebral blood flow and helps to control ICP, particularly if raised.
- Low risk of allergic reactions.
- Compatible with the other drugs mentioned.
- May cause pain on injection, hiccoughs and involuntary muscle movement.

Propofol

- Presentation: 20-ml ampoules, 10 mg/ml (1%) (50-ml syringes of 1% and 2% for infusion).
- Dose: 0.15–0.3 mg/kg but may be dramatically reduced in the injured.
- Loss of consciousness after 40–60 s, duration 3–4 min.
- Significant potential for causing hypotension, requires prior correction of any hypovolaemia.

- Reduces cerebral blood flow, helping control ICP.
- May cause pain on injection and involuntary muscle movement.

Propofol is increasingly used in trauma patients because after the initial dose, it can be administered as a continuous infusion to maintain unconsciousness, thereby avoiding inhalational agents or large doses of benzodiazepines. Infusion rates to maintain unconsciousness are variable in this group and will range from 20–60 ml/h (1%) depending upon age, weight, cardiovascular status and the concurrent administration of other drugs, particularly opioids. A purpose designed syringe pump ('Diprifusor') is available. Recovery is rapid on discontinuation of administration.

Midazolam

- Presentation: 5-ml ampoule, 2 mg/ml; 2-ml ampoule, 5 mg/ml.
- Dose: 0.1–0.2 mg/kg, this may be dramatically reduced in the critically ill and elderly.
- The time to loss of consciousness is longer than with etomidate or propofol; must be titrated against the patient's response.

Midazolam is a short-acting benzodiazepine that can be given intravenously to induce and maintain anaesthesia. Repeat doses of 2–4 mg can be given to maintain anaesthesia during ventilation.

Neuromuscular blocking drugs ('muscle relaxants'): This group of drugs are administered to abolish laryngeal reflexes, facilitate laryngoscopy and allow intubation. Once given, the patient will become apnoeic and dependent on the airway nurse and doctor to provide ventilation and secure the airway. Muscle relaxants can be divided into two groups according to their action at the neuromuscular junction: depolarizing (suxamethonium) or nondepolarizing (atracurium, rocuronium, vecuronium, pancuronium).

Suxamethonium

- Presentation: 2-ml ampoules containing 50 mg/ml .
- Dosage: bolus of 1.5 mg/kg intravenously.
- Following injection causes a transient, generalized fasciculation (twitching), followed by complete relaxation within 30–45 s.
- Duration of action of 3–5 min, due to metabolism by a naturally occurring enzyme, pseudocholinesterase.

Suxamethonium is the most rapid and profoundly acting of all neuromuscular blocking drugs following intravenous injection and unless contraindicated, remains the drug of choice in an emergency

There are a number of potential problems associated with the administration of suxamethonium:

- repeated boluses cause vagal stimulation and bradycardia. Atropine must be readily available and always administered prior to a second dose;
- may cause hyperkalaemia after major crush injuries, burns more than 24 h old, major denervation injury and certain pre-existing neuromuscular disorders;
- in penetrating eye injuries it may cause an acute rise in intra-ocular pressure, which can cause vitreous to be expelled;

- prolonged apnoea (3–24 h) in patients who do not have pseudocholinesterase (1 in 2800 of the population);
- there is a risk of triggering malignant hyperpyrexia, a rare disorder of muscle metabolism;
- it needs to be stored at 4°C, as it breaks down at room temperature.

The following two drugs reflect the authors' preferences. It is accepted that there are other valid alternatives.

Atracurium

- Presentation: 2.5 and 5-ml ampoules containing 10 mg/ml.
- Dose: 0.6 mg/kg.
- Muscle relaxation allowing intubation occurs after 90–120 s, with smaller doses the time is progressively longer.
- Duration of action is also dose dependent, lasting about 30–40 min.
- Repeated doses of 0.1–0.2 mg/kg to maintain relaxation and facilitate controlled ventilation.
- Indicated for maintenance of relaxation following intubation with suxamethonium or for the use in those situations where suxamethonium is contraindicated.
- No direct effect on the cardiovascular system, hypotension may occur after rapid administration of a large dose.
- It should be stored in the fridge as it undergoes very slow spontaneous degradation at room temperature.

Rocuronium

- Presentation: 5 and 10-ml ampoules containing 10 mg/ml.
- Dose: 0.6 mg/kg.
- Muscle relaxation allowing intubation occurs after 90 s.
- Duration of action approximately 40 min.
- Repeated doses of 0.15 mg/kg to maintain relaxation and facilitate controlled ventilation.

If the initial dose is increased to 1.0 mg/kg, the time to intubation can be reduced to around 60 s, but the duration is also significantly increased. This rapid onset makes it useful as a potential alternative in those patients where suxamethonium is contraindicated. Unfortunately, administration is associated with a relatively high incidence of anaphylactoid reactions.

2.6.5 Rapid sequence induction of anaesthesia and tracheal intubation (RSI)

Loss of the laryngeal reflexes predisposes patients to aspirating regurgitated gastric contents. As trauma delays gastric emptying, all patients should be assumed to have a full stomach, and steps taken to minimize the chances of this potentially fatal complication.

Preparation

Whenever possible, a gastric tube should be passed and aspirated to remove any liquid stomach contents, however this does not guarantee an empty stomach. Equipment

BOX 2.5 Checklist before RSI

Equipment:	As for endotracheal intubation Bag-valve-facemask system + reservoir bag Oxygen delivery apparatus Ventilator
Monitors:	BP, ECG, Pulse oximeter, end-tidal CO_2
Drugs:	Etomidate or Propofol Suxamethonium, Atropine Atracurium or Rocuronium Midazolam
Patient:	On a tipping trolley Airway in place Oxygenated Vital signs being monitored IV access in place

availability and function must be checked and drugs should be drawn up into labelled syringes (see Box 2.5). Suction is vital and should be switched on and positioned at the side of the patient's head.

Procedure

- The patient is pre-oxygenated for 2 min, by administering high flow oxygen.
- If conscious, briefly explain that they will shortly become sleepy and may feel pressure on the front of their neck.
- The chosen anaesthetic agent is injected into a fast running intravenous infusion.
- Cricoid pressure is applied as consciousness is lost.
- The suxamethonium is administered.
- After a period of 30–45 s, usually when fasciculations cease, intubation is performed.
- Once the tube is in the trachea, the cuff is inflated.
- The lungs are ventilated and tube position confirmed by monitoring for CO_2 in expired gas.
- If satisfactory, cricoid pressure can now be released and the tube secured.

If a nondepolarizing relaxant is used no fasciculations will be seen and it will be necessary to wait for between 1–2 min depending on the drug and dose administered before attempting intubation.

If by chance all ventilatory devices fail, use expired air ventilation and blow down the endotracheal tube!

The patient must be continuously monitored with emphasis on oxygen saturation, end-tidal CO_2, skin colour, blood pressure, heart rate, cardiac rhythm, airway pressures and temperature.

2.6.6 Cricoid pressure

The airway nurse should stand facing the patient's head. The tips of the thumb and index finger should be placed on the cricoid ring. This structure must be identified

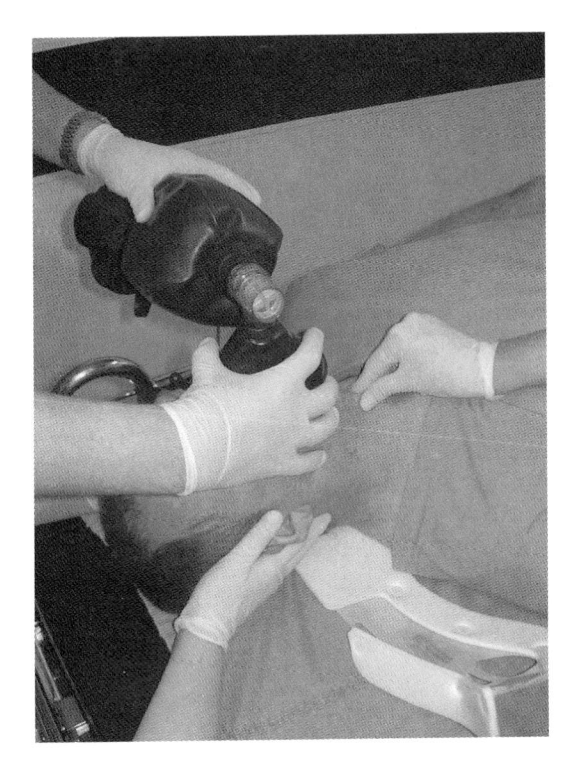

Figure 2.12 Application of cricoid pressure

beforehand if the nurse is uncertain. Direct pressure in the midline is applied as the patient loses consciousness (*Figure 2.12*). This occludes the oesophagus by squeezing it between the cricoid ring and the 6th cervical vertebrae and so prevents regurgitation and passage of air into the stomach. Cricoid pressure is still effective if a naso- or orogastric tube is in place.

If incorrectly applied, the trachea can be deviated making intubation more difficult. It should also be discontinued if the patient begins actively to vomit otherwise the oesophagus is at risk of rupturing. In this situation the patient must be quickly tipped head down, the airway cleared of vomit, the pressure released and cervical spine stabilization maintained. If there are enough personnel present, the patient can be turned in a controlled way onto their side.

Occasionally, reversal of neuromuscular block is required in the resuscitation room. This can be achieved by the intravenous administration of neostigmine along with an anticholinergic (usually glycopyrrolate). This should only be carried out by trained staff because of the associated risks.

2.6.7 Surgical airway

In some cases it may be impossible to ventilate a patient using any of the devices described above or intubate the trachea. This may result from complete obstruction of the airway due to oedema (e.g. inhalation burns) and trauma (e.g. laryngeal damage). Most of these patients will arrive in the emergency department unconscious, either a result of their initial injuries or the resulting hypoxia. In these situations a surgical airway is required urgently.

The conscious patient with an obstructed airway will tend to thrash around in a desperate desire to breathe. Where there is profuse bleeding the patient may wish to sit forward to stop the blood pooling in the pharynx and to allow unstable facial fractures to fall forward and partially clear his airway. Sedatives or muscle relaxants must not be administered without the presence of an experienced anaesthetist, as they will cause apnoea and the immediate need for an airway and ventilation. If this proves impossible, a surgical airway must be created.

Whichever technique is used, before commencing all equipment must be checked and in place, the airway cleared and secured as best as possible and a high flow of oxygen administered at all times as it is unlikely there will be complete airway obstruction.

Needle cricothyroidotomy

Also referred to as jet ventilation and consists of inserting a large bore intravenous cannula (14 g or 16 g) or purpose designed device, through the cricothyroid membrane (*Figure 2.13*) to allow intermittent delivery of oxygen. Ventilation is inadequate and results in accumulation of carbon dioxide (hypercarbia), which limits this technique to 20–30 min. During this time a definitive airway should have been created. There are several important facts to be aware of with this technique:

- Oxygenation is only achieved using a high-pressure supply, i.e. the piped (wall supply) or cylinder oxygen. An anaesthetist may use a specialized device (Sander's injector or Manujet) to deliver oxygen (*Figure 2.13*). A self-inflating bag will not generate sufficient pressure.
- Expiration occurs through the larynx, not the cannula. It is essential to ensure that gas is escaping via this route to prevent barotrauma from overinflation.

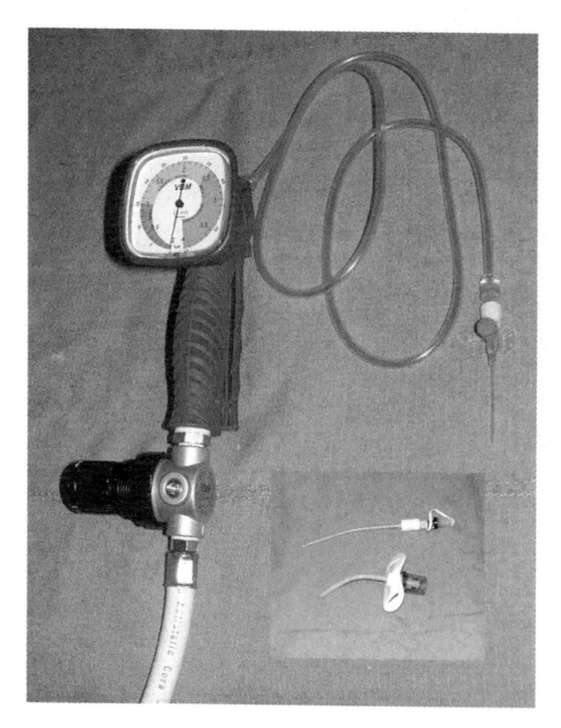

Figure 2.13 Equipment for needle cricothyroidotomy

- As a result of such high pressures, all connections between the supply and the cannula must either be luer-locked or bonded to prevent disconnection.
- Whatever system is used it should be readily available rather than constructed in haste in an emergency.

Procedure (*Figure 2.14*)

- The landmarks of the cricothyroid membrane are identified and if time permits, marked.
- When possible the skin is prepared with antiseptic solution.
- A 10-ml syringe is attached to the cannula.
- The operator stabilizes the thyroid cartilage with one hand.
- The cannula is inserted through the skin and cricothyroid membrane in a slightly caudal direction, aspirating on the syringe.
- Free flow of air into the syringe indicates that the tip of the needle has entered the trachea.
- The cannula is advanced a further 5 mm, to ensure the body of the cannula has entered the trachea, aspirating all the time.
- The cannula is advanced fully over the needle into the trachea, needle removed and a final aspiration check made.
- The assisting nurse will now need to hold the cannula in place.

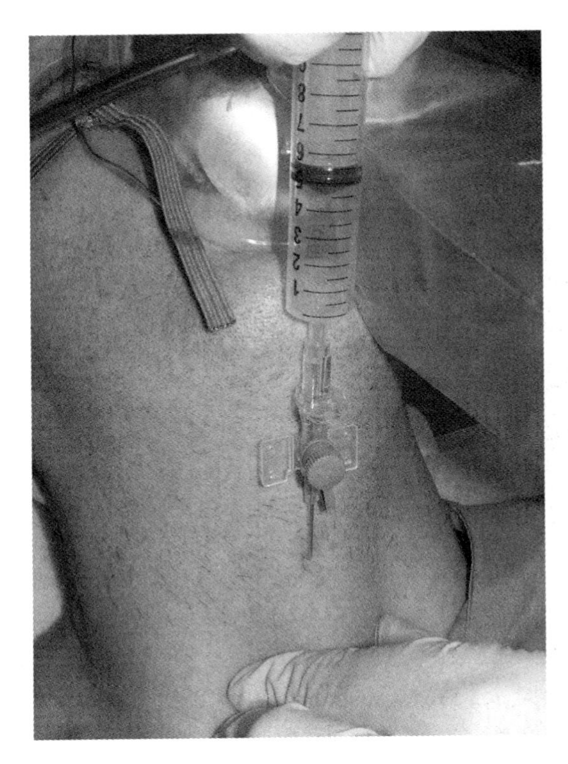

Figure 2.14 **Needle cricothryoidotomy**

- The delivery system is connected and oxygen insufflated sufficiently to make the chest rise.
- Adequacy of oxygenation is checked with a pulse oximeter.

Complications

- Barotrauma and pneumothorax due to the high airway pressure required during ventilation.
- Insertion can cause haemorrhage, oesophageal damage and surgical emphysema if positioned incorrectly.
- Kinking or obstruction of the cannula and failure of oxygenation.

Needle cricothyroidotomy is also the surgical airway of choice for patients under 12 years old.

Surgical cricothyroidotomy

In this technique, an incision is made through the skin and cricothyroid membrane into the glottis to allow the insertion of a small tracheostomy tube or tracheal tube (5–6-mm diameter) into the trachea. Although a relatively small tube is used, this is sufficient to allow both oxygenation and ventilation using standard devices, and tracheal suction to remove blood and secretions, etc. The technique is associated with significant haemorrhage from vessels dilated as a result of hypercarbia and hypoxia. If there is laryngeal trauma or an expanding haematoma within the operating field, a formal tracheostomy performed by an appropriate expert is the technique of choice.

Procedure (*Figure 2.15*)

- In the absence of trauma to the cervical spine, hyperextend the patient's head.
- The landmarks of the cricothyroid membrane are identified and if time permits, marked.
- When possible the skin is prepared with antiseptic solution.
- Infiltrate the skin over the membrane with 1% lignocaine with adrenaline (epinephrine) (1:100 000) to minimize cutaneous bleeding.

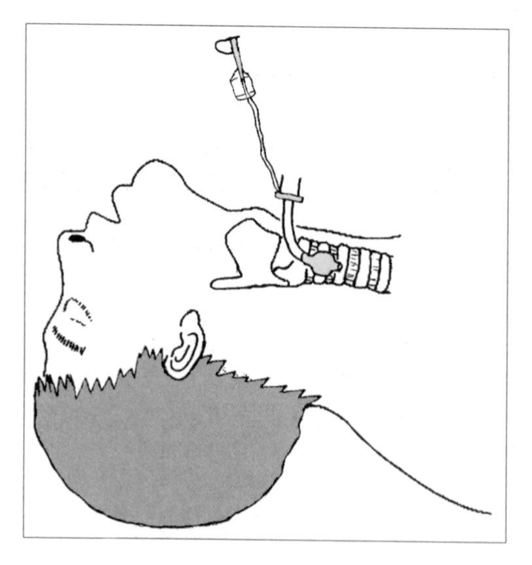

Figure 2.15 Surgical cricothryoidotomy

- The operator stabilizes the thyroid cartilage with one hand.
- A transverse incision, 2–3 cm long is made over the membrane.
- A finger is then inserted into the wound to reassess the membrane's position.
- The membrane is incised transversely.
- A channel is created with either the scalpel handle, artery forceps or a self-retaining retractor.
- The assisting nurse may need to maintain this channel if there is vigorous movement of the larynx.
- A lubricated tracheostomy tube is inserted, directed caudally into the trachea.
- The cuff is inflated and ventilation commenced.
- Correct position is confirmed by checking for CO_2 in expired gas, observing chest movement and auscultation.
- The tube is secured with sutures or tape and any blood or debris aspirated.

Complications

- Surgical damage to any of the adjacent structures.
- Haemorrhage.
- Incorrect placement of the tube, failed ventilation and surgical emphysema.

Once the airway is secure and ventilation established, a chest x-ray and an arterial blood gas sample should be taken. Small tubes are easily dislodged by the weight of any attached ventilator tubes or during movement of the patient. The airway team must take great care of the surgical airway at all times and if there is any deterioration in the patient's condition a rapid reassessment of the airway and ventilation are the first priority.

2.7 Summary

In every trauma patient, the airway must be cleared, secured, and the cervical spine stabilized, as soon as possible. Initially basic techniques are used, with more advanced procedures being carried out only if they prove to be inadequate. As the establishing of a patent airway is so fundamental to the management of the trauma patient, and the procedures potentially so varied, it is vital that only experienced members of the trauma team are given the responsibility of managing the airway.

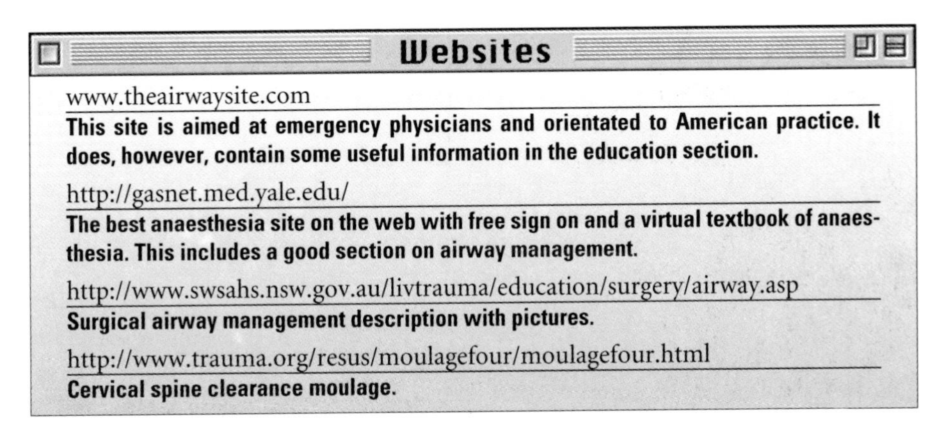

Websites

www.theairwaysite.com

This site is aimed at emergency physicians and orientated to American practice. It does, however, contain some useful information in the education section.

http://gasnet.med.yale.edu/

The best anaesthesia site on the web with free sign on and a virtual textbook of anaesthesia. This includes a good section on airway management.

http://www.swsahs.nsw.gov.au/livtrauma/education/surgery/airway.asp

Surgical airway management description with pictures.

http://www.trauma.org/resus/moulagefour/moulagefour.html

Cervical spine clearance moulage.

Further reading

1. **Bryden DC & Gwinnutt CL** (2000) Airway management: the difficult airway. *Trauma* **2:** 113.
2. **Carley SC, Gwinnutt C, Butler J, *et al.*** (2002) Rapid sequence induction in the emergency department: a strategy for failure. *Emerg. Med. J.* **19:** 109.
3. **Crosby ED, Cooper RM, Douglas MJ, *et al.*** (1998) The unanticipated difficult airway with recommendations for management. *Can. J. Anaesth.* **45**(7)**:** 757.
4. **Gwinnutt CL** (1996) *Clinical Anaesthesia*. Blackwell Science, Oxford.
5. **Gwinnutt CL & Nolan J** (In press) Trauma anaesthesia. In: Healy TEJ and Knight PR (eds): *Wylie and Churchill-Davidson's A Practice of Anaesthesia*, 7th edn. London: Arnold.
6. **Mandavia DP, Qualls S and Rokos I** (2000) Emergency airway management in penetrating neck injury. *Ann. Emerg. Med.* **35**(3)**:** 221.

3 Thoracic trauma

R Kishen, G Lomas

Objectives

The objectives of this chapter are to teach the trauma team members:

- the applied anatomy of thorax;
- the pathophysiology of ventilation and gas exchange;
- how to assess and manage thoracic injuries that are an immediate threat to life;
- how to assess and manage thoracic injuries that are a potential threat to life;
- the different investigations used in the management of thoracic trauma;
- the assessment and management of other non-life threatening thoracic injuries.

3.1 Introduction

Chest trauma is the primary cause of death in about 25% of all trauma deaths and an associated factor in a further 50%, usually as a result of hypoxia and hypovolaemia. When the heart is not involved, the mortality of isolated penetrating chest trauma is < 1%, but cardiac involvement increases mortality 20-fold. In an industrialized society, the commonest injury is to the chest wall, followed by pulmonary parenchymal injury, haemothorax, pneumothorax and flail chest. These conditions give rise to hypoxaemia and hypovolaemia, which are easily treatable with simple measures, consequently 85% of thoracic trauma victims can be successfully treated without the need for thoracic surgical intervention. Unfortunately, thoracic trauma is associated with other injuries, which may well account for the overall high mortality in these patients. This chapter will discuss the principles of management of thoracic trauma. Although the thoracic spine forms part of the thoracic cage, trauma to the spine is dealt with in Chapter 7.

3.2 Applied anatomy

3.2.1 Chest wall

The chest wall consists of a bony skeleton and associated soft tissue and acts as a cage to protect the thoracic contents. The bony skeleton comprises of 12 semicircular ribs on either side, which are attached to the thoracic vertebrae posteriorly and, anteriorly through the costal cartilages to the sternum, except for ribs 11 and 12 that are free anteriorly. The sternum consists of a short upper manubrium, a larger body and a small xiphoid process and protects the heart and the great vessels that lie directly posterior to it while giving attachment to various neck, abdominal and pectoral muscles.

The skeletal elements are covered with muscles, fascia, subcutaneous tissue and skin. The inside of the rib cage is lined by the parietal pleura (see Section 3.2.4).

Overlying the upper part of the rib cage are the clavicles and scapulae. A fracture of the 1st or 2nd ribs usually indicates significant energy transfer, for example a fall from height or high-speed impact. This should alert the trauma team to look for other associated injuries. When several ribs are fractured in two places, the chest wall will show *paradoxical movement* during respiratory cycle, i.e. the broken section will be pulled inwards during inspiration and bulge out during expiration; this is called *a flail segment*. This will result in inadequate ventilation and is usually associated with an underlying lung contusion. The combination inadequate ventilation and lung injury will lead to severe hypoxaemia. The neurovascular bundle lies along the lower border of each corresponding rib, a fact that is important to remember when inserting a chest drain in order to avoid unnecessary injury. The area inferior to the axillae, usually the 5th intercostal space, is the thinnest portion of the chest wall and an ideal site for insertion of chest drains.

3.2.2 Diaphragm

This is the main muscle of respiration and consists of a central tendon with radially orientated muscle fibres forming two domes (right and left) or hemidiaphragms. Several structures traverse the diaphragm: the aorta, the thoracic duct, the azygos vein, the oesophagus, the vagus nerves and their branches and the vena cava. During normal quiet breathing, the diaphragm moves about 1.5–2 cm but this can increase to 10 cm during deep breathing. During deep exhalation, the dome of diaphragm can ascend to the 5th intercostal space, an important point to remember while inserting chest drains. This also explains diaphragmatic and intra-abdominal injuries following penetrating injuries high on the chest wall.

3.2.3 Trachea and bronchi

The trachea extends from the cricoid cartilage, at the level of 6th cervical vertebra to the carina. On each side lie the jugular veins, common carotid arteries and the vagus nerves. It bifurcates at the level of lower border of 4th or upper border of 5th thoracic vertebra, into the main bronchi, the right being shorter, straighter and less angulated in relation to the trachea than the left. The right main bronchus lies posterior to the right main pulmonary artery while the left main bronchus is adjacent to the aortic arch, posterior to the left atrium. The trachea is loosely fastened in the neck and superior mediastinum and can be displaced laterally by external pressure.

3.2.4 Lungs and pleurae

The right lung has three lobes: upper, middle and lower, divided by transverse and oblique fissures. The left lung has two lobes, upper and lower, divided by the oblique fissure (*Figure 3.1*). Both lungs are divided into bronchopulmonary segments corresponding to the bronchial branches of the right and left pulmonary arteries. Both lungs are drained by superior and inferior pulmonary veins.

The surface of lungs and the inner surface of the chest wall are lined by a thin pleural membrane, the visceral and parietal pleura, respectively and in the healthy state there

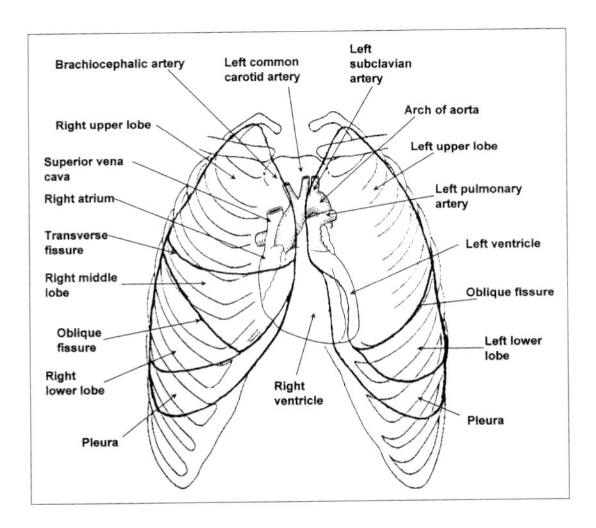

Figure 3.1 **The thoracic contents**

is only a potential space between the two layers. The opposing forces of the chest wall (pulling out) and the elastic recoil of the lungs (pulling in) cause a negative pressure in this potential space that keeps the lung from collapsing. If there is a break in either membrane, then air and/or fluid can enter the cavity and a 'space' is created. If air enters the cavity a *pneumothorax* exists. If a 'one-way valve' forms into the pleural cavity, then air enters but cannot leave and results in a potentially life-threatening condition of *tension pneumothorax*. Accumulation of blood in the pleural cavity is called a haemothorax.

3.2.5 Mediastinum

This contains all the thoracic viscera except the lungs and extends from the spine posteriorly to the sternum anteriorly, with the heart occupying the middle mediastinum. The heart is invested by the pericardium – a tough, nonelastic membrane that is attached to the diaphragm inferiorly and extends along the two branches of the pulmonary artery as well as the ascending aorta. If blood collects between the pericardium and heart, the chambers of the heart are compressed and cardiac output is reduced.

The thoracic aorta is divided into an ascending part, the arch and the descending part. The main branches of the aorta are innominate artery, which divides into right subclavian and right common carotid arteries just behind the right sternoclavicular joint, the left common carotid and left subclavian arteries which arise further downstream (separately) from the arch just before it becomes the descending aorta. The descending part continues downwards, behind the heart to pass through the diaphragm into the abdominal cavity.

The oesophagus lies in the posterior mediastinum and extends from the pharynx in the neck to the gastro-oesophageal junction and is extrapleural. The thoracic duct ascends through the aortic hiatus into thorax and lies on the right side of the vertebral bodies. It empties into the venous system at the junction of the left subclavian and internal jugular vein.

The major consequences of thoracic trauma are disruption of pulmonary and cardiac function, resulting in hypoxaemia and hypotension respectively, that either jointly or separately cause reduced oxygen delivery to the tissue, hypoperfusion, organ failure and death. For clarity the two disturbances are considered separately, but there is considerable overlap and disturbance of one system may profoundly affect the function of the other.

3.3 Pathophysiology

The main functions of the lungs are oxygenation of blood and removal of carbon dioxide. To achieve this:

- adequate air has to reach the alveoli (ventilation);
- an adequate circulation is required around the alveoli (perfusion);
- transfer of gases must occur in both directions between the alveoli and blood (diffusion).

If there is no problem with diffusion, oxygenation of the blood is primarily a function of the inspired oxygen concentration and removal of carbon dioxide is a function of alveolar ventilation. Any disruption of one or more of these processes can lead to hypoxaemia or hypercarbia.

3.3.1 Ventilation

The amount of air taken into the lungs with each breath is the tidal volume (V_T) and during quite periods of breathing is normally about 7–8 ml/kg (about 500 ml in a 70 kg adult). The volume of air inspired into (or expired from) the lungs each minute is the minute volume and under normal circumstances is approximately 7 l/min (500 ml/breath at a rate of 14 breaths/min; *Figure 3.2*).

Not all of the tidal volume takes part in the respiratory gas exchange. Only about 70% of V_T (350 ml) reaches the alveoli; the rest fills the mouth, trachea and the bronchi. This is called the dead space or more accurately *anatomical dead space*, as it is not involved with gas exchange. Failure of gas exchange also occurs in areas of lung that are ventilated but not perfused with blood. When added to the anatomical dead space, this is called the *physiological dead space*. In health, these are almost identical as most areas of the lung are both ventilated and perfused. The volume of ventilation that actually takes part in the gas exchange is called *alveolar ventilation*, and is approximately 5 l/min (350 ml × 14 breaths/min).

At the end of a normal expiration there is a considerable volume of gas remaining in the lungs, termed the *Functional Residual Capacity (FRC)*. This is the result of the two opposing forces between the chest wall (outwards) and the lung (inwards). Approximately 15% of the FRC is replaced with fresh gas during each tidal volume breath. The FRC acts as a reservoir, keeping alveoli open at the end of expiration and ensuring that sudden changes in gas composition within the lungs and blood are avoided.

3.3.2 Perfusion

The lungs are perfused (Q) with approximately 5 l blood/min (*Figure 3.2*). The pulmonary circulation is a low-pressure system and, as a consequence, gravity influences the flow of blood in different parts of the lungs. In turn this effects oxygenation of the

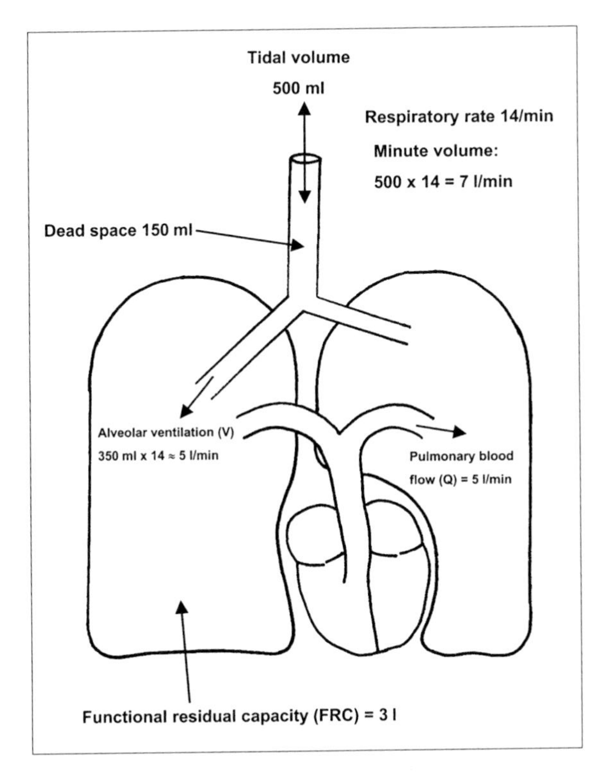

Figure 3.2 Normal volumes and flows

blood circulating in that part. In the erect position, apical alveoli are therefore less well perfused than basal alveoli, giving rise to dead space (see above). In turn the basal alveoli are overperfused in relation to ventilation and this leads to some of the blood not taking up oxygen nor giving up carbon dioxide. This latter effect is termed *shunting* (the blood is literally shunted past alveoli with no effect) and in health this amounts to less than 5% of the cardiac output.

3.3.3 Diffusion

Gas exchange occurs by diffusion a process dependent upon:

- partial pressure gradient of the gas;
- solubility of the diffusing gas;
- the thickness of this membrane;
- area of the membrane across which diffusion is taking place.

The partial pressure of a gas is dependent on the percentage it contributes to a mixture, multiplied by the total pressure. For example, oxygen comprises 21% of the atmosphere (pressure 100 kPa), therefore the partial pressure of oxygen in air is $21/100 \times 100 = 21$ kPa.

Gases diffuse down a partial pressure gradient (i.e. from high to low). As the partial pressure of oxygen in the alveoli is high and in the pulmonary capillary blood low, oxygen diffuses from alveoli to blood. Conversely, carbon dioxide diffuses from blood to alveoli. However, carbon dioxide is 20 times more diffusible than oxygen so despite a lower gradient, diffuses across the alveolar–capillary membrane far more rapidly.

The alveolar–capillary membrane is ideally suited for diffusion as it is only 0.0005 mm thick and has a large surface area (50 m^2). It follows then, that an increase in the thickness of this membrane (e.g. pulmonary oedema) or a reduction in its size (collapse, consolidation, pneumothorax, etc.) will impair diffusion, particularly of oxygen and cause hypoxaemia.

3.3.4 Ventilation/perfusion ratio

Under normal conditions, ventilation (*V*, 5 l/min) and perfusion (*Q*, 5 l/min) are well matched (despite minor variations at the extremes of the apices and bases) and the ventilation/perfusion ratio (*V/Q*) is approximately 1 (*Figure 3.3*). Oxygen in the alveoli diffuses into blood, saturating all the haemoglobin molecules and, as a result, the partial pressure of oxygen in the blood (PaO_2) leaving the lungs is approximately 13 kPa. In addition a very small amount of oxygen is dissolved in the plasma.

If ventilation exceeds perfusion, for example in shock (low cardiac output, $V/Q > 1$), there is not enough blood circulating to accept all the oxygen available. Oxygen is 'wasted' as once the haemoglobin is fully saturated the arterial content cannot be increased any further, except for a small increase in oxygen directly dissolved in plasma.

Conversely, when perfusion exceeds ventilation, for example, a lung contusion (reduced ventilation, $V/Q < 1$) there is an inadequate amount of oxygen fully to

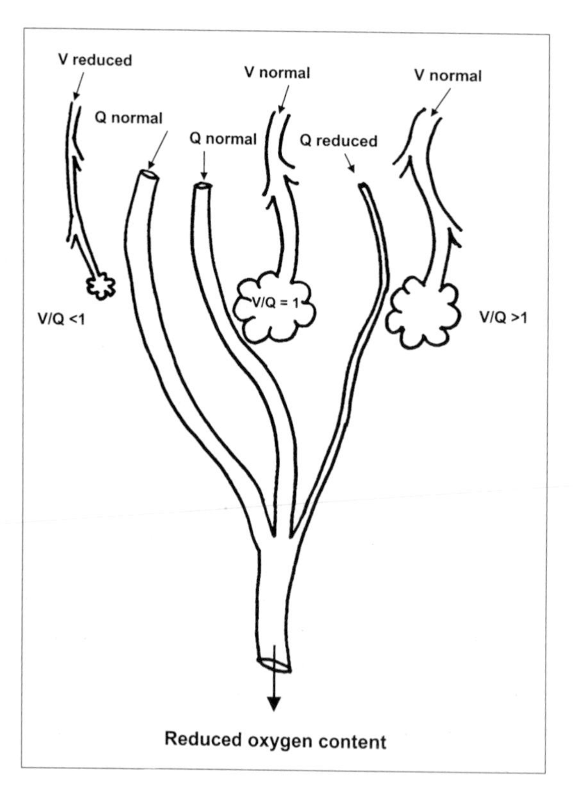

Figure 3.3 Three different V/Q ratios

saturate the haemoglobin. Consequently there is a reduced oxygen content in the blood leaving these areas of the lung. This has the same effect as 'shunting' described earlier, that is, the blood seems to have 'bypassed' the lung without being oxygenated.

After trauma areas of normal, high and low V/Q co-exist in the lungs and the final oxygen content of arterial blood depends upon the combined influence of all three. The small rise in oxygen dissolved in plasma from areas of high V/Q cannot compensate for the larger deficit in the oxygen content from areas of low V/Q. As the latter tend to predominate this results in hypoxaemia. Once 30% or more of the blood in the pulmonary circulation passes through areas of low V/Q, the hypoxia cannot be corrected by simply increasing the oxygen content of the inspired gas. Not surprisingly, V/Q mismatch is responsible for many deaths in trauma victims.

3.4 Assessment and management

This follows the well-defined categories for all trauma victims used throughout this book, remembering that the primary survey and resuscitation are simultaneous events.

3.4.1 Primary survey and resuscitation

This follows the same plan as described in Section 1.6.1, with the aim of identifying and correcting any immediately life-threatening conditions. With respect to thoracic trauma there are six conditions that fall into this category:

- airway obstruction;
- tension pneumothorax;
- open chest wound;
- flail chest;
- cardiac tamponade;
- massive haemothorax.

Airway

Airway obstruction has been covered in Section 2.4. Members of the team responsible for the airway must assess, clear and secure the airway using whatever techniques are appropriate, whilst maintaining in-line cervical immobilization. A high-inspired oxygen concentration should be delivered. The position of trachea, any neck injuries or distended neck veins are looked for and noted, before the reapplication of the collar.

Breathing

The patient's chest is exposed and inspected for bruising, penetrating wounds, intercostal indrawing, abnormal chest movements and the rate, depth and pattern of breathing are carefully observed. Rapid shallow breathing usually accompanies chest injury or developing hypoxia. Paradoxical chest wall movement during respiration (indrawing of the chest wall during inspiration and vice versa) suggests a flail segment. Both sides of the chest are percussed and the note compared. Hyperresonance suggests a pneumothorax, while a dull note indicates a haemothorax, or the possibility of a ruptured diaphragm. Finally, the chest is auscultated on both sides, high in the axillae, to assess adequacy and equality of air entry.

Tension pneumothorax

This is caused by air entering the pleural cavity by a 'one-way' valve during inspiration (spontaneous or controlled ventilation) and failing to escape. It may be due to rupture of an emphysematous bulla or direct lung trauma. Normally, the pleural cavity has a negative pressure with respect to atmospheric pressure, but if air accumulates over a period of time, the pressure becomes positive. This causes mediastinal shift, which in turn reduces venous return, cardiac filling and tamponade of either or both ventricles. These effects dramatically reduce cardiac output causing hypotension and hypoperfusion. Compensatory mechanisms of increased catecholamine release and adrenergic discharge cause a tachycardia and peripheral vasoconstriction to try to maintain cardiac output and perfusion of the vital organs. If the tension is not relieved, the compensation will ultimately fail causing 'irreversible' shock. The diagnosis is clinical not radiological and made by finding the signs shown in Box 3.1.

If a tension pneumothorax is suspected, it must be dealt with immediately by needle decompression (needle thoracocentesis) followed by the insertion of a chest drain (see later).

BOX 3.1 Signs of tension pneumothorax

- Anxiety
- Tachypnoea/respiratory distress
- Shock (hypotension and tachycardia)
- Hyperresonance and decreased air entry in the same hemithorax
- Deviation of the trachea (late)
- Engorged neck veins if no hypovolaemia
- Cyanosis (very late)

Needle thoracocentesis

Needle decompression of a tension pneumothorax is an emergency life-saving procedure; there is no time for 'skin prep' or local anaesthetic! It converts a tension pneumothorax into a simple pneumothorax (*Figure 3.4*).

- A large bore cannula (14 or 16 g) is inserted in midclavicular line in the 2nd intercostal space just above the upper margin of the lower (3rd) rib.
- Some advocate use of a syringe attached to the cannula, but in reality, it does not matter.
- Upon removing the cap of the cannula, a rush of air is a positive sign, confirms the diagnosis and usually results in significant improvement of the patient's cardiovascular and respiratory status.
- After removing the inner metal needle, the cannula may be fixed in place by adhesive tape.
- Preparations must be made for a definitive chest drain, as these cannulae are notorious for either getting blocked by blood clots, getting bent or falling out, thus causing a recurrence of a tension pneumothorax.

In case of a misdiagnosis of tension pneumothorax (when there is no rush or passage of air), the clinicians will appreciate that a pneumothorax has now been created and needs to be dealt with as in simple pneumothorax.

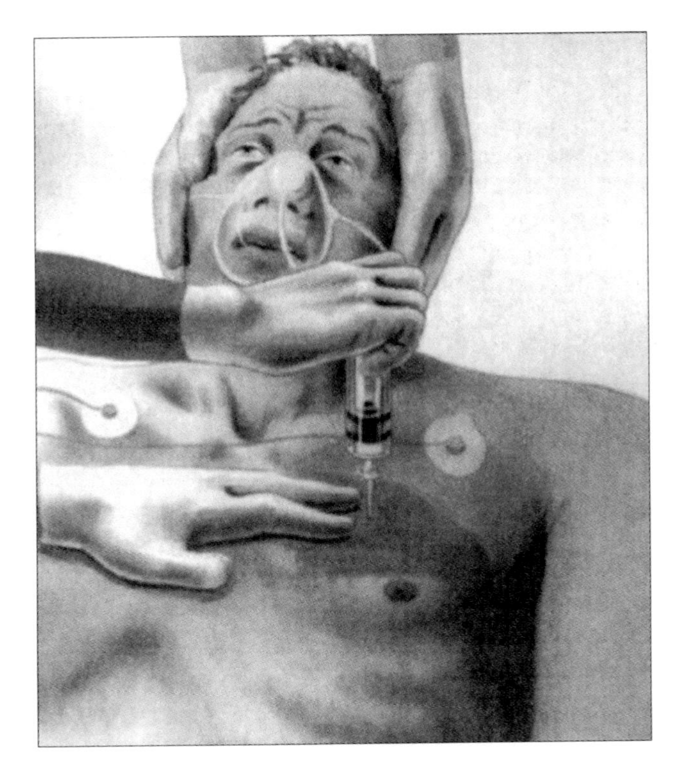

Figure 3.4 Needle thoracocentesis

Open chest wound

This results in a pneumothorax on the same side as the injury. If the wound size is greater than two-thirds the diameter of the trachea, then air will preferentially enter the pleural cavity via this route during inspiration, compromising ventilation and causing hypoxia. Untreated the lung will eventually collapse. In some situations air can enter via the wound but not escape (sometimes referred to as a 'sucking chest wound'). This may be due to the shape of the wound or an inadequate dressing. A tension pneumothorax will then develop rapidly. The immediate management consists of removing any completely occlusive dressing to allow air to escape. A new dressing, taped on three sides, should be applied whilst preparation is made for the insertion of a chest drain via a separate route. The wound can then be formally redressed.

Flail chest (*Figure 3.5*)

This occurs when more than one rib is fractured at more than one site. If conscious, the patient will be in severe pain, with rapid shallow ventilation. Examination of the chest wall may reveal crepitus, abrasions or paradoxical movement of the flail segment. Early on, the flail may be splinted and paradoxical movement only seen as the victim becomes exhausted. Management consists of high-flow, warmed, humidified oxygen, adequate fluid resuscitation and early administration of analgesia. This usually consists at this stage of iv opioids. Intercostal or epidural analgesia should be considered during the secondary survey, depending on the expertise available. Some patients (see Box 3.2) will require more aggressive management, as an increased inspired oxygen concentration

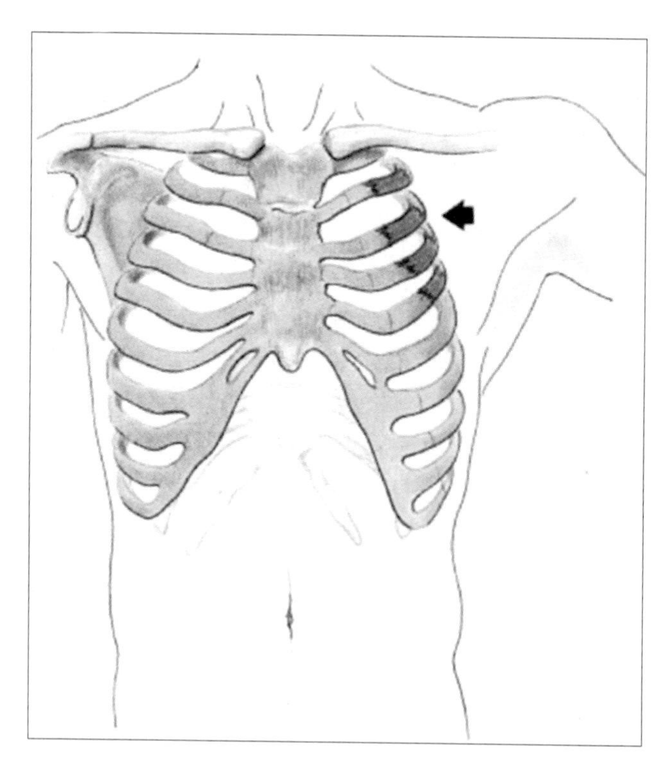

Figure 3.5 Diagram of flail chest – more than one rib fractured at more than one site

BOX 3.2	Indications for tracheal intubation and ventilation
	• Falling PaO_2 or $PaO_2 < 7$ kPa breathing air • $PaO_2 < 10$ kPa on high flow oxygen • Increasing $PaCO_2$, or > 6 kPa • Exhaustion, respiratory rate > 30 breaths/min • Associated head or abdominal injury

fails to compensate for the progressive deterioration of ventilation and increasing hypoxia. This will require tracheal intubation and controlled ventilation. In all patients arterial blood gases need to be monitored frequently to assess respiratory function.

Circulation

The circulation doctor must make a quick assessment of the patient's colour, capillary return and presence of radial, femoral and carotid pulses, while the nurse measures the pulse rate, blood pressure, pulse pressure and temperature. Organ perfusion is initially assessed by the level of consciousness and (later) by urine output. The heart is auscultated and attention is paid to the presence of any murmurs. Neck veins will have been examined whilst the neck collar was off. Two large (14–16 g) peripheral intravenous cannulae should be inserted and, from one, 20 ml blood taken for investigations and cross-match or typing. Assuming a tension pneumothorax has already been ruled out or treated, shock may be due to either of the following conditions.

Cardiac tamponade

This should be suspected in any victim with a penetrating wound of the chest, neck or upper abdomen as these may involve the heart (*Figure 3.6*). A penetrating wound of the heart may result in bleeding into the 'intact' pericardial sac (smaller injuries of the pericardium may seal with a clot). The accumulated blood in the pericardial sac restricts ventricular filling during diastole, thus reducing the stroke volume during systole. This in turn results in a low cardiac output. As mentioned earlier, compensatory mechanisms come into play to maintain cardiac output (by increasing heart rate) and perfusion pressure (by increasing peripheral vascular resistance). If the pressure within the pericardial cavity is not released, cardiac output keeps falling and the compensatory mechanisms are not enough to maintain organ perfusion. Profound hypotension results, which in turn causes further myocardial injury (as a consequence of reduced coronary perfusion). If not relieved promptly, the patient will die from grossly inadequate cardiac function and perfusion. The signs of cardiac tamponade are shown in Box 3.3, but are only seen in approximately one-third of trauma patients.

BOX 3.3 Signs of cardiac tamponade

- Beck's triad
  - Shock
  - Raised jugular venous pressure (JVP) (impaired return to the right ventricle)
  - Decreased heart sounds (difficult in the resuscitation room)
- Pulsus paradoxus $>$ 10 mmHg fall in pressure during inspiration
- Kussmaul's sign – raised JVP on inspiration

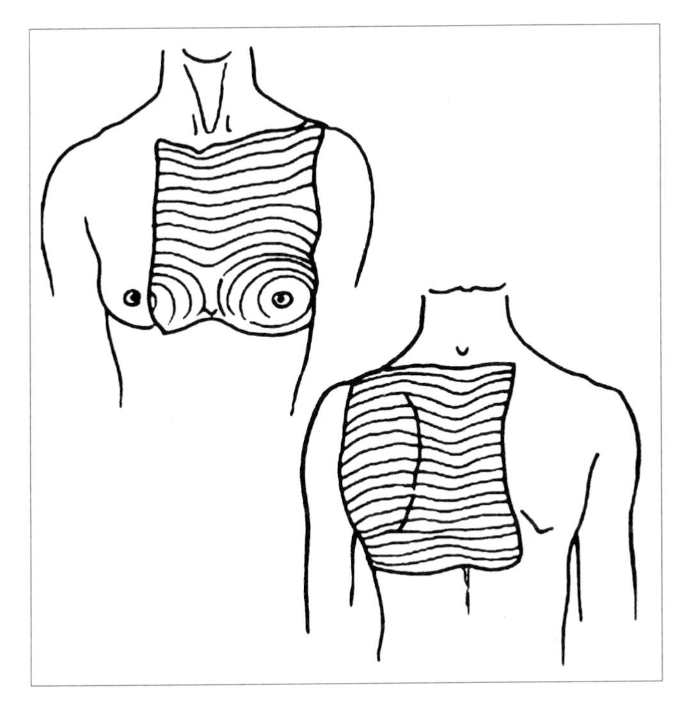

Figure 3.6 Sites of wounds associated with cardiac tamponade

Initial management consists of augmenting venous return to maintain cardiac output by elevating the patient's legs and increasing the rate of intravenous infusion. Emergency treatment consists of attempted pericardiocentesis while arrangements are made for a thoracotomy, a procedure that should only be carried out by trained staff.

Pericardiocentesis

- If time permits, prep and drape the skin, infiltrate local anaesthetic, ensure ECG monitoring.
- The skin is punctured 1–2 cm below and left of the xiphoid process, using a long needle and cannula, at an angle of 45°.
- While aspirating continuously, the needle is advanced towards the tip of the left scapula.
- The ECG monitor may show an injury pattern (ST depression or elevation) and dysrhythmia (ventricular ectopics) indicating that the needle has advanced too far and is now touching the myocardium.
- Withdraw the needle until a normal ECG is restored.
- Once in the pericardial sac, as much blood as is possible should be withdrawn.
- As the pressure on myocardium decreases and its filling increases, the myocardium may move towards the needle tip and an injury pattern may be seen again.
- The cannula is taped in place, the metal needle is removed from within it and a three-way tap attached.
- Should the signs of tamponade recur, the pericardial sac can be reaspirated.

Cardiac tamponade is definitively treated by surgery to repair the cardiac laceration and evacuate clotted blood in the pericardial sac.

Massive haemothorax

This condition is defined as greater than 1.5 l blood in the thoracic cavity or continuing drainage of more than 200 ml/h for 4 h. It is usually secondary to a laceration of either the intercostal or internal mammary arteries. Accumulation of blood in the pleural cavity compresses the lung, impairs ventilation and causes hypoxia, while at the same time causing hypovolaemia. It may also occur following injury to one of the great vessels in the mediastinum, for example, a tear of the pulmonary hilum. Such injuries are commonly fatal unless victims reach hospital very rapidly and undergo emergency thoracotomy. The signs of a massive haemothorax are shown in Box 3.4. Immediate management will consist of securing venous access and commencing fluid resuscitation, with the early requirement for blood. Venous access must precede insertion of a chest drain as the latter may precipitate circulatory collapse, making cannulation extremely difficult. Once the chest drain has been inserted and the diagnosis con-

BOX 3.4 Signs of a massive haemothorax

- Shock
- Dull to percussion over the affected hemithorax
- Decreased air entry in the hemithorax
- Raised JVP

firmed, the appropriate surgeon must be informed as some of these patients will need a thoracotomy to control the bleeding.

Once the six immediately life-threatening conditions have been eliminated or resolved the primary survey should proceed along the lines already discussed.

Insertion of a chest drain

A chest drain is inserted in the 5th intercostal space just anterior to the mid-axillary line.

- The patient's arm is abducted and the 5th intercostal space identified, the 4th or even 6th space may be chosen if there is an injury at the site of 5th space.
- The chest is cleaned and the area draped.
- Local anaesthetic is infiltrated into the skin, subcutaneous tissue, down to the pleura keeping just above the upper margin of the lower rib so as not to injure the neurovascular bundle.
- A 3–4 cm transverse incision is then made along the upper margin of the rib through the anaesthetized area.
- The track is continued through the intercostal muscles using blunt dissection down to the pleura.
- The pleura is then pierced just above the upper margin of the rib using a curved clamp.
- The operator then inserts a finger along the track into the pleural cavity and sweeps around the space to detect the presence of any adhesions or bowel (in case of a ruptured diaphragm).
- Having removed the metal trocar, a clamp is put across the distal end of the drain and used to direct it through the incision into the pleural cavity.
- Fogging and condensation caused by warm air escaping down the drain confirms placement in the pleural cavity.
- The proximal end of the drain is then connected to a suitable underwater seal. There may initially be a rush of air out into the underwater seal but this usually settles down and a raised fluid level in the tubing suggests establishment of intra-pleural negative pressure and nearly resolved pneumothorax.
- The chest drain is then secured by anchoring sutures, and an appropriate dressing.
- A chest radiograph, taken after the placement of the chest drain, confirms the tube placement and resolution of the pneumothorax (*Figure 3.7*).

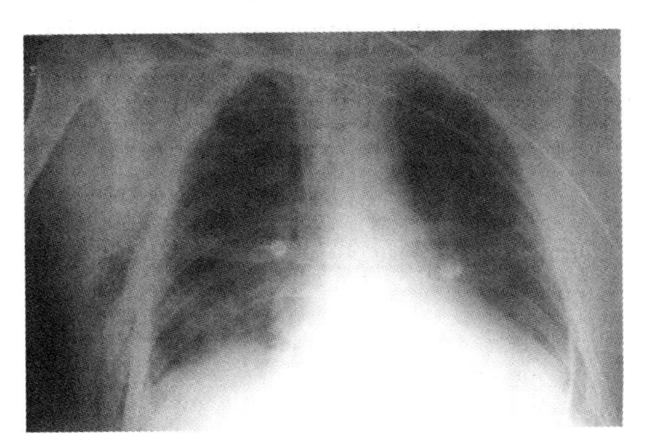

Figure 3.7 Chest x-ray with bilateral chest drains *in situ*

- The circulation nurse must continue to monitor the chest drain to ensure it is swinging with ventilation and to note any blood loss.

Emergency room thoracotomy

This is a controversial topic and debate has not resolved the question yet. This strategy is a desperate attempt to save a patient who is in immediate danger of dying. It has been claimed that under such circumstances, with an extremely poor prognosis, this procedure should never be undertaken. Recently, it has been suggested that the procedure is justified in patients with penetrating trauma, who displayed vital signs at the scene, where there is no alternative and the patient is rapidly deteriorating, but that those patients who do not have vital signs at the scene and patients with blunt injuries who have no vital signs on arrival in the emergency department should not undergo emergency room thoracotomy. The patients who most benefit from this procedure are those with penetrating cardiac injury who decompensate upon or just before arrival in the emergency room. Because of the risks of damage to the thoracic organs, this procedure must only be performed by a doctor with appropriate training.

3.4.2 Secondary survey

Only once the patient's condition has been stabilized and all the immediately life-threatening conditions described above have been treated or eliminated, a detailed head-to-toe examination is carried out in the manner described in Section 1.6.2. The aim at this stage is to identify the potentially life-threatening injuries (see Box 3.5) and begin a plan for definitive care for this patient. It also includes investigations, for example x-rays, ECG and arterial blood gases. Further invasive monitoring may require the patient to be transferred to a specialist area like an intensive care unit. If this happens before the secondary survey has been completed, this must be reported and recorded. Other sophisticated investigations may be warranted as a result of the findings on preliminary chest radiograph, for example CT scan, magnetic resonance imaging (MRI) or angiography. It is also important to remember that many of the conditions sought in the secondary survey may develop relatively slowly and if the secondary survey is performed soon after the patient presents, signs or symptoms may be minimal or absent.

It must be emphasized that should a patient's condition deteriorate during the secondary survey, it is essential to return to primary survey and resuscitation in case a new life-threatening condition has developed or an already existing one has been missed! Secondary survey should once again proceed (or be completed) once the threat to life has been satisfactorily dealt with.

BOX 3.5 Potentially life-threatening thoracic conditions

- Pulmonary contusion/laceration (parenchymal injuries)
- Myocardial contusion
- Ruptured diaphragm
- Aortic dissection
- Ruptured oesophagus
- Airway rupture

Pulmonary contusion/laceration (parenchymal injuries)

There is a high incidence (> 50%) of pulmonary parenchymal injuries seen in thoracic trauma. The primary effect of these injuries is on patients' oxygenation.

Pulmonary contusion

These are due to direct impact from forces that cause thoracic trauma causing haemorrhage in the underlying lung tissue. There are almost always associated rib fractures and often an accompanying pneumothorax or haemothorax. The contusion is usually, but not always, localized to the area directly adjacent to rib fractures (*Figure 3.8*). On examination ventilation is often rapid and shallow, there may be bruising or abrasions on the chest wall and tenderness on palpation. Percussion and auscultation may be normal, particularly early after the insult. As the disease progresses, respiratory distress ensues and ventilation becomes more difficult. Serial arterial blood gas analysis is essential – the PaO_2 gradually falls as the ventilation/perfusion mismatch increases. It is very important carefully to assess the chest radiograph for evidence of lung contusion, bearing in mind that this may occur away from the area of the chest wall involved in direct impact. A series of radiographs may be needed as the condition may evolve over hours or even days. Management consists initially of warmed, humidified oxygen, careful fluid resuscitation and observation, preferably in a critical care area.

Larger contusions cause respiratory failure and hypoxaemia of various degrees and many patients will require mechanical ventilation. The criteria used to determine the need for ventilation will vary between units; an example is given in Box 3.6.

One of the most controversial questions in the management of pulmonary contusions is fluid therapy. Fluid requirement varies from patient to patient and also depends upon loss of blood from other injuries. The contused lung tissue is also prone to damage by fluid overload. However, fluid and blood resuscitation is mandatory if

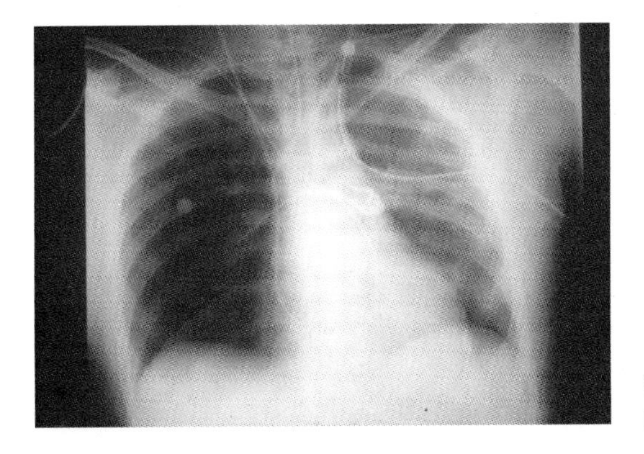

Figure 3.8 Chest x-ray showing pulmonary contusion

BOX 3.6 Indications for ventilation following pulmonary contusion

- Elderly
- Decreased level of consciousness
- Associated long bone fractures
- Increasing $PaCO_2$
- Decreasing PaO_2
- General anaesthesia required for surgery
- Transfer
- Renal failure
- Severe pre-existing lung disease

the consequences of hypoperfusion are to be avoided. Recommendations for fluid infusions in such patients are varied; it is the authors' view that fluid management in such patients needs to be guided by invasive haemodynamic monitoring with a pulmonary artery catheter (PAC), oesophageal Doppler or transoesophageal echocardiography (TOE) (see Section 3.5). Recently, attention has been drawn to the technique of small volume resuscitation with hypertonic saline (7.5%), which effectively supports the haemodynamic profile of these patients without the disadvantages of administering large fluid volumes.

Pulmonary lacerations

Pulmonary lacerations are usually the consequence of penetrating thoracic trauma but they can also be produced by blunt injuries with a heavy impact. These injuries are invariably accompanied by a pneumothorax, haemothorax or haemopneumothorax. The injury is managed using the principles already described. About 5% of these patients will require formal thoracotomy, especially if there is persistent bleeding, persistent pneumothorax and haemoptysis or for evacuation of clotted haemothorax or failure of the lung to re-expand. Most patients can be managed by suturing of lacerations at operation; occasionally a lobectomy or pneumonectomy may be required.

Myocardial contusion

Myocardial contusion has been reported to occur in 30–70% of cases of thoracic trauma. This wide variation in incidence is probably due to the lack of a 'gold standard' for its definitive diagnosis, and the high incidence quoted probably reflects the incidence of ECG changes of ischaemia and arrhythmia without myocardial dysfunction seen after blunt thoracic trauma. Frank infarction may co-exist with contusion along with rib and sternal fractures. The mechanism of injury is usually compression of the heart between the sternum and spine. This injury may be seen in severe frontal impact road traffic accidents, falls from heights, crush from falling masonry as well as iatrogenically after cardiopulmonary resuscitation. Right, left or biventricular cardiac failure may also occur.

Measurement of enzymes like creatinine kinase is not very helpful but toponin I has been suggested to be specific for myocardial contusion. Echocardiogram, particularly TOE, is a useful bedside investigation in detecting hypokinesia, abnormal wall motion, ruptured papillary muscle and valvular abnormalities following cardiac trauma.

Treatment of myocardial contusion is supportive. This includes rest, oxygenation, restoration of haemodynamic normality and careful monitoring. Serial ECGs to monitor the ischaemic changes, serial enzyme measurements, continuous monitoring in High Dependency Unit (HDU) or Intensive Care Unit (ICU) and invasive monitoring by PAC and inotropic support may all be required; the latter especially in patients with deteriorating haemodynamic parameters. Arrhythmias can develop late in this condition and careful monitoring and use of antiarrhythmic drugs has reduced mortality. In severe cases of cardiac decompensation, intra-aortic balloon pump (IABP) or ventricular assist devices (VAD) may be needed.

Ruptured diaphragm

This may arise as a result of either blunt or penetrating trauma (*Figure 3.9*). Blunt injuries to the abdomen or thorax that produce a sudden rise in pressure may cause a burst type of injury resulting in irregular tears, with herniation of abdominal viscera into the thoracic cavity causing respiratory embarrassment and occasionally an acute abdomen due to strangulation of bowel loops through the tear. The commonest causes of diaphragmatic injuries are automobile accidents; side impact collisions cause three times more diaphragmatic disruption than frontal impacts. The left hemidiaphragm is more prone to injury than the right, probably because of the protective effect of the liver. Consequently, right-sided injuries can be very severe and usually involve the liver.

Where the diaphragm is injured by penetrating trauma, 75% of cases are associated with intra-abdominal injury, whilst 20% of penetrating injuries of the thorax will involve the diaphragm. Again the left side is more involved than the right, probably because most assailants are right handed! As the diaphragm is always moving, these small penetrating wounds do not heal spontaneously and will enlarge over a period of time and may result in herniation of the abdominal contents years later.

Many of these injuries are asymptomatic at presentation; the most suggestive sign of a diaphragmatic injury is the proximity of the penetrating wound. On examination, breath sounds may be decreased over the affected hemithorax and occasionally bowel sounds may be heard in the chest. Often the first suspicion comes from the appearance of the chest x-ray. The injured hemidiaphragm is elevated and there may bowel in the pleural space. If a gastric tube has been inserted, this may be visible above the diaphragm. If diagnostic peritoneal lavage is performed, this may be positive if there is an intra-abdominal injury and, if a chest drain is in the same hemithorax, the lavage fluid may appear in the drain.

Diaphragmatic injuries may also be diagnosed with contrast gastrointestinal studies, ultrasonography and abdominal/thoracic CT. Occasionally, pneumoperitoneography and radiolabelled peritoneography may be required. Diaphragmatic ruptures, however small, never heal spontaneously. They should always be surgically repaired.

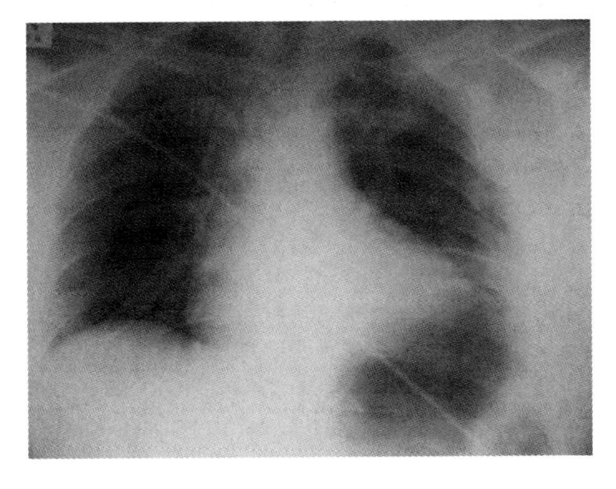

Figure 3.9 X-ray of ruptured diaphragm

Aortic disruption/great vessel injury

These are found in victims of high-speed road traffic accidents and falls from great heights and 85% of these injuries are due to blunt trauma. These injuries manifest in a variety of ways: from various degrees of shock to profound haemodynamic disturbances. The majority (80–90%) of the patients die at the scene of the accident from massive blood loss. Of the patients reaching hospital alive, only 20% will survive without operation. The mortality remains high even after surgery.

In cases of aortic disruption, the clinical presentation depends upon the site of injury. Patients with injury to the intrapericardial portion of the ascending aorta will usually develop a cardiac tamponade. Extrapericardial ascending aortic injury produces a mediastinal haematoma and a haemothorax, usually on the right side. Injury to the aortic arch may remain undiagnosed initially if the adventitia remains intact and the damage is contained in the form of a mediastinal haematoma. Rapid deceleration is believed to be responsible for dissection of the aorta. This occurs in the region of the ligamentum arteriosum, just distal to the origin of left subclavian artery as the aorta is relatively firmly fixed at this point. These patients show transient hypotension, which responds well to fluid therapy and further clinical signs may be absent. This may delay the diagnosis with catastrophic results should the aorta rupture completely. Thus a high index of suspicion and judicious use of appropriate investigations cannot be overemphasized.

Aortic disruption should always be suspected in patients with profound shock and who have no other external signs of blood loss and in whom mechanical causes of shock (tension pneumothorax and pericardial tamponade) have been excluded. In a patient who has suffered rapid deceleration, upper body hypertension (relative to lower body) should immediately arouse a suspicion of trauma to the aorta. Symptoms (if the patient is conscious) may include severe retrosternal pain, pain between the scapulae, hoarseness of voice (pressure from haematoma on recurrent laryngeal nerve), dysphagia (compression of the oesophagus) and paraplegia or paraparesis (reduced perfusion of the vessels supplying the spinal cord). There may also be ischaemia or infarction of other areas, for example limbs and abdominal organs. There may be accompanying fractures of ribs or sternum as well. There are several features that may be seen on a plain chest x-ray that are indicative of the possibility of thoracic aortic (see Box 3.7).

With these symptoms and signs, investigations for aortic injury and consultation with thoracic surgeon are mandatory as delay may mean profound hypotension and death. The definitive investigation of choice is angiography or a CT scan of the aortic arch, the choice depending on local policy. Survival in patients who have their injury

BOX 3.7 Radiological features suggesting dissecting thoracic aorta

- Widened mediastinum
- Pleural cap (apical haematoma), especially on the left
- Compression and downward displacement of left main bronchus
- Fractured first or second ribs
- Trachea shifted to right
- Blunting of the aortic knuckle
- Raised right main bronchus
- Left haemothorax with no obvious rib fractures or other cause
- Deviation of the nasogastric tube to the right

repaired surgically and who have remained haemodynamically stable during the repair is 90%.

Oesophageal injury

Oesophageal injuries are uncommon, as the organ is well protected in the posterior mediastinum. The cervical oesophagus is more prone to injury as a result of penetrating trauma and following crush injury. The thoracic oesophagus may rupture following a severe blow to the epigastrium. On examination there is often shock and severe pain out of proportion to the apparent injuries. Pain on swallowing suggests oesophageal injury and must be investigated. A left-sided pneumothorax or effusion in the absence of trauma or rib fractures should raise suspicions. Surgical emphysema or signs of peritonitis, depending on site of rupture, may develop with time. Patients should be kept nil by mouth and the oesophageal injury should be surgically repaired, ideally within 12 h. A cervical oesophagostomy is performed to prevent soiling of the mediastinum, along with a gastrostomy. Surgical repair and restoration of oesophageal continuity is undertaken when mediastinal infection has settled and the patient is stable. Mediastinitis is a very severe form of infection and may rapidly progress to multiple organ dysfunction syndrome (MODS).

Airway rupture

Most patients with major airway injuries die at the scene due to asphyxia, intrapulmonary haemorrhage or aspiration of blood. However, survival is possible if the transection of the airway, even a major airway, is sealed off by soft tissue. These injuries produce severe surgical emphysema, pneumothorax, pneumomediastinum, haemothorax, pneumopericardium or even pneumoperitoneum. Diagnosis is by high index of suspicion, evidence of pneumothorax, pneumomediastinum and confirmed by airway endoscopy. Injuries may be overlooked even on endoscopy if the vision is blocked by blood in the airway and complications increase if not properly diagnosed. Fractures, especially scapular, clavicular or ribs 1–3 indicate high impact injury and airway injury must always be suspected in such patients. Treatment of these injuries is almost always surgical. An urgent consultation with a thoracic surgeon is mandatory in all such cases.

3.5 Imaging and investigations in thoracic trauma

3.5.1 Chest radiograph

This is the most important basic investigation performed in a patient with thoracic trauma and is mandatory in these patients. Although an erect posterioanterior (PA) view is the best option, in practice, anterioposterior (AP) view with the patient lying in supine position is often all that is possible.

Fracture of first three ribs indicates a high-energy transfer and should prompt a search for other underlying injuries, for example, an aortic injury or severe pulmonary contusion. Fractures of the lower ribs should prompt a search for injury to the abdominal organs, spleen and the kidneys. Other fractures may also be obvious, sternum, clavicle and or scapula, which may suggest the presence of a flail segment. It has been suggested that only 50% of rib fractures are evident on initial chest radiographs.

When a pneumothorax is suspected, a chest radiograph in full expiration is ideal as the reduced air in the lungs provides a better contrast between the air in the pleural cavity and the lung parenchyma. Pneumothoraces are identified by a rim of complete translucency on the lateral side of the lung, without any lung markings distally. A rim of about 1 cm on the radiograph corresponds to a pneumothorax of 10% of total lung volume. In the treatment of pneumothoraces, the chest radiograph is only a guide; the treatment of the pneumothorax itself is dependent on the clinical condition of the patient. Surgical emphysema does not need a chest radiograph for diagnosis but its presence may make diagnosis of a pneumothorax difficult.

A haemothorax, in an erect radiograph, can be diagnosed by obliteration of the costophrenic angle (requiring presence of 300–400 ml of blood). In supine patients, this amount of blood may not be immediately obvious. Careful observation of the chest radiograph may reveal presence of increased density in one hemithorax (massive haemothorax will result in a unilateral whiteout). A haemopneumothorax will have a classic air–fluid level.

Pulmonary parenchymal injuries may be masked by the presence of a pneumothorax, a haemothorax or both along with other pathology (rib fractures, etc.). The appearances range from a small infiltrate, through an involved lung segment to a complete white out. The condition usually evolves insidiously over a period of time and serial radiographs are important in this respect. Lung lacerations are accompanied by pneumothoraces or small opacities denoting lung haemorrhage and haematomas. Lung haematomas can also be difficult to diagnose and they may appear as pulmonary infiltrates because of the extravasation of blood into the surrounding lung tissue.

Blast injuries can give rise to diffused bilateral infiltrates in the lung field, often with associated pneumothoraces and/or pneumomediastinum. A similar picture is seen in patients with traumatic asphyxia but here the radiographic appearance is due to diffused interstitial haemorrhages along with pulmonary oedema.

Injuries to trachea and bronchi are suspected in the presence of fractures to first 2–4 ribs and the presence of mediastinal emphysema, pericardial air and subcutaneous emphysema. These injuries can be difficult to diagnose and a quarter of the chest radiographs in these patients are reported as normal.

3.5.2 Computerized tomography (CT)

CT is becoming increasingly used in the assessment of patients with major trauma as the information obtained is often very specific and there is a growing expertise available. The disadvantages of CT are delay in organizing the procedure and transport of the patient to a specific area, often away from a resuscitation room. Hence this procedure can only be performed in stable patients in whom the life-threatening conditions have been effectively managed. The recent innovations in CT technology ('spiral CT') make CT imaging of trauma victim easier and quicker; this is becoming popular in many countries as the imaging of choice in trauma victims.

Notwithstanding the disadvantages, valuable information may be obtained about occult (or difficult to diagnose) pneumothoraces (*Figure 3.10*), mediastinal haematomata, small haemothoraces and pericardial fluid. One such small haemothorax is the 'pleural cap' or minimal apical haemothorax; the presence of which should prompt the clinicians to look for injuries such as a ruptured diaphragm or aortic arch injury.

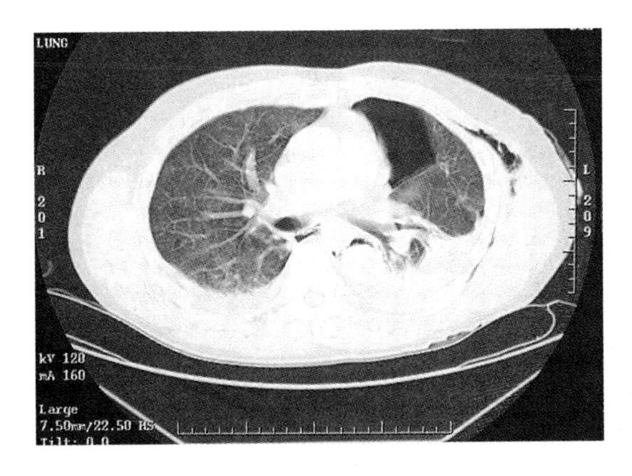

Figure 3.10 CT scan of chest showing pneumothorax

The most significant contribution of CT scanning is in the diagnosis and identification of aortic and great vessel injury. It also distinguishes other causes of 'widened mediastinum' (congenital abnormalities, anatomical variations) from that caused by aortic injury. In a recent study, 22% of aortic injuries were diagnosed only after CT imaging. CTs also detect small haematomas that may not be obvious on chest radiographs and the presence of such, especially in the mediastinum, may indicate the need for an aortogram to rule out aortic injury.

CT may help identify pericardial fluid (where it compares favourably with echocardiography). Pericardial fluid surrounding the base of the heart is a strong indication of myocardial injury and efforts must be directed in this direction if this is found.

3.5.3 Magnetic resonance imaging (MRI)

MRI offers a number of potential advantages over CT; solid structures can be differentiated from blood vessels and fluid collections without the use of intravenous contrast; image quality is superior and there is also no danger of radiation. However, at present the scans take considerably longer, therefore isolating critically ill patients for a variable length of time. Furthermore, most currently used ventilators and monitoring are not compatible with the strong magnetic field of MRI scanners. MRI is currently being evaluated in diagnosis of cardiac injuries as well as small diaphragmatic injuries.

3.5.4 Endoscopy

Several forms of endoscopy are used in thoracic trauma, some of which may be performed in the emergency or intensive care departments by the patient's bedside.

Bronchoscopy may be the only diagnostic tool useful in the diagnosis of life-threatening injuries such as tracheal or bronchial tears. It is indicated in thoracic trauma victims when there is:

- haemoptysis;
- subcutaneous emphysema without obvious pneumothorax;
- persistent pneumothorax;

- persistent pneumomediastinum;
- massive air leaks through a chest tube (suspicion of ruptured bronchus).

Oesophagoscopy is indicated in the diagnosis of oesophageal injury, often when contrast swallows are negative in the presence of clinical suspicion of oesophageal injuries. Oesophagoscopy may also be indicated in patients with such injury but who cannot swallow contrast (unconscious or sedated patients on ventilators).

3.5.5 Echocardiography

Two types of echocardiography are available today; *transthoracic echocardiography (TTE)* and *TOE*. Whereas TTE is commonly available in the UK, TOE may not be available in all institutions.

TTE can provide useful information about the ventricular septal and wall movement abnormalities (hypokinetic segments), valvular integrity and presence of pericardial effusion as well as mural thrombi. TTE can also calculate ventricular ejection fraction (a measure of overall ventricular function). TOE is a more accurate instrument in the diagnosis of cardiac abnormalities and useful in patients when large areas of surgical emphysema or mediastinal emphysema preclude effective examination by TTE. TOE provides information about valvular injuries, intracardiac shunts, septal defects and great vessel injuries. Its rapid, safe and its diagnostic ability by the bedside makes TOE a very useful diagnostic tool in suspected aortic injuries.

3.5.6 Angiography

Angiography is still considered the 'gold standard' in imaging for suspected aortic or great vessel injury in thoracic trauma or any other vascular trauma. A widened mediastinum on the initial chest radiograph is regarded as a standard indication for angiography, despite a high false-positive rate. Various forms of vessel injury may be identified, for example, laceration (from penetrating trauma), avulsion, internal flap formation, obstruction (from blunt trauma). Rarely, an aortogram may appear completely normal (sometimes in blast injury) despite the presence of a serious injury as the injury may not have breached the intima.

3.5.7 Other investigations

ECG, cardiac enzyme analysis and arterial blood gases (ABG) are nonspecific but easy bedside procedures and give valuable information about cardiorespiratory dysfunction and may alert the clinician to evolving problems. New Q waves or heart block on ECG usually indicates a significant myocardial injury. It has been estimated that about a third of ECGs have signs of myocardial injury but often go unnoticed. Serial ECGs may be more useful. Assay of cardiac enzymes is useful, bearing in mind that creatinine kinase (CK) is a nonspecific enzyme and may be elevated in muscular (noncardiac muscle) injury and MB (myocardial band) fraction is more specific for myocardial injury. Recently, troponin has been considered to be more specific for myocardial injury with troponin I more specific for myocardial contusion. ABGs, like chest radiographs, are mandatory for any trauma victim but more specifically for thoracic trauma. These will not be further discussed here; these are covered in many excellent reviews and texts.

3.6 Other injuries in thoracic trauma

3.6.1 Rib fractures

Rib injuries and fractures are common in thoracic trauma. Multiple rib fractures are usually associated with contusion of the underlying lung to a varying degree. Apart from injury to the underlying lung, pain from rib fractures impairs breathing by restricted movement and inadequate cough. This in turn leads to accumulation of secretions, infection, collapse and consolidation and, sometimes, frank respiratory failure. Consequently, most patients with more than two fractured ribs will need admission to hospital for analgesia and monitoring of respiratory function. Patients with isolated rib injuries, or the elderly with osteoporosis who may suffer 'simple' isolated rib fractures with little or no injury to the underlying lung parenchyma, will require adequate analgesia. Strapping of the chest wall as a form of 'therapy' has now been abandoned.

Despite genuine concerns about opiates, especially in the elderly, their careful use is beneficial especially when combined with supervision and monitoring, adequate humidification of oxygen and chest physiotherapy. A useful way of administering opiate analgesia is by patient-controlled analgesia (PCA), in consultation with acute pain service (see Section 16.3.3). Problems of inadequate analgesia should be vigorously pursued and may need consultation with senior medical staff. There is no justification for allowing patients to breathe and cough inadequately for want of adequate analgesia.

Should these simple measures prove unsatisfactory, alternative methods of pain relief should be considered. These include epidural analgesia, intercostal nerve block (see Section 16.3) and intrapleural analgesia. Epidural analgesia consists of the administration of a continuous infusion of local anaesthetic agent, sometimes containing an opioid (morphine or fentanyl), into the epidural space via a fine catheter inserted percutaneously. It is a specialized technique, particularly in the thoracic vertebral region, and should only be administered by those with experience and preferably with the involvement of the acute pain service. Because of the risk of complications, particularly hypotension, such patients should be cared for in a high dependency area. Epidurals are contraindicated in presence of an open wound in the midline posteriorly at the intended site of the epidural, thoracic vertebral column fractures, infection at or close to the site of epidural and coagulation abnormalities.

Alternative modalities of providing analgesia are via indwelling intrapleural or paravertebral catheters. This form of therapy has been used when epidurals are contraindicated because of open wounds, fractures of the thoracic spine or coagulopathy. Details of these techniques are beyond the scope of this text.

3.6.2 Simple pneumothorax

Patients with a simple pneumothorax will present with sharp pain in the chest, particularly on inspiration (rib fractures present in the same way). Respiratory distress varies in degree, depending upon the extent of pneumothorax, accompanying rib fractures and the presence or absence of lung contusion. A pneumothorax may be suspected from bruising or a penetrating wound and decreased movement of the ipsilateral chest wall. Hyperresonant percussion note may be present on the affected side and breath sounds may be decreased or absent. There may be tachycardia but if there has been no loss of blood, the patient is not usually hypotensive.

3.6.3 Haemothorax

This may be diagnosed on an erect chest film and should be drained, as a radiologically visible haemothorax comprises at least 500 ml. This will also allow monitoring of the rate of blood loss from the pleural cavity. Large size drains are necessary otherwise the blood will clot in the drain. Failure of the haemothorax to drain may also suggest clotted blood in the pleural cavity or a collection of subpleural blood. In either case, a thoracotomy will eventually be required to drain the clots and/or blood. Continued blood loss from a chest drain (about 100 ml/h) may indicate a clotting abnormality, usually due to dilutional thrombocytopenia or diluted coagulation factors following large blood transfusions. These should be treated accordingly.

3.6.4 Air embolism

Four percent of patients with major thoracic trauma are said to have air embolism associated with bronchopulmonary-venous fistulae. This is a life-threatening problem occurring either in blunt or penetrating trauma but usually in the later condition. Unfortunately, this condition is not easy to diagnose. It can affect the left or right sides of the heart. Left-sided embolism usually presents as sudden cardiovascular collapse shortly after initiation of mechanical ventilation as air is forced into the pulmonary vein by positive pressure. Expansion of the intravascular space by fluid resuscitation, increasing systemic arterial pressure by inotropes (and/or vasopressors), ventilation with 100% oxygen and reduction of tidal volume of the ventilator to reduce intra-thoracic pressure are the holding measures until a thoracotomy can be organized. Mortality remains high, particularly with the neurological consequences of air entering the cerebrovascular system.

Right heart air embolism can occur when there is an open venous channel above right heart. Trauma to pelvis, abdominal viscera, inferior vena cava and to the thorax itself are causes of right-sided air embolism. In patients with patent foramen ovale, paradoxical left heart embolism may follow right-sided air embolus.

3.6.5 Myocardial ischaemia and infarction

Penetrating trauma involving coronary arteries may induce sudden, fatal myocardial infarction. If there is significant bleeding from the artery, cardiac tamponade may occur. Associated hypovolaemia makes cardiac injury worse and increases mortality. Blunt trauma may occasionally cause coronary artery injury and infarction, either directly or by torsion of the heart; in such cases, left anterior descending artery is the commonest vessel involved. In most cases, the injury is limited to intimal damage but complete occlusion has been described which is usually fatal. Myocardial infarction is usually managed conservatively. Occasionally, isolated coronary artery injuries may require coronary artery bypass grafting. Thrombolysis in cases of myocardial infarction in trauma is usually contraindicated as there are other injuries present precluding the use of these agents.

3.6.6 Thoracic duct injury

Usually occurs from blunt trauma due to a fall, compression, hyperextension or hyper-flexion spinal injuries. It presents itself as a pleural effusion subsequently found to be chyle (chylothorax), which may occur soon after the injury or may be delayed. Milky white fluid draining from the chest drain is highly suspicious and analysis of the fluid showing chylomicrons will confirm the diagnosis. Consultation with a thoracic or general surgeon is essential in management of these patients as there are varying opinions as to the best course of management for these patients.

3.7 Summary

Thoracic trauma is common and contributes directly to death in about a quarter of all trauma deaths. Most deaths are due to hypoxaemia and hypovolaemia, both conditions that should be aggressively treated. Most of the thoracic injuries (85%) can be managed with simple measures of oxygenation, fluid and blood resuscitation and chest tube placement. Surgical intervention is required in but a few patients.

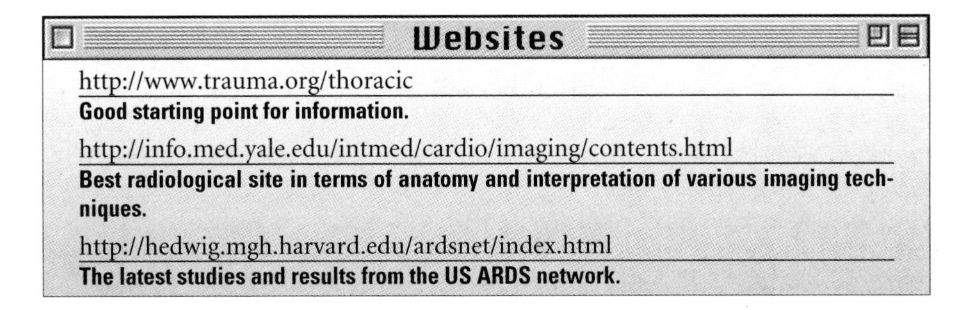
Websites

http://www.trauma.org/thoracic
Good starting point for information.

http://info.med.yale.edu/intmed/cardio/imaging/contents.html
Best radiological site in terms of anatomy and interpretation of various imaging techniques.

http://hedwig.mgh.harvard.edu/ardsnet/index.html
The latest studies and results from the US ARDS network.

Further reading

1. **American College of Surgeons Committee on Trauma** (1997) *Advanced Trauma Life Support Course for Doctors.* American College of Surgeons, Chicago, IL.
2. **Hanowell LH & Grande CM** (1994) Perioperative management of thoracic trauma. *Seminar Anaesth.* 13(2): 89.
3. **Hyde JA, Shetty A, Kishen R, *et al.*** (1998) Pulmonary trauma and chest injuries. In Driscoll P and Skinner D (eds): *Trauma Care: Beyond the Resuscitation Room.* London: BMJ Books, p. 35.
4. **Hyde JAJ, Rooney SJ & Graham TR** (1996) Fluid management in thoracic trauma. *Hospital Update* 22: 448.
5. **Kearny PA, Smith DW & Johnson SB** (1993) Use of transoesophageal echocardiography in the evaluation of traumatic aortic injury. *J. Trauma* 34: 696.
6. **Langanay T, Verhoye J-P, Corbineau H, *et al.*** (2002) Surgical treatment of acute traumatic rupture of the thoracic aorta: a timing of reappraisal? *Eur. J. Cardio-thor. Surg.* 21: 282.
7. **Moore PG, Kien ND & Safwat AM** (1994) Perioperative management of cardiac trauma. *Seminar Anaesth.* 13(2): 119.
8. **Richens D, Field M, Neale M, *et al.*** (2002) The mechanism of injury in blunt traumatic rupture of the aorta. *Eur. J. Cardio-Thor. Surg.* 21: 288.
9. **West JB** (1990) *Respiratory Physiology – The Essentials.* Baltimore: Williams & Wilkins.

4 Shock

A McCluskey

Objectives

The objectives of this chapter are that members of the trauma team should understand the:

- definition and classification of shock;
- normal determinants of cardiac output, arterial blood pressure and regional organ perfusion;
- importance of oxygen delivery and consumption;
- causes of shock;
- normal cardiovascular response to hypovolaemia;
- initial management of the shocked patient.

4.1 Definition

Shock is an expression used frequently but inexactly by lay people and the media. Medically, the term is defined as *inadequate oxygen delivery to vital organs* and it is in this restricted sense that the word is used throughout this book.

4.2 Classification

Circulatory shock embodies a number of diverse pathophysiological cardiovascular disorders with distinctive aetiologies (see Box 4.1) and is associated with systemic arterial hypotension. Although cardiac output is usually decreased in shock associated with major trauma, it may be normal or even increased in neurogenic and septic shock.

BOX 4.1 Classification of shock

Type	*Examples of causes*	*Effect on cardiac output*
Hypovolaemic	Haemorrhage, dehydration	Decreased
Cardiogenic	Acute myocardial infarction, myocardial contusion, cardiac tamponade	Decreased
Neurogenic	High spinal cord injury (usually above T5)	Decreased
Septic	Pneumonia, intra-abdominal catastrophe, as a late complication of major trauma	Normal or increased
Anaphylactic	Acute allergic reaction (type I hypersensitivity)	Decreased

Regardless of the aetiology, regional perfusion of organs and tissues at the cellular level is impaired, leading to cellular hypoxia, dysfunction and eventually cell death.

4.3 Cardiovascular physiology

To appreciate the rationale of appropriate treatment of the shocked patient, it is necessary to understand the normal physiological control of cardiac output, arterial blood pressure and regional organ perfusion.

For the reader who is particularly interested, the formulae for calculating the various physiological variables discussed are listed in Appendix 4.1 at the end of this chapter.

4.3.1 Cardiac output

Cardiac output (CO) is defined as the volume of blood ejected by each ventricle each minute and is the product of the volume of blood ejected with each heartbeat (stroke volume, SV) and the heart rate (beats/min) and is expressed in litres per minute. It is influenced by changes in either stroke volume or heart rate:

$$\text{Cardiac Output} = \text{Stroke Volume} \times \text{Heart Rate}$$

To enable meaningful comparisons between patients of different sizes, the term cardiac index (CI) is often used. This is cardiac output divided by body surface area and is measured in litres per min per m^2:

$$\text{CI} = \text{CO/body surface area}$$

Factors affecting stroke volume

The three principal determinants of stroke volume are:

A. preload;

B. myocardial contractility;

C. afterload.

Preload

The force with which a muscle contracts is dependent on its resting length (*Figure 4.1*); the more it is stretched beyond its normal resting length before it is stimulated to contract, the more forcefully it contracts. Because of the internal molecular structure of muscle fibres there is an upper limit to this relationship and above a critical (optimal) length the force of contraction decreases.

This property also applies to the myocardial muscle fibres (*Figure 4.2*), which are stretched during diastole by the blood returning from the venous circulations; this is termed the preload. The more the myocardial fibres are stretched during diastole, the more forcibly they will contract during systole and the more blood will be expelled into the systemic and pulmonary circulations, providing that the optimal level is not exceeded (Starling's Law). Clearly, it is not possible to measure the length of individual myocardial fibres, but an estimate may be obtained by measuring either ventricular volume or pressure at the end of diastole. In routine clinical practice it is more common to measure pressure.

- Central venous pressure (CVP) gives an estimate of right ventricular end diastolic pressure (RVEDP).

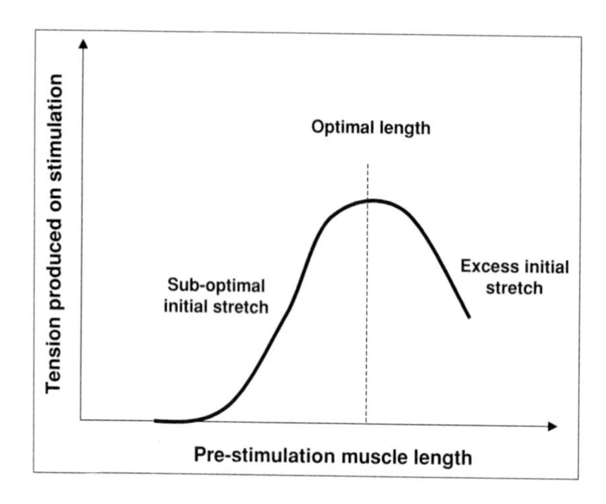

Figure 4.1 Starling curve – single muscle

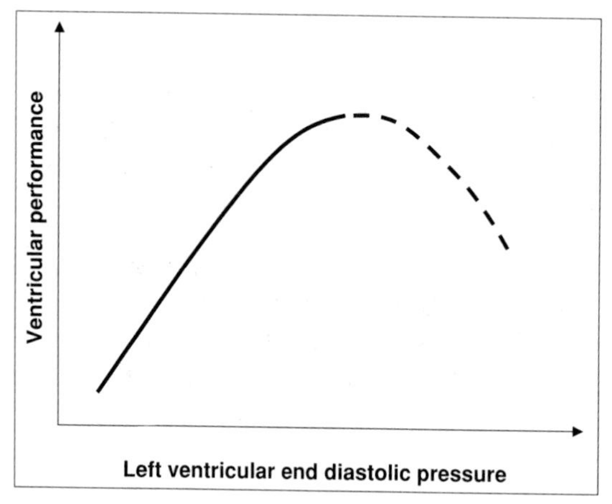

Figure 4.2 Starling curve – LVEDP

- Pulmonary artery occlusion pressure (PAOP) or wedge pressure gives an estimate of left ventricular end diastolic pressure (LVEDP).

The main physiological determinants of venous return to the heart are blood volume and venous tone. The systemic venous system acts as a reservoir for up to 50% of the circulating blood volume. The amount at any one time is dependent on the calibre of the vessels, which is controlled primarily by the sympathetic nervous system. A change from minimal to maximal venous tone may increase the venous return by approximately 1 l/min.

An increase in venous filling (preload) will only lead to an increase in stroke volume and cardiac output if it is kept below a critical level

Myocardial contractility

This is the force with which myocardial fibres contract for a given degree of stretch, the most important determinant of which is stimulation by the sympathetic nervous system. Substances affecting myocardial contractility are termed *inotropes*, and they can be either positive or negative in their actions. In a clinical context, the term is usually taken to refer to a substance with a positive inotropic effect, that is, one that produces

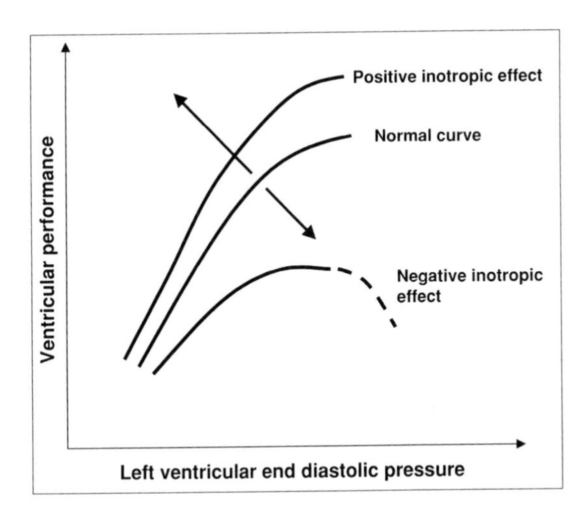

Figure 4.3 Starling curve – LVEDP with positive/negative inotropic effects

a greater rate and force of contraction for a given resting length (proportional to end diastolic volume or pressure). This action can be represented as shifting the Starling curve to the left (*Figure 4.3*). Adrenaline, noradrenaline and dopamine are naturally occurring catecholamines with positive inotropic actions.

Substances with negative inotropic effects cause a decrease in contractility, i.e. the Starling curve shifts to the right. Drugs being taken by the patient, e.g. antidysrhythmics, or administered acutely, e.g. anaesthetic and sedative agents, and severe hypoxia and acidosis may also have a negative inotropic effect.

Afterload

During ventricular systole, the pressure within the left and right ventricles increases until it exceeds the pressure in the aorta and pulmonary artery respectively. The aortic and pulmonary valves open and blood is ejected. The resistance faced by the ventricular myocardium to ejection of the blood is termed the afterload.

- Left ventricular afterload is due to the resistance offered by the systemic arterial blood vessels (and aortic valve) and is termed the *systemic vascular resistance* (SVR).
- Right ventricular afterload is due pulmonary blood vessels (and pulmonary valve) and is termed the *pulmonary vascular resistance* (PVR).

When afterload is reduced (whilst maintaining preload), the ventricular muscle shortens more quickly and extensively, thus increasing the stroke volume

Factors affecting heart rate

Normally, heart rate is determined by the rate of intrinsic spontaneous depolarization of the sinoatrial node. In the resting state this rate averages 60–100/min, depending on the age and level of physical fitness of the patient. An increase in heart rate is mediated by the sympathetic nervous system and is termed a *positive chronotropic effect*. Conversely, the parasympathetic nervous system (via the vagus nerve) causes a decrease in heart rate, a *negative chronotropic effect.* The resting heart is usually subject to dominant vagal activity.

An increase in heart rate usually leads to an increase in CO (see Section 4.3.1) and occurs largely as a result of shortening diastole. As ventricular filling (and perfusion of the myocardium) occurs during diastole, excessive heart rates reduce stroke volume and cardiac output decreases. In a 'normal', fit individual, stroke volume is relatively unaffected between 40 and 150 beats/min. This range may be considerably reduced by age and disease so that a heart rate well within this range may not be tolerated.

An increase in the heart rate will only lead to an increase in cardiac output if it is kept below a critical level

In summary the main factors affecting the cardiac output of the left ventricle are listed in Box 4.2.

BOX 4.2 Factors that affect left ventricular cardiac output

- Preload (or LVEDP)
- Myocardial contractility
- Afterload (or SVR)
- Heart rate

4.3.2 Systemic arterial blood pressure

This is the pressure within the arterial blood vessels:

- *systolic pressure* is the maximum pressure generated in the large arteries during each cardiac cycle;
- *diastolic pressure* is the minimum;
- *pulse pressure* is the difference between systolic and diastolic pressures;
- *mean arterial pressure* is the average pressure during the cardiac cycle and is approximately equal to the diastolic pressure plus one-third of the pulse pressure.

Mean arterial pressure (MAP) is dependent on cardiac output and systemic vascular resistance and is therefore affected by all the factors discussed above.

$$\text{MAP} = \text{CO} \times \text{SVR}$$

Arterial blood pressure is normally tightly controlled by neural, humoral and metabolic mechanisms to maintain adequate perfusion pressure and blood flow to organs and tissues. Following a fall in arterial blood pressure a number of mechanisms operate to restore pressure:

- baroreceptors located in the aortic arch, carotid sinus and heart send impulses to the vasomotor centre within the brainstem;
- the vasomotor centre increases sympathetic nerve activity to the heart, arteries, veins, adrenal medulla and other tissues;
- sympathetic activity results in vasoconstriction of most arteries and veins together with increased myocardial contractility and heart rate;
- selective arteriolar and precapillary sphincter constriction of nonessential organs (e.g. skin, gut) operates and helps to maintain perfusion of vital organs (e.g. brain, heart);

- cardiac output and SVR rise in an attempt to restore arterial blood pressure back towards its homeostatic set point;
- sympathetic stimulation of arterioles supplying skeletal muscle actually causes vasodilatation (acting through β_2 receptors), an appropriate response for 'fight or flight';
- reduction in renal blood flow is detected by specialized cells within the juxtaglomerular apparatus of the kidney releasing renin which leads to the formation of angiotensin II (a vasopressor and stimulator of aldosterone production);
- aldosterone secreted from the adrenal cortex and antidiuretic hormone (vasopressin) released from the pituitary, increase reabsorption of sodium and water by the kidney, reducing urine volume to help maintain the circulating volume.

In addition, insulin and glucagon are released which promote the supply and utilization of glucose by the cells. The liver also attempts to enhance circulating volume by releasing osmotically active substances that increase plasma oncotic pressure, thus reducing the osmotic gradient causing extravasation of fluid from the circulation through leaky capillaries.

Clearly, if either CO or SVR decrease in isolation, arterial blood pressure will decrease. Normally, a fall in one results in an increase in the other to maintain arterial blood pressure. However, following major trauma, if hypovolaemia is severe enough, arterial blood pressure may still be below normal even though sympathetic activity increases causing positive inotropic and chronotropic effects on the heart, and arterial and venous constriction. Clinically, the patient is pale, cold and clammy with a weak or absent peripheral pulse.

4.3.3 Regional organ perfusion

Blood flow through many organs, particularly the kidneys and brain, remains almost constant as a result of a process termed *autoregulation*. Smooth muscle within arteriolar walls and precapillary sphincters is responsive to a variety of stimuli; locally produced metabolic products such as K^+ and H^+ ions, CO_2, hypoxia and increase in temperature cause a direct relaxant effect on the arterioles. Arteriolar calibre increases, thereby increasing blood flow as necessary to the cells. Hypotension also causes dilatation to maintain flow, while hypertension causes vasoconstriction in an attempt to protect the organs from high pressure.

4.3.4 Oxygen delivery

The delivery of oxygen (DO_2) to the tissues is dependent on:

- transfer from pulmonary alveoli into blood flowing through the pulmonary capillaries;
- transport to the tissues in the blood;
- release to the tissues.

Transfer from alveoli to blood

The factors affecting this, namely ventilation, perfusion, diffusion and V/Q ratios have already been discussed in Section 3.3.

Transport to the tissues

The amount of oxygen transported from the lungs to the tissues in arterial blood (DO_2) is dependent on the oxygen content of arterial blood (CaO_2) and the cardiac output and is normally 500–720 ml/min/m^2:

$$DO_2 = CaO_2 \times CO$$

The oxygen content of arterial blood (CaO_2) depends on the haemoglobin concentration and its saturation with oxygen. The vast majority (98.5%) of oxygen carried in the blood is bound to haemoglobin (a clinically insignificant amount is dissolved in plasma). The relationship between the PaO_2 and oxygen uptake by haemoglobin is not linear but assumes a sigmoid curve (*Figure 4.4*), with haemoglobin virtually fully saturated at a PaO_2 of 13 kPa (100 mmHg), the normal healthy state. Increasing the PaO_2 further therefore has little effect on oxygen transport. At a PaO_2 below 8 kPa (60 mmHg) saturation falls precipitously reducing content. The affinity of haemoglobin for oxygen at a particular PaO_2 is increased by an alkaline environment, low PCO_2, a low concentration of 2,3 diphosphoglycerate (2,3 DPG) in the red cells, carbon monoxide and a fall in temperature (e.g. shifting of the curve to the left). The opposite of these factors reduces the affinity and shifts the curve to the right (see later).

Although increasing haemoglobin increases the oxygen carrying capacity of blood, this will also increase blood viscosity. In turn this impedes blood flow, increases myocardial workload and SVR, thus negating any advantage. The normal haemoglobin concentration is somewhat above the point for optimal oxygen transport and a modest reduction will reduce viscosity and myocardial work, improve flow through the microcirculation and therefore increase oxygen transport. It is certainly seldom necessary to strive for a haemoglobin concentration above 10 g/dl (haematocrit 30%) during resuscitation and levels as low as 8 g/dl are often well tolerated.

The factors affecting cardiac output have already been described.

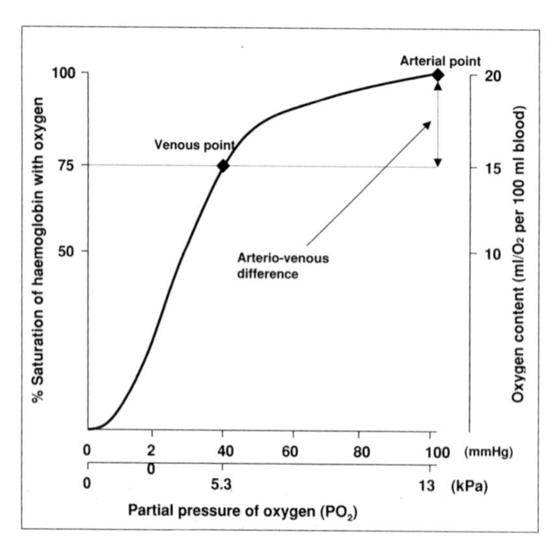

Figure 4.4 Oxygen dissociation curve

Oxygen release to the tissues

At tissue level, there is a partial pressure gradient driving oxygen from capillaries to cells:

- the PaO_2 of blood at the proximal end of capillaries is approximately 13 kPa;
- at the distal capillaries the PO_2 has equilibrated with the interstitium, approximately 4.3 kPa;
- intracellular PO_2 normally averages only 3–3.5 kPa and may fall as low as 0.8 kPa;
- a PO_2 of 0.1–0.6 kPa is required for full support of all oxidative intracellular metabolic processes.

Any metabolic activity that increases demand for oxygen results in local changes that act to allow O_2 to be released more readily (shifting the curve to the right).

To help remember these factors, think of an athlete during a race. The active muscles require more oxygen than when they are at rest. Due to the increased metabolism they generate lactic acid, CO_2 and heat, all of which will assist in the release of oxygen from haemoglobin

4.3.5 Oxygen consumption

In the normal resting subject, total consumption of oxygen per minute (VO_2) is 100–160 ml/min/m^2 and remains constant over a wide range of oxygen delivery (normal value of DO_2 500–720 ml/min/m^2; *Figure 4.5*). The tissues are taking up only 20–25% of the oxygen delivered to them and this is termed the *oxygen extraction ratio* (OER). Normally there is great potential for the tissues of the body to extract more oxygen from the circulating blood if required.

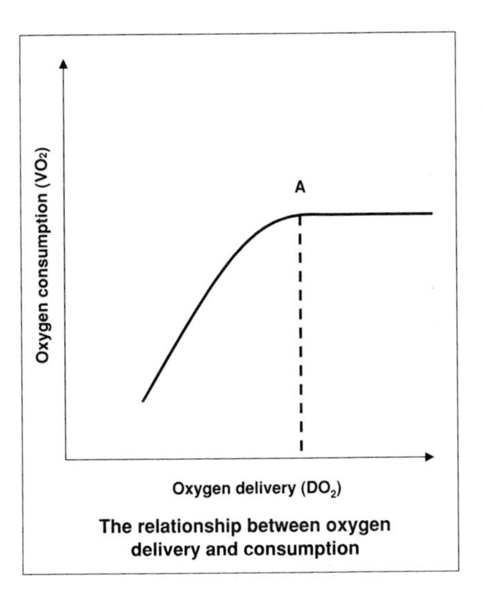

Figure 4.5 Graph showing relationship between oxygen delivery and consumption

Trauma results in an early increase in oxygen consumption, despite the fact that the delivery of oxygen falls because of a reduction in haemoglobin and cardiac output (see above). Initially, the increase in consumption is achieved by increasing the extraction of oxygen, but this mechanism only operates while the delivery of oxygen is greater than approximately 300 ml/min/m^2. Below this level the tissues cannot increase oxygen extraction any further – oxygen extraction is at its maximum. Oxygen consumption therefore progressively falls because it is now directly dependent on the rate of oxygen delivery to the tissues – *supply dependency* is said to operate.

4.4 Cellular effects of shock

Patients cannot remain indefinitely in a state of shock: they either improve or die. Shock can be viewed as 'a momentary pause on the way to death'. This pause gives the trauma team time and opportunity to prevent further deterioration and, ultimately, death.

If shock persists, cells rely on anaerobic metabolism that results in an intracellular lactic acidosis causing dysfunction and eventually cell death. Autolysis occurs and damaged intracellular components are released into the circulation with toxic effects. Hypoperfusion of the gastrointestinal tract impairs its normal function as a mucosal barrier and may allow absorption (translocation) of the normal gut flora into the circulation. Septic shock develops and may trigger the development of multiple organ failure. This condition is one of the commonest causes of late death after trauma. The likelihood of multiple organ failure supervening is increased if resuscitation and correction of circulatory shock is inadequate or delayed.

4.5 Causes of shock

Although there are a number of causes of shock, after trauma there is usually a hypovolaemic component. This is also the most easily managed and should be identified and treated before it is attributed to other causes.

4.5.1 Hypovolaemic shock

In the trauma patient, haemorrhage may be overt, when its volume is often overestimated or occult, and underestimated. Occult haemorrhage occurs into the cavities of the thorax, abdomen and pelvis, or in potential spaces, for example, the retroperitoneal space and muscles and tissues around long bone fractures. Intravascular volume is also lost as a result of leakage of plasma through damaged capillaries into the interstitial spaces, accounting for up to 25% of the volume of tissue swelling following blunt trauma.

The rate of venous return to the heart is dependent on the hydrostatic pressure gradient between the peripheral veins and right atrium of the heart. Hypovolaemia (tension pneumothorax or cardiac tamponade) will reduce this gradient and venous return to the heart, thereby decreasing cardiac output and arterial pressure. External compression on the thorax or abdomen may have a similar effect in obstructing venous return. In relatively young, fit patients, the compensatory mechanisms described earlier may minimize the effects on cardiac output and arterial pressure following acute haemorrhage up to 1–1.5 l blood (i.e. approximately 20–25% total blood volume

BOX 4.3 Blood volumes

- Adult: 70 ml per kilogram ideal body weight (approximately 5 l in 70 kg person)
- Child: 80 ml per kilogram ideal body weight

– see Box 4.3). Tolerance may be much less than this in the elderly and those with cardiovascular comorbidity.

4.5.2 Cardiogenic shock

In cardiogenic shock due to myocardial trauma and/or ischaemia, the compensatory sympathetic response is often ineffective in restoring cardiac output and arterial blood pressure. The dysfunctional left ventricle is unable to increase its contractility and cardiac output fails to be maintained despite the development of an increasing tachycardia. Attempts to maintain arterial blood pressure in the face of a low cardiac output occur as a result of a massively elevated SVR. Unfortunately, both tachycardia and increased afterload raise myocardial oxygen demand and a vicious circle develops with further myocardial ischaemia and dysfunction.

4.5.3 Neurogenic shock

The sympathetic outflow is from the spinal cord between the levels T1–L3. The vasoconstrictor supply to the blood vessels arises from all these levels, and the heart receives its sympathetic innervation from levels T1–T4. A spinal cord injury will impair the sympathetic outflow below the level of the injury: the higher the lesion, the more pronounced the disturbance. Lesions above T4 will result in generalized vasodilatation (reduced SVR), at the same time denervating the heart and preventing any increase in stroke volume and rate to try and maintain cardiac output. The clinical picture is one of severe hypotension, low cardiac output, relative bradycardia and systemic vasodilatation. The trauma team must therefore learn to recognize those clinical situations in which cardinal signs of acute hypovolaemia are absent as a result of a spinal cord injury preventing the lack of a sympathetic response.

4.5.4 Septic shock

Septic shock is caused by circulating toxins which have a multitude of effects including:

- profound systemic vasodilatation;
- impaired tissue autoregulation;
- poisoning of cells whose capacity to metabolize oxygen is impaired despite satisfactory oxygen delivery;
- extravasation of plasma through leaky capillaries causing hypovolaemia and oedema formation.

Trauma victims may develop septic shock after resuscitation from acute haemorrhagic shock due to release of toxic mediators from damaged or ischaemic tissues (e.g. cytokines, complement, kinins, prostaglandins, leukotrienes) or translocation of bacteria into the circulation from the gut flora following breakdown of the normal gastrointestinal mucosal barrier.

In patients with pre-existing ischaemic heart disease or poor cardiovascular reserve, and in all patients in the advanced stages of sepsis, the situation is aggravated by toxins exerting negative inotropic effects on the myocardium. The relatively high cardiac output typical of septic shock is now compromised and a vicious cycle develops, accelerating the demise of the patient.

(Further details on the pathophysiology of septic shock is beyond the scope of this book. Several references are listed in the Further Reading section for the interested reader.)

4.6 Estimating volume loss and grading shock

Shock may be graded clinically according to several basic and easily measured physiological variables:

- delayed capillary refill;
- skin colour and temperature;
- heart rate;
- blood pressure;
- respiratory rate;
- conscious level;
- urine output.

These physiological variables can be used to subdivide hypovolaemic shock into four categories (Box 4.4) and so enable a reasonable estimate of the loss of circulating volume to be made.

BOX 4.4 Categories of hypovolaemic shock

	I	II	III	IV
Blood loss (litres)	< 0.75	0.75–1.5	1.5–2.0	> 2.0
Blood loss (% BV)	< 15%	15–30%	30–40%	> 40%
Heart rate	< 100	> 100	> 120	140 or low
Systolic BP	Normal	Normal	Decreased	Decreased ++
Diastolic BP	Normal	Raised	Decreased	Decreased ++
Pulse pressure	Normal	Decreased	Decreased	Decreased
Capillary refill	Normal	Delayed	Delayed	Delayed
Skin	Normal	Pale	Pale	Pale/cold
Respiratory rate	14–20	20–30	30–40	> 35 or low
Urine output (ml/h)	> 30	20–30	5–15	Negligible
Mental state	Normal	Anxious	Anxious/confused	Confused/drowsy
Fluid replacement	(Colloid)	Colloid	Blood	Blood

Diastolic blood pressure rises in grade 2 shock without any fall in the systolic component, reducing the pulse pressure as a result of vasoconstriction. A narrow pulse pressure with a normal systolic blood pressure is an important sign.

4.6.1 Limitations to estimations of hypovolaemia

Blindly using the grading scheme shown in Box 4.4 could potentially lead to gross over- or underestimation of the blood loss in some groups of patients (see Box 4.5).

BOX 4.5 Patients with a risk of over- or underestimation of blood loss

Type of patient:
- Elderly (decreased cardiovascular reserve)
- Drugs/pacemaker
- Pregnancy
- Athlete

Environment/pre-hospital:
- Hypothermia
- Delay in resuscitation
- Type of injury

Management must be based on the response to treatment of individual patients and is not narrowly focused on trying to attain isolated 'normal' physiological parameters.

The elderly patient

The elderly usually have a reduced cardiorespiratory reserve and are less able to compensate for acute hypovolaemia than a younger (fitter) trauma victim. Loss of smaller volumes of blood will produce a drop in blood pressure and therefore reliance on blood pressure alone can lead to an overestimation of blood loss. Patients with a low fixed cardiac output (e.g. aortic stenosis) behave similarly. As a corollary to this, it should also be noted that very young patients will compensate for hypovolaemia extremely well and hypotension is a late sign and presages impending cardiovascular collapse (see Section 12.4.1).

Drugs and pacemakers

Various drugs may alter the physiological response to blood loss, a good example being β-blockers. Even after losing over 15% of the circulating volume, these drugs prevent the development of a tachycardia and also inhibit the normal sympathetic positive inotropic response. This could lead to an underestimation of blood loss if relying unduly on heart rate. Similarly, hypotension will develop with loss of smaller volumes of blood by the same mechanisms.

An increasing number of patients have pacemakers fitted each year. Depending on their complexity and sophistication, these devices may only pace the heart at a constant rate (approximately 70–100 beats/min), irrespective of volume loss or arterial blood pressure. Therefore they may give rise to errors in estimation of acute blood loss.

The pregnant or athletic patient

The pregnant patient will undergo a variety of physiological changes which may complicate the assessment of blood loss including increased blood volume, increased heart rate and respiratory rate. For more details see Chapter 13 on trauma in pregnancy.

The resting heart rate in a trained athlete may be less than 50 beats/min. Therefore a compensatory tachycardia indicative of significant acute blood loss may be less than 100 beats/min. An increase in blood volume of 15–20% as a consequence of training may constitute a further possible reason for underestimation of blood loss.

The patient with hypothermia

Hypothermia (core temperature < 35°C) will reduce arterial blood pressure, pulse and respiratory rate in its own right, irrespective of any blood loss. If this is ignored, hypovolaemia may be overestimated. It has also been found that hypovolaemic, hypothermic patients are often 'resistant' to appropriate fluid replacement. Estimation of the fluid requirements of these patients may therefore be very difficult and invasive haemodynamic monitoring is often required (see Section 15.4.1).

Delay in resuscitation

The longer the time the patient spends without resuscitation (especially in the young), the longer the normal compensatory mechanisms will have to work. This will lead to improvements in blood pressure, respiratory rate and heart rate. Underestimation of blood loss may then occur.

4.7 Assessment and management of the shocked patient

Successful treatment of shock does not simply equate to the restoration of a normal arterial blood pressure as satisfactory oxygen delivery to the tissues is dependent on other factors including cardiac output and autoregulation of capillary networks.

4.7.1 Primary survey and resuscitation

The same plan described in Section 1.6.1 is used, with members of the team carrying out their tasks simultaneously.

The first priority is for the airway nurse and doctor to clear and secure the patient's airway and ensure adequate ventilation with a high inspired oxygen concentration to optimize oxygen uptake and delivery. At the same time, the spinal column in general, and the cervical spine in particular, should be immobilized if the mechanism of trauma suggests the potential for injury. The remaining five immediately life-threatening respiratory problems need to be excluded or treated if they are present.

Shock is presumed to be due to hypovolaemia until proved otherwise. Team members responsible for circulation should stem overt bleeding by direct pressure while two large bore peripheral iv lines (14 or 16 g) are inserted. Short, wide cannulae should be used as flow is inversely proportional to length and directly related to radius (see Box 4.6).

Immediately following successful venous cannulation, 20 ml blood is taken for estimation of serum electrolytes, full blood count (FBC), grouping and cross-matching and pregnancy test in females of appropriate age. At the same time, the circulation nurse should begin monitoring the patient, measuring and recording the vital signs (see Box 4.7).

BOX 4.6 Relationship between cannula length, radius and flow

Cannula size	*Flow rate (ml/min)*
14 g short	175–200
14 g long	150
16 g short	100–150
16 g long	50–100

BOX 4.7	Vital signs that must be monitored in trauma patients

- Heart rate, arterial blood pressure, pulse pressure
- Respiratory rate
- Capillary refill time
- Urine output
- Glasgow Coma Scale score
- ECG via chest leads (rhythm and waveform)
- Peripheral oxygen saturation
- Temperature, core and peripheral

By the time the cannulae are in place, the team leader should have quickly assessed the patient to try and differentiate between shock due to controlled and uncontrolled haemorrhage. In the former, satisfactory haemostasis can be achieved and it should be possible to resuscitate the patient prior to any urgent surgery being performed. When haemorrhage is controllable, the following fluid regimen can be used:

- grade 2 shock or worse, 1 litre of fluid is rapidly infused, 500 ml via each cannula;
- where there has been over 30 min delay in resuscitation, 2 l should be administered, with at least 1 l of crystalloid to compensate for the interstitial fluid volume loss;
- further infusions of colloid or blood may be given according to the response;
- aim to maintain the haematocrit (packed cell volume) at 30–35% so that oxygen delivery is optimized;
- in grade 1 shock, 0.5 l of fluid is infused *slowly*, further fluids are given according to subsequent assessment.

There is currently some debate regarding resuscitation of patients with uncontrolled haemorrhage, i.e. when haemostasis has not been achieved. This situation is usually due to ongoing haemorrhage in a major body cavity. Although aggressive resuscitation with rapid infusion of a large volume of fluid tends to raise arterial pressure, there may be adverse effects including dislodgement of thrombus formation and a dilutional coagulopathy. These factors then lead to further haemorrhage necessitating even greater fluid resuscitation – a vicious circle develops making optimization of such patients difficult if not impossible. The priority in these patients is emergency surgical haemostasis. Fluid resuscitation prior to surgery should be limited to achieving an arterial blood pressure sufficient to maintain organ viability in the short term. Although precise values cannot be given, a systolic blood pressure of 80–90 mmHg is a good target. Evidence from animal and clinical studies suggests that mortality may be reduced by allowing this so-called *permissive hypotension*. For example, mortality from ruptured abdominal aortic aneurysm decreased from 70% to 23% when preoperative fluid therapy was restricted to maintaining a systolic blood pressure of 70 mmHg. The evidence for this approach is far from conclusive in acute hypovolaemic shock generally. Thus it is not possible to be didactic regarding when to accept that optimization of an individual patient is unachievable by infusion of fluids alone and when to recommend emergency surgery in the presence of permissive hypotension. The choice of which approach to take is unfortunately a complex one and requires an experienced team leader aware of the potential pros and cons of either approach to make an appropriate decision.

In uncontrolled haemorrhage it may be necessary to restrict preoperative fluid resuscitation to facilitate rapid surgical haemostasis

The arguments for and against crystalloid and colloid infusions are described in Appendix 4.2 at the end of this chapter. Red cell replacement is a secondary consideration, becoming more important with progressively larger blood loss (remember the advantageous effect of a reduced haematocrit on blood viscosity and flow). In the majority of trauma cases who require blood in the resuscitation room, type-specific blood is used, i.e. the recipient and donor blood are checked for ABO and Rhesus compatibility. Most laboratories can provide this within 10 min. Occasionally, exsanguinating haemorrhage will require immediate administration of blood. In these cases, uncross-matched blood (O negative) is used initially until typed blood is available.

Coagulation abnormalities may occur after massive blood loss as a result of dilution of clotting factors by administered fluids, the release of tissue factors and minimal amounts of clotting factors in stored blood. They should be treated precisely, using information gained by a regular assessment of the patient's clotting status rather than blindly treating any bleeding problem with platelets and fresh frozen plasma.

All fluids given to trauma patients should be warmed before administration to prevent iatrogenic hypothermia. A simple way of achieving this is to store them in a warming cupboard, thereby eliminating the need for warming coils which increase resistance to flow and slow the rate of fluid administration.

Accurate measurement of urine volume will obviously require the insertion of a urinary catheter and the volume is then recorded whenever the other vital signs are measured.

4.7.2 Venous access

In adults, there are two alternatives if a peripheral site for venous access is not available:

- central line;
- venous cutdown.

For both, an aseptic technique must be used along with infiltration of local anaesthesia when appropriate.

Central line

This technique involves the insertion of an appropriate cannula (14 or 16 g) into a central vein, usually the subclavian, internal jugular or femoral vein, using the Seldinger technique (see below). The procedure should be carried out only by experienced staff because it has potential for damaging the vein and neighbouring structures. One of the circulation nurses should prepare the equipment listed in Box 4.8. The anatomy of the central veins is shown in *Figure 4.6*.

The Seldinger technique

Using a needle attached to a syringe, the central vein is initially punctured percutaneously, confirmed by the ability to aspirate blood. The syringe is removed, the flexible guidewire passed down the needle, 4–5 cm into the vein and the needle carefully withdrawn leaving the wire behind. The dilator is then loaded onto the wire and whilst

BOX 4.8 Equipment required for central venous cannulation

- Skin preparation solution
- Swabs
- Sterile sheets
- Sterile gowns and gloves for the nurse and doctor
- Local anaesthetic
- Syringe and needle for administering the anaesthetic
- Scalpel and blade
- Suture and sterile scissors
- Central line pack:
  - Syringe
  - Large bore needle
  - Guidewire
  - Dilator
  - Cannula
- Three-way tap
- Giving set attached to intravenous fluid for infusion
- Opsite™ or other transparent adhesive sterile dressing
- Monitor and appropriate connecting tubing

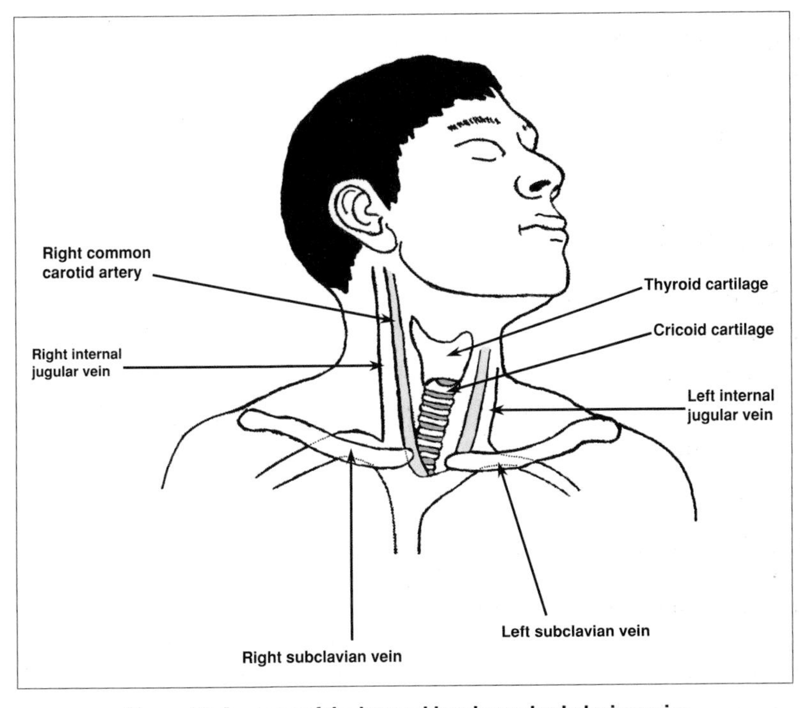

Figure 4.6 Anatomy of the internal jugular and subclavian veins

holding the proximal end of the wire, advanced into the vein. A small incision in the skin may be required to facilitate insertion of the dilator. The dilator is withdrawn leaving the wire in the vein and then the cannula is introduced into the vein in a similar manner. The wire is then removed, the syringe reattached and blood aspirated to confirm the cannula lies in the vein. If difficulty is encountered inserting the wire, the needle and wire must be withdrawn together to avoid damaging the wire on the needle tip.

The subclavian vein

This vein can be cannulated via both the supra- and infraclavicular approach. The following is a brief description of one of many approaches to the vein.

(i) The patient is placed supine, arms at his side, head turned away and if safe 10° head down.

(ii) The operator stands on the same side as that to be punctured and identifies the midclavicular point and the suprasternal notch.

(iii) The needle is inserted 1 cm below the midclavicular point, advanced horizontally, postero-inferior to the clavicle towards the 'tip' of a finger in the suprasternal notch, aspirating on the syringe.

(iv) When the needle tip enters the vein, usually at a depth of 4–6 cm, blood is easily aspirated, the syringe is removed and the cannula introduced as described above.

(v) The cannula is secured, a sterile dressing applied and a chest x-ray taken to exclude a pneumothorax and confirm correct positioning of the cannula.

Complications

- Pneumothorax.
- Haemothorax.
- Puncture of the subclavian vein.
- Injury to mediastinal structures.
- Air embolism.
- Infection.

Internal jugular vein

The following is a brief description of one of many approaches to the vein. The right side is usually chosen as there is a straight line to the heart, the apical pleura is not as high, and the main thoracic duct is on the left.

(i) The patient is supine, head turned slightly away from the side of approach and if safe 10° head down.

(ii) The carotid artery is identified at the level of the thyroid cartilage with the tips of the fingers of the left hand.

(iii) With the fingers still marking the position of the artery, the needle is introduced 0.5 cm lateral to the artery, towards the medial border of the sternomastoid muscle, aspirating on the syringe.

(iv) When the needle tip enters the vein, usually at a depth of 2–3 cm, blood is easily aspirated, the syringe is removed and the cannula introduced as described above.

(v) The cannula is secured, a sterile dressing applied and a chest x-ray taken to exclude a pneumothorax and confirm correct positioning of the cannula.

(vi) If the vein is not entered on first attempt, a further attempt can be made slightly more laterally.

Complications
- Puncture of the carotid artery.
- Pneumothorax.
- Air embolism.
- Infection.

Femoral vein

Access to this vein may be easier during resuscitation, however sterility is more difficult to maintain. Because of the risk of deep vein thrombosis, the cannula should be used for the minimum time possible.

- The patient is placed in a supine position and the inguinal ligament identified.
- Locate the femoral artery just below the ligament.
- With a finger on the artery, the needle is introduced 1 cm medially at an angle of 45° cranially, aspirating on the syringe.
- The vein is usually entered at a depth of 3–4 cm and the syringe is removed and the cannula introduced as described above.
- Secure the cannula and apply a sterile dressing.

Complications
- Arterial puncture.
- Deep vein thrombosis.
- Infection.
- Injury to the femoral nerve.

Venous cutdown

An alternative method is to cut down onto the long saphenous or medial basilic vein. The circulating nurse will need to be familiar with the equipment and procedure described in Box 4.9.

If the saphenous vein is to be used, identify the medial malleolus; if the medial basilic vein is used, identify the medial epicondyl of the humerus.

BOX 4.9 Equipment required for a venous cutdown

- Skin preparation solution
- Swabs
- Sterile sheets
- Sterile gowns for the nurse and doctor
- Local anaesthetic
- Syringe and needle for administering the anaesthetic
- Scalpel and blade
- Suture and sterile scissors
- Small haemostats
- Cannula
- Giving set attached to intravenous fluid for infusion
- Opsite™ or other transparent adhesive sterile dressing

- A 3-cm incision is made through the skin and subcutaneous tissues, either:
  - 2 cm anterior and superior to the medial malleolus;
  - 2–3 cm lateral to the medial epicondyl at the flexion crease at the elbow.
- Using blunt dissection, a 2-cm length of vein is freed from local structures and two sutures passed beneath the vein.
- The distal end of the vein is tied off, leaving the suture full length to allow traction on the vein while the proximal suture is looped around the vein but not tied.
- Using either a scalpel or scissors, a small incision is made in the vein, taking care not to divide the vein totally, and the cannula introduced. Alternatively, the vein can be cannulated under direct vision using a cannula over needle type device.
- The proximal suture is then tied to secure the cannula.
- Blood should be aspirated to confirm correct placement, but this is not always possible. A freely running infusion without any signs of extravasation is an acceptable alternative.
- Close the skin around the cannula with interrupted sutures and apply a sterile dressing.

Complications
- Venous thrombosis.
- Haematoma.
- Infection.
- Transection of the vein or local artery or nerve.

The intraosseous route may be used in children if it is not possible to cannulate a peripheral vein. This technique is described in Appendix 4.3.

The rest of the primary survey is completed as previously described in Section 1.6.1. At the end, the nursing and medical team leaders must ensure that the required tasks have been or are being carried out. An arterial blood sample may be sent at this stage. Acidosis is invariably a result of anaerobic metabolism in poorly perfused tissues. Appropriate management consists of increasing cardiac output by fluid administration, optimizing PaO_2 and reducing PCO_2 to ensure adequate delivery of O_2 to the tissues. Sodium bicarbonate is reserved for cases of immediately life-threatening acidosis where the pH approaches 7.0. In such cases it is preferable to have the patient intubated and hyperventilated so that the generated CO_2 may be rapidly excreted via the lungs.

4.7.3 Secondary survey

After the detailed head-to-toe assessment of the patient has been carried out, the team should have a reasonable estimation of the blood loss and its source. They should also know the patient's allergic history, current medication, past medical history, time of last meal and the mechanism of injury (remember 'AMPLE' in Section 1.6.2).

Pain relief is usually necessary to relieve suffering, increase the patient's ability to compensate for any hypovolaemia and to decrease myocardial workload by reducing catecholamine secretion. In the conscious patient, morphine in 1–2 mg increments (best achieved by diluting 10 mg of morphine to 10 ml of normal saline) can be administered intravenously until satisfactory analgesia is achieved. An appropriate dose of an antiemetic agent (e.g. metoclopramide 5–10 mg, ondansetron 4–8 mg) should also be given. There is a wide therapeutic dose range for morphine amongst patients, depending on their age, premorbid fitness, comorbidity and physical status postinjury. Consequently, a wide dose range may be required to achieve satisfactory analgesia (see Section 16.3). Analgesia should never be given by the intramuscular route: initially there is only limited systemic uptake due to the poor perfusion of the patient's muscles but once perfusion has improved after resuscitation, a large bolus of opioid analgesia may be absorbed rapidly into the bloodstream with profound effects on conscious level, respiration and arterial blood pressure.

In the time it takes an efficient trauma team to reach this stage in the resuscitation, the first litre of colloid will have been given to the patient. The original estimated blood loss can therefore be compared with the patient's response to the fluid volume provided. Essentially, there are three outcomes with regard to the change in the patient's condition after reassessment.

The patient is improving

This suggests that the intravascular volume deficit is less than 20% and that the rate of fluid input is greater than the rate of fluid loss. Such patients may require blood later but one can afford to wait for a full cross-match. The circulation nurse should closely monitor vital signs and inform the team leader of any sudden deterioration (see below).

The patient initially improves, then deteriorates

In these cases the rate of bleeding has increased, either because of a new source of bleeding or loss of haemostasis at the original site. The latter may occur with the rise in blood pressure following resuscitation. The majority of these patients will require surgery and early involvement of the appropriate surgical team. Blood is also required, the choice being between typed or uncross-matched, unless fully cross-matched blood has already been prepared. The decision will depend on the clinical state of the patient (as above).

The patient does not improve

These patients are either bleeding faster than blood or other fluids are being supplied or they are not suffering from hypovolaemic shock alone. The former group of patients will have lost over 40% of their blood volume and therefore require urgent surgery with ongoing fluid resuscitation.

Shock may also be due to a cardiogenic, neurogenic or septic cause, either alone or in combination with hypovolaemia. Aspects of the history, examination and vital signs are essential to distinguish between these possibilities.

Cardiogenic shock

Cardiac tamponade and tension pneumothorax should be rapidly excluded because these conditions can quickly kill the patient (see Section 3.4.1). If heart failure is suspected, it is essential to discover the past medical history and current medication. In addition to the more usual signs of shock, there may be evidence of chest trauma, dysrhythmias, crackles on auscultation of the chest or a raised CVP suggested by engorged jugular veins. These patients are also less able to compensate for any hypovolaemia and their management is complex. Early involvement of the Intensive Care team is essential as invasive haemodynamic assessment using a pulmonary artery flotation catheter

(PAC) is usually required. This enables the filling pressure of the left side of the heart and cardiac output to be estimated along with a combination of mechanical ventilation, vasodilators, inotropes and expansion of circulating volume to increase CI and DO_2 to satisfactory levels.

Neurogenic shock

Patients with neurogenic shock will have a history and physical findings suggestive of spinal cord damage (see Section 7.3.2). It is important that these patients are neither under- nor overtransfused. The former may lead to poor perfusion of the spinal cord and exacerbate injury, the latter to pulmonary oedema. In patients with no previous heart or lung disease, the CVP and LVEDP have a close correlation. Therefore in the early stages, CVP will be useful in estimating fluid requirements and response to treatment. However, the patient may require more intensive and accurate fluid monitoring at a later stage on the ICU.

Septic shock

It takes time to develop septic shock and so these patients are often transfers from other hospitals or those who have suffered a bowel perforation some hours previously. Early signs are a wide pulse pressure and warm skin due to dilated peripheral blood vessels and the cardiac output may be in the normal range or even raised. The patient is often agitated, pyrexial and hypoxic due to the development of acute respiratory distress syndrome (ARDS). Coagulopathies such as disseminated intravascular coagulation are often associated with septic shock. This abnormality may be life-threatening and manifests initially as blood oozing from wounds and cannula sites. The management of these patients is generally the domain of the Intensivist, but the Trauma Team should be able to recognize the signs and symptoms of septic shock to allow them to participate in the care of patients who may arrive in the resuscitation room following transfer from another hospital.

4.8 Summary

All members of the trauma team must recognize and initiate treatment in shocked patients as early as possible. They must also constantly monitor and reassess appropriate physiological variables. Any subsequent deterioration needs to be detected quickly and treated appropriately. As the patient improves, other problems may become apparent.

Appendices

Appendix 4.1: Invasive monitoring

Recent studies have cast some doubt on the validity of the assumption that it is possible to manipulate the haemodynamic and oxygen transport status of critically ill patients into 'survivor mode' goals, derived from the median values of survivors of critical illness (see Box 4.10). It seems achievement of survivor goals reflects an unmasking of the physiological reserve capacity required to survive critical illness.

BOX 4.10 Optimal goals in securing adequate oxygen transport (normal ranges in brackets)

- Cardiac index (CI) > 4.5 l/min/m_2 (2.8–3.6 l/min/m_2)
- Oxygen delivery (DO_2) > 600 ml/min/m_2 (500–720 ml/min/m_2)
- Oxygen consumption (VO_2) > 170 ml/min/m_2 (100–160 ml/min/m_2)
- Pulmonary artery occlusion or wedge pressure (PAOP) 18 mmHg (5–15)
- Mixed venous oxyhaemoglobin saturation (S/O_2) > 70% (70–75%)
- Whole blood lactate concentration = < 2 mmol/l (< 2 mmol/l)

Patients without such reserve capacity cannot be made to achieve the goals by manipulation of their treatment. Thus whilst rigid adherence to these goals is no longer practised in most ICUs in the UK, most intensivists nevertheless aim as far as reasonably practicable to achieve supranormal indices, guided by regular assessment of acid-base status and SvO_2.

Most of the indices monitored require the prior insertion of a multilumen, pulmonary artery catheter (PAC).

Cardiac output (CO)

The CO is measured using a thermodilution technique (an application of the indirect Fick principle) by rapidly injecting 10 ml of cold crystalloid solution into the right atrium via a proximal lumen of the PAC. This causes a reduction in blood temperature, monitored at the tip of the catheter by the thermistor. The reduction in temperature is inversely proportional to the extent of dilution of the injectate which is itself directly proportional to the CO. More sophisticated (and expensive) PACs are now available that use a variation of the thermodilution principle to provide a continuous readout of CO. The distal portion of the catheter proximal to the thermistor is surrounded by a heating coil that warms the blood slightly as it flows past, causing the temperature detected by the thermistor to rise.

Left ventricular end diastolic pressure (LVEDP)

The LVEDP cannot be measured directly and is estimated from the pulmonary artery occlusion or wedge pressure (PAOP). This is the pressure at the tip of the PAC with the balloon inflated and wedged against the walls of the pulmonary artery. As distal flow is interrupted, there is a direct communication between the tip and the left atrium. At end diastole, the pressure within the left atrium approximates to the LVEDP which itself is usually an accurate reflection of left ventricular (LV) preload. Normal values range between 5–15 mmHg.

Systemic vascular resistance (SVR)

The SVR is a derived variable and not directly measured. It is calculated from the mean arterial pressure (MAP), the central venous pressure (CVP) and the cardiac output (CO) (see Box 4.11). It is usually increased in hypovolaemic and cardiogenic shock and decreased in septic, anaphylactic and neurogenic shock.

BOX 4.11	Calculating the systemic vascular resistance
	MAP = Diastolic pressure + 1/3 (systolic pressure – diastolic pressure) SVR = (MAP – CVP) × 80/CO (normal range = 800–1400 dyne/s/cm^5)

Oxygen content of arterial blood

Accurate measurement of haemoglobin oxygen saturation (SaO_2), PaO_2 and haemoglobin concentration [Hb] are needed to calculate the oxygen content of arterial blood (CaO_2), which includes both oxygen bound to haemoglobin plus that dissolved in plasma.

The amount bound to Hb = [Hb] (g/dl) × SaO_2 (expressed as a decimal fraction) × 1.34

(when fully saturated, 1g Hb binds 1.34 ml O_2)

$$\text{The amount dissolved in plasma} = PaO_2 \times 0.003$$

(i.e. 0.003 ml/dl oxygen dissolves in plasma for each mmHg PaO_2.)

Therefore:

$$CaO_2\ (\text{ml/dl}) = ([Hb]\ (\text{g/dl}) \times SaO_2 \times 1.34) + (PaO_2 \times 0.003)$$

It can be seen that the amount of oxygen dissolved in plasma physiologically is only 1–2% of the total and is relatively insignificant.

Delivery of oxygen

The delivery of oxygen to the tissues (DO_2) is dependent on the content of oxygen in the blood (CaO_2) and the rate at which blood is reaching the tissues (CO).

$$DO_2\ (\text{ml/min}) = CO \times CaO_2 \times 10\ (\text{normal value 500–720 ml/min})$$

The factor of ten is needed to express CaO_2 in units of ml/l.

DO_2 is often indexed to body surface area in the same way as CO when it is designated $DO_{2\ INDEX}$. $DO_{2\ INDEX}$ is calculated from the CI and CaO_2.

Consumption of oxygen

In order to assess the oxygen consumption (VO_2) of the cells and tissues of the body, it is necessary to measure the amount of oxygen left in venous blood returning to the heart. If this is low (less than approximately 70%), it indicates that the tissues are extracting larger amounts of oxygen than normal from arterial blood as it passes through the capillary network (i.e. the oxygen extraction ratio is high) from which it may be deduced that regional blood flow through the tissues is suboptimal.

The metabolic activity of organs and tissues differs and hence the oxygen extraction ratio varies. However, pulmonary artery blood is a homogeneous mixture of the venous blood returning from all the organs and tissues and a sample of blood is taken from the distal lumen of a PAC which lies in the pulmonary artery. This is often termed a mixed venous sample. Some modern types of PAC incorporate a miniature oximeter within the tip of the catheter, thereby permitting a continuous readout of mixed venous oxygen saturation.

The oxygen content of a mixed venous blood sample (CvO_2) is calculated using an analogous formula to that used to calculate the CaO_2:

$$CvO_2\ (ml/dl) = ([Hb]\ (g/dl) \times SvO_2 \times 1.34) + (PvO_2 \times 0.003)$$

SvO_2 and PvO_2 represent the oxygen saturation and oxygen partial pressure of the mixed venous sample. VO_2 is also often indexed to body surface area in the same way as CO when it is designated $VO_{2\ INDEX}$.

Appendix 4.2 Colloids versus crystalloids

Much has been written about which type of fluid is most appropriate in treating shocked patients. Advocates for colloids argue that rapid replacement of intravascular volume is of primary importance. The proponents of crystalloids consider that fluid is required to restore the deficit from the entire extracellular space (e.g. intravascular and interstitial spaces).

Colloids

Colloid solutions are usually isotonic and can be used to replace an intravascular loss up to 1 l, on a 1:1 basis. Greater degrees of blood loss usually require packed cells to be added so that the haematocrit does not fall below 30%. Colloids are either plasma derivatives (5% albumin and human plasma protein fraction (HPPF)) or plasma substitutes (gelatins, dextrans, hydroxyethyl starches).

The two gelatin preparations in common use are Haemaccel and Gelofusine. They are derived from alkaline hydrolysis of bovine collagen. The average molecular weight of the molecules is approximately 30–35 000 daltons and they have a half-life within the circulation of 2–4 h during which time the gelatin is eliminated completely by filtration in the renal glomeruli and hepatic metabolism. These fluids do not adequately replace the interstitial loss but they do produce less tissue oedema than crystalloids. However cardiac failure has been reported more often in patients receiving inappropriately large volumes of colloids. Haemaccel has a higher calcium and lower sodium concentration than Gelofusine and the former may therefore produce flocculation (clumping) of red cells if Haemaccel and blood are administered via the same giving set.

Dextrans are polysaccharides produced with differing ranges of molecular weight, that is, used to describe the solution, for example Dextran 70 (average molecular weight 70 000 daltons). This is the only type used for trauma resuscitation. Although the clinically effective intravascular half-life of dextran 70 is about 6 h, higher molecular weight components can be detected days or even weeks later. Dextran solutions also interfere with both cross-matching and coagulation due to effects on platelet function and fibrin formation. Although dextran diluted blood can still be used for cross-matching purposes, it is more time consuming for the laboratory and as a consequence, dextran solutions tend not to be used during resuscitation.

Another type of colloid solution are the hydroxyethyl starches. Hetastarch (Hespan, 6% starch in isotonic saline) has an average molecular weight of 450 000 daltons. Accordingly it has a much longer circulatory half-life than the gelatins and the clinical effect may even extend beyond 24 h. Care must therefore be taken to avoid fluid overload when blood is added later to restore the haematocrit. Pentastarch differs only from hetastarch in its degree of hydroxyethylation. It is available as 6% and 10% solutions in normal saline and has an average molecular weight of 250 000 daltons.

Both gelatin and starch colloid solutions have a low incidence of acute allergic reaction.

Crystalloids

The most commonly used crystalloid solutions are Hartmanns solution (Ringer's lactate) and 0.9%N (physiologically normal) saline. The former may be preferred because it contains a lower concentration of sodium and chloride ions and may therefore reduce the risk of producing hyperchloraemic acidosis in the shocked patient. Hartmanns solution is closer to the ionic composition of extracellular fluid. It contains lactate ions that are metabolized in the liver to produce bicarbonate, although this process may be inhibited in the shocked patient.

Both crystalloids have an intravascular half-life of only 30–60 min before they diffuse throughout the extracellular fluid compartment. Over 60% of the volume infused is taken up by the interstitium under normal conditions and this may be increased to 90% in the shocked patient. Consequently at least three times the estimated intravascular loss has to be infused as crystalloid to maintain intravascular volume. This becomes a major problem when there is large volume loss (grade 3 or 4 shock). It is difficult to infuse such large volumes of crystalloid quickly (> 5 l) and tissue oedema may result. This is of particular importance in acute brain and lung injury when further cerebral swelling or pulmonary oedema may be produced. Renal complications may also occur, particularly in elderly patients receiving large volumes of crystalloids. The advantages of using crystalloids over colloids are that they restore intracellular and interstitial fluid loss, they are cheap, convenient, have an extremely low incidence of allergic reactions and a long shelf-life. Despite the problems associated with the use of large volumes of crystalloid, fluid resuscitation using only Hartmanns solution and blood is a technique commonly used in the USA.

Recently hypertonic-hyperosmotic crystalloid solutions have been advocated for initial resuscitation of hypovolaemia. Although it is suggested that they may be superior to isotonic crystalloid or colloid solutions, they are not in routine use in the UK.

When deciding on fluid replacement, the most appropriate fluid for the affected body space should be chosen. Blood should be given as early as possible for patients in grade 3 or 4 shock. For lesser grades there is mainly an intravascular loss initially. Therefore in this situation the primary fluid is colloid. (Crystalloid, in adequate volumes, can be given as a substitute.) At a later stage, crystalloids will be needed to replace the interstitial loss.

Appendix 4.3: Intraosseous infusion

This technique is carried out when it is not possible to cannulate a peripheral vein in a child and the expertise to cannulate a central vein is unavailable. It is simple to learn and has a low incidence of complications. Osteomyelitis and local soft tissue infection may occasionally occur when the needle has been left in place for several days or a hypertonic solution has been infused.

Ideally a purpose-designed intraosseous infusion needle should be used, but spinal and bone marrow aspiration needles are suitable alternatives. Whichever type is available, the needle must have a trocar to prevent it becoming obstructed as it traverses the bony cortex. The commonest site for needle insertion is 2–3 fingerbreadths below the tibial tuberosity on the anteromedial surface of the tibia.

A leg without a fracture proximal to the insertion site is chosen and the site cleaned. The needle is then pushed into the bone at 90° to the skin's surface. Steady pressure is maintained until there is a sudden fall in resistance, indicating that the needle is in the bone marrow. This position must be checked by first removing the trocar and aspirating marrow and, secondly, noting a free flow of fluid into the bone without the development of a visible subcutaneous leak.

The aspirated marrow should not be discarded but instead sent for blood typing. The choice and quantity of fluid needed to resuscitate children is described in Section 12.4.1.

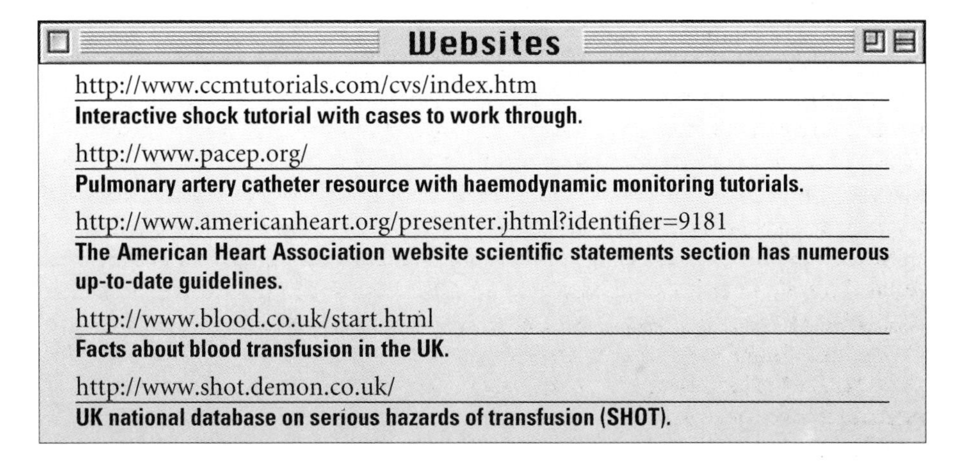
Websites

http://www.ccmtutorials.com/cvs/index.htm

Interactive shock tutorial with cases to work through.

http://www.pacep.org/

Pulmonary artery catheter resource with haemodynamic monitoring tutorials.

http://www.americanheart.org/presenter.jhtml?identifier=9181

The American Heart Association website scientific statements section has numerous up-to-date guidelines.

http://www.blood.co.uk/start.html

Facts about blood transfusion in the UK.

http://www.shot.demon.co.uk/

UK national database on serious hazards of transfusion (SHOT).

Further reading

1. **Buckley R** (1992) The management of hypovolaemic shock. *Nursing Standard* **6:** 25.
2. **Cohen J & Glauser M** (1991) Septic shock: treatment. *Lancet* **338:** 736.
3. **Edwards J** (1990) Practical application of oxygen transport principles. *Crit. Care Med.* **18:** S45.
4. **Edwards J, Nightingale P, Wilkins R, *et al.*** (1989) Haemodynamic and oxygen transport response to modified gelatin in critically ill patients. *Crit. Care Med.* **17:** 996.
5. **Glauser M, Zanetti G, Baumgantner J, *et al.*** (1991) Septic shock: pathogenesis. *Lancet* **338:** 732.
6. **Little R** (1989) Heart rate changes after haemorrhage and injury – a reappraisal. *J. Trauma* **29:** 903.
7. **Nolan JP & Parr MJA** (1997) Aspects of resuscitation in trauma. *Br. J. Anaesth.* **79:** 226.
8. **Scalea T, Simon H, Duncan A, *et al.*** (1990) Geriatric blunt multiple trauma: improved survival with early invasive monitoring. *J. Trauma* **30:** 129.
9. **Secher N, Jensen K, Werner C, *et al.*** (1984) Bradycardia during severe but reversible hypovolaemic shock in man. *Cir. Shock* **14:** 267.
10. **Shoemaker W** (1985) Critical care. *Surg. Clin. N. Am.* **4:** 65.
11. **Sinkinson C (ed.)** (1990) Septic shock: where are we now? *Em. Med. Reports* **11:** 177.
12. **Thompson D, Adams S, Barrett J, *et al.*** (1990) Relative bradycardia in patients with isolated penetrating abdominal trauma and isolated extremity trauma. *Ann. Em. Med.* **19:** 268.

5 Abdominal and pelvic trauma

A Sen, M Scriven

Objectives

The objectives of this chapter are that members of a trauma team understand the following:

- applied anatomy of abdomen and pelvis;
- importance of the mechanism of injury;
- principles of management for abdominal trauma.

5.1 Introduction

Abdominal trauma causes significant mortality and morbidity, despite recent advances in diagnostic and therapeutic possibilities. Unrecognized injuries to the abdomen present diagnostic challenges and are, therefore, a cause of preventable death.

The reasons behind these problems are:

- the abdomen constitutes a large part of the trunk and yet is relatively unprotected;
- the main effects of abdominal injury are bleeding and peritoneal contamination from the hollow viscera. The early manifestations of these are often subtle and there may be no external markers of such injury;
- the main presenting symptom is pain. The main signs are those of peritoneal irritation. These are often masked by an alteration of mental state, consumption of drugs and/or alcohol and painful distracting injuries elsewhere;
- for the reasons outlined above clinical assessment alone is unreliable. The clinician's index of suspicion must be high and must dictate the need for specialized investigations.

It is important to have a clear understanding of the clinical anatomy of the abdomen, the mechanism of injury and the specialized investigations available in order to make an early diagnosis.

In managing patients with abdominal trauma the decision about the need for early laparotomy is critical. It is less important to know the precise nature of the intra-abdominal injury; this can be confirmed at operation. If there are signs of shock and abdominal injury, early laparotomy should be undertaken as part of the resuscitative efforts. Signs may be of intra-abdominal bleeding or peritonitis. In those in whom there is no immediate indication for laparotomy but a high degree of suspicion, transfer for specialized investigations, such as CT scanning, should only be done when the patient is haemodynamically normal and stable. The whole trauma team, including those involved in the pre-hospital phase, must be involved in the management of these patients with the aim of minimizing preventable death.

A suggestive mechanism of injury should lead to a strong suspicion of abdominal trauma

5.2 Applied anatomy

In the following sections the applied anatomy is combined with a discussion of the nature of injuries and their management.

5.2.1 The abdomen

The abdomen is bounded by the muscles of the diaphragm above and those of the pelvic floor below. The pelvic brim divides the abdomen from the pelvis, although the two are contiguous. Posteriorly are the vertebral column and paravertebral muscles. Anterolaterally are the bony rib cage, the abdominal muscles and the bony pelvis, from above downwards.

The contents of the abdomen occupy the following regions:

- peritoneal cavity;
- retroperitoneum;
- pelvis.

Organs that are largely covered with peritoneum (see below) are called intraperitoneal and those which are not extraperitoneal. The pelvis contains both intraperitoneal and extraperitoneal structures. The retroperitoneum contains extraperitoneal structures and is continuous below, with the extraperitoneal part of the pelvis (*Figure 5.1*).

Peritoneum

The peritoneum is a continuous serous membrane that covers certain organs in the abdomen. It is a closed sac and so has two layers that contain a potential space containing a small volume of serous fluid. The visceral layer covers the organs and the

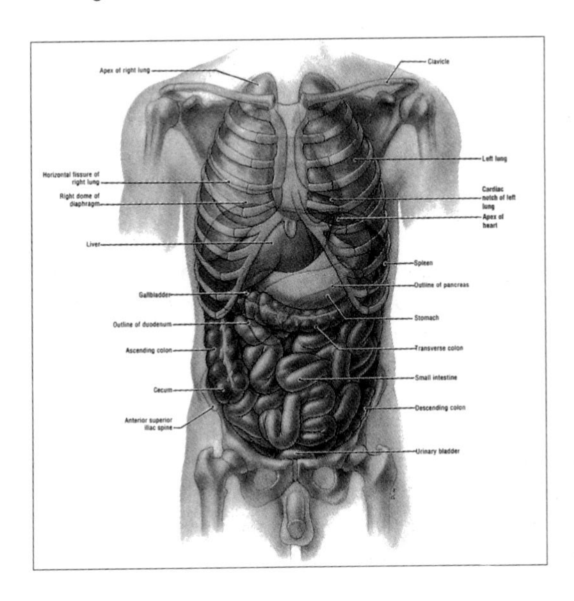

Figure 5.1 Boundary and content of abdomen. *Grant's Atlas of Anatomy* (1991) 9th edn. Agur AMR and Lee MJ (eds). Reproduced with permission from Lippincott, Williams & Wilkins.

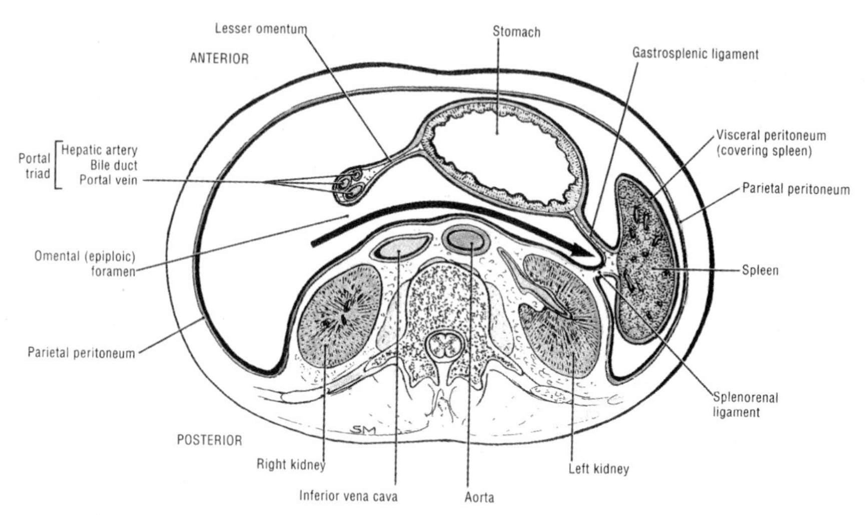

Figure 5.2 Arrangement of peritoneal pouches. ***Grant's Atlas of Anatomy*** **(1991) 9th edn Agur AEM and Lee MJ (eds). Reproduced with permission from Lippincott, Williams & Wilkins.**

parietal layer lines the abdominal wall. These two layers are closely applied to each other, and the cavity itself only becomes apparent when fluid collects in it. Such fluid may be blood, bowel content or urine. Fluid tends to accumulate in certain deep pockets in a supine patient, which may be examined by imaging. Identification of fluid in the hepatorenal space (of Morrison), the rectovesical space (of Douglas) or the space between left diaphragm and spleen may be very important in managing patients with abdominal trauma (*Figure 5.2*).

Chemical or bacterial irritation of the peritoneum leads to peritonitis, which eventually causes clinical features such as severe pain, muscle guarding and rebound tenderness. These symptoms and signs are often subtle in early peritonitis and may appear too late to be relied upon for diagnosis.

Obvious signs of peritoneal irritation may be a late feature of abdominal trauma – such signs should lead to early laparotomy as part of the resuscitative efforts

The peritoneal cavity can be considered in three parts when reviewing possible injuries in trauma patients. The upper *intrathoracic* part is contained within the bony rib cage and the lower *pelvic* part within the bony pelvis. The *abdominal* part is between these two. The intrathoracic part may extend up to the nipple line in peak expiration so that lower chest trauma can lead to injury to intraperitoneal organs as well as those of the chest. Equally, intraperitoneal structures in the pelvis, mainly the small intestines, may be damaged by trauma to the pelvis.

Contents of peritoneal cavity

Intrathoracic
- Diaphragm
- Liver
- Spleen
- Stomach

Abdominal
- Small intestine
- Large intestine
- Omentum

Pelvic
- Intestines
- Bladder
- Uterus and ovaries

Some of these structures are only partly intraperitoneal. For instance, the colon is retroperitoneal in its ascending and descending parts but intraperitoneal in its transverse and sigmoid parts. In other structures their containment within the peritoneum may vary. For instance the urinary bladder extends more and more into the peritoneal cavity as it distends. Rupture into the peritoneum is thus more common when the bladder is distended and injured by a compressing force.

Diaphragm

On each side the diaphragm forms a dome-shaped muscular structure separating the thorax from the abdomen. The muscular root fans out from attachments to the upper three lumbar vertebrae, becoming tendinous over the dome. Peripherally it is attached to the sternum and ribs. Diaphragmatic injury occurs in only 3% of all abdominal trauma.

There is a physiological pressure gradient across the diaphragm. A sudden increase in this gradient can cause rupture of the diaphragm with consequent herniation of the abdominal contents into the chest. A considerable force is needed to do this and there are, therefore, a number of significant associated injuries. Splenic trauma occurs in 25% of patients and pelvic disruption in 40%. Other associated injuries include long bone fractures and closed head injury.

Diaphragmatic injury is more common in penetrating trauma especially where there are penetrating left thoraco-abdominal wounds

Diagnosis can be difficult although a penetrating chest injury should alert clinicians to the possibility. The typical features – disproportionate chest/abdominal pain, dyspnoea, reduced air entry/dullness to percussion at the bases – are often equivocal in the resuscitation room.

Radiographic signs indicating the presence of abdominal structures in the chest, for instance bowel gas patterns or gastric tube, are diagnostic. Change to the contour of the diaphragm is an indicative but not diagnostic radiographic sign. Other modalities including ultrasonography, CT scanning and diagnostic peritoneal lavage are all unreliable. Diagnostic laparoscopy has recently been shown to be accurate and reliable in stable patients, where there is no clear indication for laparotomy.

At laparotomy for trauma a diaphragmatic injury should always be sought by careful examination. A tear may not be obvious particularly as herniation through a defect may be prevented by positive pressure ventilation. Repair should be undertaken at operation. A carefully sited nasogastric tube and titrated opiate analgesia are of great benefit pre-operatively.

Liver

The liver is situated in the right upper quadrant of the abdomen and is almost entirely covered by the abdominal rib cage. It is mostly intraperitoneal, very vascular and is connected to the inferior vena cava by large hepatic veins. Liver injury may be associated with biliary tree damage and/or massive bleeding.

After the spleen, the liver is the second commonest abdominal organ damaged in blunt or penetrating trauma. Bleeding may remain undetected and is an important cause of preventable death. Systems exist to grade liver injury to help decide the most appropriate management. They depend on the size of haematomata and the degree of parenchymal disruption.

The presence of hypovolaemic shock, in the absence of an alternative source, should be assumed to be due to hepatic or splenic injury

Liver injury may only be diagnosed at laparotomy for nonspecific signs of intra-abdominal bleeding or peritonitis. It is, however, important to recognize that some severe disruptive injuries are best managed conservatively as surgery may lead to sudden overwhelming haemorrhage. Liver damage may be reparable in some cases although in severe cases the liver may need to be packed and arrangements made for transfer to a specialist centre, with the packs in situ.

Haemodynamically normal and stable patients may be investigated by bedside ultrasonography or CT scanning. The latter has the advantage of accurate delineation of the extent of liver damage, which is vital for nonoperative management.

Gall bladder and biliary tract

These organs are located under the right lobe of liver and so are commonly damaged in association with the liver (50%) and sometimes the pancreas (17%). Clinical features depend on the presence of blood or bile in the peritoneum. Endoscopic retrograde cholangiopancreatography (ERCP) may be necessary to evaluate damage, where there is no clear indication for laparotomy. The patient must be haemodynamically normal and stable to tolerate the transfer and procedure. Surgical treatment of extrahepatic biliary damage can involve cholecystectomy and biliary drainage, diversion or reconstruction.

Spleen

The spleen lies under the seventh to eleventh ribs in the left upper quadrant of the abdomen. It is a very vascular organ and forms part of the reticulo-endothelial system. Patients who have had their spleen removed are prone to particular infections such as those caused by pneumococci. This is especially so in children.

Failure to diagnose and promptly treat splenic injury is a significant cause of preventable death following trauma, as massive bleeding can occur

As with the liver, splenic injury may only be diagnosed at laparotomy done for signs of intra-abdominal bleeding following trauma. Where there is no immediate indication for laparotomy there are few specific clinical signs to help. The early signs of intraperitoneal bleeding may be subtle and hidden by painful distracting injuries such as rib fractures. Left upper quadrant pain, left lower rib fractures or changes to the contour of the left hemidiaphragm on plain radiography are suggestive but nonspecific features. Ultrasonography or CT scanning may show the injury and can help to determine whether nonoperative intervention is appropriate. Diagnostic laparoscopy may be useful in assessing a stable patient with penetrating abdominal trauma.

Where splenic injury is found in a haemodynamically normal and stable patient careful investigation and observation may suggest that a conservative approach is appropriate. Preservation of the spleen to reduce the long-term risks of sepsis is the aim. Grading scales exist to aid this decision-making. Patients treated conservatively must be very carefully observed.

When an injured spleen is found at laparotomy it can be removed or, in some cases, carefully preserved. Where the latter approach is used, very careful observation should be instituted to detect any signs of complication arising in the spleen.

Stomach

The stomach is a flat hollow viscus in the epigastrium and left upper quadrant, which is rarely injured as a result of blunt trauma. The clinical features are usually, therefore, of a penetrating injury with peritonitis, due to leakage of gastric contents into the peritoneal cavity. Blood in the gastric aspirate or free gas on chest radiography may help to confirm the diagnosis. CT scan is insensitive. Any patient with peritonitis following trauma should undergo surgical exploration. Diagnosis may only be established at such an operation. Surgical repair of the stomach is the rule.

Small intestine and colon

The small intestines (jejunum and ileum) are entirely within the peritoneal cavity. Injuries to them are similar to those of the intraperitoneal colon (e.g. the transverse and sigmoid colon) and may result from blunt or penetrating trauma.

Rapid deceleration injuries while wearing restraints (e.g. seatbelt) may cause compression for bowel loops and consequent rupture, by a closed loop mechanism. Tears may occur to the bowel itself or to its mesentery. The latter can cause intestinal ischaemia and is a cause of late rupture. Occasionally mesenteric tears are associated with massive bleeding. The flexion/distraction nature of this mechanism of injury means that there is an association with transverse vertebral body fractures in the thoracolumbar spine (Chance fractures).

Intestinal perforation from either penetrating or blunt injury leads to peritonitis from leakage of intestinal content. As outlined above, such peritonitis may be easy to miss in the early stages. CT scanning even with oral contrast may not be reliable in the early stages. The treatment of intestinal injury is surgical repair at exploratory laparotomy under prophylactic antibiotic cover.

Retroperitoneum

Injury to structures in the retroperitoneum may be difficult to detect. Unless there is communication with the peritoneal cavity there are no signs of peritoneal irritation and diagnostic peritoneal lavage is negative. Haematomata will often become contained with arrest of bleeding, due to a combination of hypotension and local tamponade. Injuries may be easier to detect if there is rupture into the peritoneal cavity.

The retroperitoneum is continuous with the extraperitoneal part of the pelvis, containing the rectum, bladder and pelvic vessels (see Box 5.1).

Pancreas

The pancreas lies horizontally across the body of the first lumbar vertebra, with its tail in contact with the splenic hilum. It may be injured by either penetrating or blunt trauma. In 60% of cases, injury results from a high-speed impact against the steering

BOX 5.1 Contents of retroperitoneum/extraperitoneal pelvis

- Pancreas
- Duodenum
- Colon – ascending and descending
- Aorta/pelvic arteries
- Inferior vena cava/pelvic veins
- Kidneys, ureter and bladder
- Rectum

wheel. The consequences of injury include acute pancreatitis and leakage of pancreatic exocrine enzymes into the peritoneal cavity.

The most common symptom is abdominal pain, which may be unexpectedly severe. If there is a clear indication for laparotomy the pancreas must always be carefully examined at the time. If there is no clear indication for laparotomy diagnosis of pancreatic injury may be very difficult. The clinical signs are often nonspecific and serum amylase may be normal in the early stages. Similarly CT with dual contrast (intravenous and oral) has a high false-negative rate, despite being the imaging modality of choice. Sequential measurement of serum amylase and CT scanning may be helpful. If there is any suspicion of pancreatic duct injury endoscopic retrograde cholangiopancreatography (ERCP) should be considered.

The patient's condition and the extent of damage will determine whether conservative or operative intervention is appropriate. Operative treatment may involve drainage, repair or excision of the pancreas.

Duodenum

The first part of duodenum lies in continuity with the stomach in the peritoneal cavity and the remaining three parts are in the retroperitoneum. Penetrating trauma causes about three-quarters of duodenal injuries. Impact from a steering wheel or bicycle handle bar is the commonest form of blunt injury. The diagnosis may be difficult and is helped by free air under diaphragm or blood in the gastric tube. A double contrast CT (oral and intravenous) is usually confirmatory.

As with many injuries within the abdomen, confirmation may only be possible at laparotomy carried out for nonspecific reasons. The duodenum should be carefully inspected in all cases and surgical repair undertaken.

Colon and rectum

Injuries to the intraperitoneal segments of the colon are considered above. Injuries of the retroperitoneal colon and the rectum usually result from penetrating trauma. Unless there is faecal contamination of the peritoneal cavity and consequent peritonitis, the diagnosis may be very difficult. The diagnosis may, thus, be made late as a result of abscess development.

If suspected, a soluble contrast enema or CT with triple contrast (oral, rectal and intravenous) may help. Surgical repair of the colonic injury is the rule. Such repair often necessitates the formation of a temporary colostomy/ileostomy, proximal to the injury.

Aorta and vena cava

These vessels lie on the vertebral column as they pass through the abdomen. They are entirely retroperitoneal and are continuous with the pelvic vessels in the extraperitoneal parts of the pelvis. Major injury to these vessels occurs in about 10% of blunt trauma to the abdomen and 25% of gunshot wounds.

Injuries may present with bleeding or secondary thrombosis. Bleeding can present late as arterial false aneurysms. Injuries from the vena cava or aorta are very dangerous although caval bleeding may be less profuse.

The presenting symptoms or signs are those of abdominal pain, shock from bleeding or ischaemia of the lower limbs or kidneys. Signs of retroperitoneal haemorrhage may be present although this may not be so early on. Such signs include flank bruising (Grey Turner sign).

The diagnosis may only be established at operation. Pre-operatively either portable ultrasonography or contrast CT scanning can aid diagnosis. Contrast CT is preferable to intravenous urography for assessment of renal involvement but great care must be exercised in such patients to ensure that transfer only takes place when the patient is haemodynamically normal and stable. Many patients are best managed by immediate transfer to the operating theatre for direct repair.

Kidneys

The kidneys lie on the posterior abdominal wall at the level of twelfth thoracic and upper three lumbar vertebrae. They are surrounded by renal fascia and are well protected by muscle and bone behind and the peritoneal cavity in front. Blunt injuries are commoner and are often associated with injuries to adjacent organs – in particular the spleen and liver. Isolated renal damage may result from penetrating injury to the flank.

Haematuria is the most consistent feature of renal trauma, but its degree may not correlate well with the severity of injury. Although a perinephric haematoma is common, haemorrhage is rarely life threatening, except where a renal pedicle has been avulsed.

In a stable haemodynamically normal patient, contrast CT is 98% accurate for detailed imaging of renal trauma, including vascular and parenchymal injury. An (intravenous pressure) IVP is a suitable but less comprehensive alternative. Perinephric haematoma may also be visualized by ultrasonography.

Most renal trauma is managed conservatively, even in the presence of gross haematuria. Surgical repair is reserved for persistent haemorrhage, urinary extravasation or vascular pedicle injury.

Ureters

The ureters lie behind the peritoneum on the psoas major muscle as they run along the transverse process of the vertebrae.

Unlike the kidneys, ureteric damage from blunt or penetrating trauma is uncommon. Surgical repair or reconstruction is the rule for damaged ureters. As with injuries to the retroperitoneal colon late diagnosis may occur due to secondary abscess formation.

Bladder

The urinary bladder is a pelvic organ that may stretch to the umbilicus when full. It lies in the extraperitoneal part of the pelvis but indents the peritoneal cavity as it distends. Rupture may occur into the peritoneum or outside it. Compression injuries will often lead to intraperitoneal rupture and, thus, the clinical features of peritonitis. Blunt trauma may lead to a penetrating injury as a result of perforation by fragments of fractured pelvic bones. This accounts for 80% of bladder injuries. This sort of injury usually results in extraperitoneal extravasation of urine, which is difficult to diagnose. Secondary pelvic sepsis may allow late diagnosis of these injuries when they are missed.

Bladder rupture is suspected in all cases of gross haematuria and pelvic fracture. Urinary extravasation may be palpable as a boggy perineal swelling. A retrograde cystogram is more accurate than excretory urography or diagnostic peritoneal lavage (see below) for the detection of bladder injury.

Indwelling catheter drainage may suffice for most bladder ruptures, with surgical repair reserved for extensive lacerations. Most intraperitoneal ruptures require laparotomy for peritonitis and surgical repair.

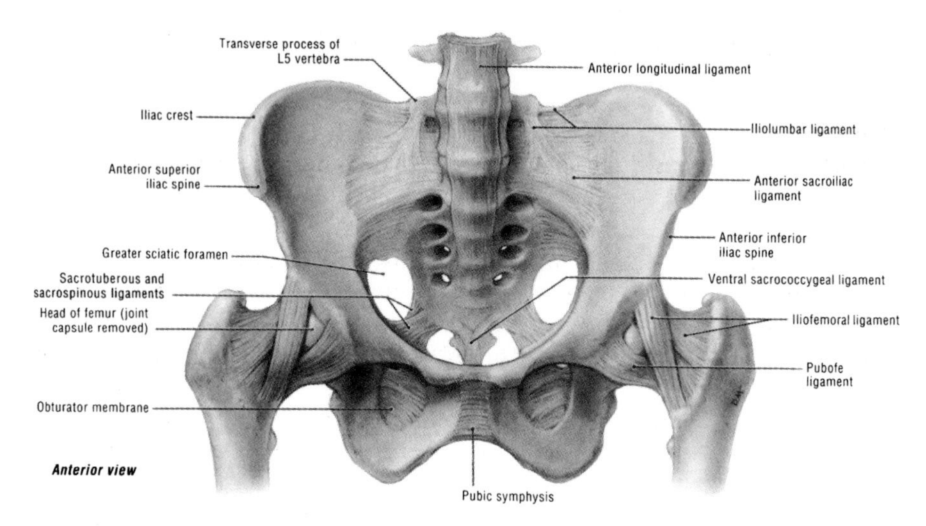

Figure 5.3 Structure of the pelvis. *Grant's Atlas of Anatomy* (1991) 9th edn. Agur AMR and Lee MJ (eds). Reproduced with permission from Lippincott, Williams & Wilkins.

Urethra

The short female urethra is rarely injured. In contrast, the male urethra may be injured above or below the urogenital diaphragm. Above the urogenital diaphragm extravasation occurs into the extraperitoneal pelvis. Injuries below lead to urine collecting in the scrotum and lower abdomen (*Figure 5.3*).

Urethral injury occurs in 10% of pelvic fractures and therefore is often associated with injuries to other body regions. Isolated injury can occur as a result of blunt trauma to perineum, for instance a fall astride a hard object.

The diagnosis is suspected from a suggestive history, inability to pass urine, blood at the urethral meatus and a high prostate on rectal examination. The site of rupture may be identified by leakage of contrast in ascending urethrography. Urinary leakage leads to local sepsis either in the pelvis or superficial tissues.

If suspected, no attempt should be made to pass a urinary catheter until urological advice is sought. Suprapubic urinary drainage is often adequate for healing. Major disruptions require surgical repair.

Pelvis

Most injuries to the pelvic contents have been covered in the previous sections. Injuries to the uterus and ovaries are very unusual and are not covered further.

The bony pelvis is composed of three strong bones – the two innominate bones connected to each other anteriorly and to the sacrum posteriorly (*Figure 5.3*). Very strong ligaments over the sacro-iliac joints contribute significantly to the stability of the pelvis. For the joints to be disrupted these strong ligaments must be torn. With separation of the bones pelvic vessels are torn and may bleed profusely. The bleeding is largely venous, extraperitoneal and often life threatening. The reported mortality of such open pelvic fractures is around 40–50%.

Other structures may also be injured, in particular the sciatic nerve in 30% of lateral sacral fractures and the urethra and bladder in a high proportion of pubic fractures or pubic symphysis separation (diastasis).

Control of haemorrhage and restoration of circulating blood volume are the urgent immediate goals of management.

Pelvic fractures

Most pelvic fractures arise from compression and may, thus, be classified as AP or lateral compression injuries. Three subtypes of each of these are described, depending on disruption at the pubic symphysis and/or sacro-iliac joints. By opening the pelvis and therefore increasing its volume, the AP compression injuries are associated with more significant haemorrhage with about 20% requiring over 15 units of blood transfusion.

Clinical assessment of pelvic injury is unreliable even in the conscious patient. Stress testing for pelvic stability ('springing of pelvis') is best avoided as it may exacerbate soft tissue injury within the pelvis and increase bleeding. Pelvic injury should be suspected in multiply injured patients and injuries involving high velocity. Plain AP pelvic radiography should be undertaken in the resuscitation room early in the management of such patients.

Control of haemorrhage is achieved by reducing pelvic volume and restoring stability. Simple measures such as tying strong sheets across the pelvis may suffice initially. Application of an external fixator may be needed early. If these measures fail angiography and selective embolization may be needed. This is needed in about 20% of cases and is successful in 90% of cases where the source can be identified.

5.3 Mechanism of injury

Knowledge of the mechanism of injury is important in the management of multiply injured patients. The distribution of potential injuries can be predicted and therefore anticipated – this may be of vital importance to avoid missing fatal injuries. In the early assessment of patients as much information as possible about the mechanism of injury must be collected from those who first attended the scene.

The broad types of mechanisms of injury are *blunt* and *penetrating*. This may not cover all injuries but is very useful in predicting the injury pattern, particularly with abdominal injuries where clinical features are so unreliable. Knowledge of the mechanism of injury may suggest that a particular organ may be injured. With some organs the nature of the injury is the same whatever the mechanism, for instance the spleen. In other organs the mechanism of injury may allow prediction of the type of injury. The diaphragm may have an enormous defect as a result of blunt trauma whereas a penetrating injury may cause a very small tear.

Finally, it should be appreciated that one mechanism of injury may lead to another. For instance, blunt trauma to the bony pelvis may lead to penetrating trauma of the bladder from the fractured bone.

5.3.1 Blunt abdominal trauma (BAT)

This is the commonest (98%) mechanism of abdominal injury in the UK. It usually arises from Road Traffic Accidents (RTA) or falls. Abdominal damage results from deceleration or compression forces on solid organs and shear effects or closed-loop phenomenon on mesentery and bowel. The application of blunt force to the abdomen is usually over a wide area, with the exception of localized blows to the renal angle (assault) or anterior abdomen (for example bicycle handlebars).

Injuries to the chest and pelvis should suggest that a significant abdominal injury is highly likely, given that much of the contents of the abdomen are within either the bony chest or pelvis. Equally, wherever there is evidence of hypovolaemia or its consequences, abdominal injuries should be suspected and sought.

In cases of blunt injury to the trunk, if the chest and pelvis are injured, the abdomen must be considered injured, unless proven otherwise

The spleen, liver and kidneys are the commonest solid organs injured by blunt trauma. The hollow viscera may rupture due to the closed loop phenomenon – in particular the small intestine and bladder. The mesentery may be torn by shear forces in falls, leading to bowel ischaemia.

There may be minimal evidence of injury over the exterior of abdomen in blunt trauma. The diagnosis of visceral damage is notoriously difficult, as clinical assessment of abdomen is extremely unreliable. Painful distracting injuries and an altered mental state compound these difficulties. If the conventional clinical signs of peritonitis – tenderness, guarding, absent bowel sounds – are present laparotomy is indicated. Often they are not and the use of special investigations is necessary where injury is suspected but there is no clear indication for laparotomy.

Blunt injury to the pelvis causes haemorrhage with associated skeletal and visceral damage. Plain radiography of the pelvis in the resuscitation room is necessary in all multiply injured patients. Pelvic fractures confirm severe forces and necessitate a search for other major injuries and for aggressive resuscitative measures.

5.3.2 Penetrating abdominal trauma (PAT)

Penetrating trauma accounts for a high proportion of abdominal trauma in the USA and other countries such as South Africa. In the UK such injuries are much less common.

Injuries can result from low velocity objects, such as a knife, or high velocity objects, most commonly gunshot. The pattern of injury resulting from knife-like injuries may be fairly predictable given the entry site. The injury will, of course, not respect anatomical boundaries. Gunshot injury may result in a path of traverse that is neither straight nor short. Abdominal injuries may thus arise from remote entry points. Furthermore, damage in these injuries may be more extensive due to the cavitation effect of high velocity missiles. This results from the pressure wave that spreads radially from the missile trajectory. The cavity is larger than the bullet and contaminated by debris sucked in the path, both of which require extensive debridement.

The pattern of injury arising from stab wounds to the abdomen may, to some extent, be predicted from the entry site. The abdomen is divided into anterior, posterior, flank and lower chest areas to allow for this. The anterior area is bordered by the anterior axillary lines laterally and the nipple line above. The posterior area is bordered by the posterior axillary lines laterally and the tips of the scapulae above. The flanks are the areas between these. The lower chest area is a special area overlapping with these areas, lying between the nipple line and the costal margin.

Stabs wounds in the anterior and flank areas are more likely to penetrate the peritoneum. Local exploration of such wounds, by a surgeon, may clearly demonstrate no such penetration. If there is doubt diagnostic peritoneal lavage or double contrast CT may help. Laparoscopy and ultrasound have limited benefits for assessment of these patients. If all such wounds are explored by laparotomy up to half will not show any significant injury. Stab wounds to the lower chest area, nipple line to costal margin, may damage thoracic and/or abdominal structures.

The incidence of serious internal damage is much higher for gunshot wounds to the abdomen. The presence of hypotension or signs of peritonism should mandate laparotomy. As outlined above, the pattern of such injuries is unpredictable and usually extensive. A low threshold for laparotomy is appropriate. Diagnostic peritoneal lavage and laparoscopy are not reliable in such injuries.

5.4 Assessment and management

The initial assessment and management of all trauma patients should follow the protocol of primary survey, resuscitation, secondary survey and definitive care for reasons explained elsewhere. It is helpful for the trauma team leader to have a clear idea of the mechanism of injury and the pre-hospital status of the patient early on.

5.4.1 Primary survey

The purpose of the primary survey is to identify and treat life-threatening injuries rapidly (see Section 1.6.1). The threat from abdominal trauma is haemorrhagic shock related to occult blood loss. After treating airway and breathing, the abdomen, along with chest, pelvis and long bones, are the four areas to be assessed for source of haemorrhage. In addition shock may be due to peritonitis from perforation of hollow viscera.

The questions to ask in cases of abdominal trauma are:

- is the abdomen the source of the patient's shock?
- is a surgeon needed to control bleeding or peritonitis?

Shock should be assessed and treated according to the priorities described in Section 4.6. The key elements are control of haemorrhage and restoration of circulating blood volume.

Identifying the abdomen as the source of shock may be difficult. If the patient fails to respond to the initial fluid resuscitation and an abdominal source of shock is suspected immediate laparotomy should be the rule. It is crucial to understand that resuscitation may include laparotomy and that correction of hypovolaemia may not be possible before surgical control of bleeding. This control may include the application of an external fixator to stabilize pelvic fractures.

If the patient is haemodynamically normal and stable, the primary survey is completed and the abdomen re-evaluated as part of secondary survey. Continual re-evaluation is very important.

5.4.2 Secondary survey

A head-to-toe examination looking to identify potentially life-threatening injuries is now performed as described in Section 1.6.2. The abdomen is assessed for possible internal damage using the system of LOOK – LISTEN – FEEL.

Look

The patient must be completely exposed and the abdominal surface inspected for wounds, bruising and imprints from contact – for example, tyre marks. This must include the back and the perineum during an early log roll of the patient. Care must be taken to prevent hypothermia.

Listen

Auscultation of the abdomen to detect bowel sounds adds very little to the assessment, and may be very difficult in the resuscitation room.

Feel

The abdomen should be gently palpated to assess distension, tenderness and guarding. All these signs may be subtle or totally absent in the early stages. Percussion may elicit rebound tenderness more reliably than direct palpation. Remember: injuries to the chest or the pelvis can produce abdominal signs.

Rectal or vaginal examination should be performed to detect the presence of blood and bony fragments, assess the prostate and anal sphincter tone. This can be done supine or during the log roll. Rectal examination is mandatory before urinary catheterization.

As explained above, the practice of 'springing' the pelvis to elicit instability is best avoided. On suspicion of a pelvic injury, a plain x-ray is the quickest and safest way to establish the diagnosis.

Clinical assessment of abdomen by itself is unreliable. Abdominal visceral injury cannot be ruled out by a normal examination.

A nasogastric tube helps decompress the stomach and may identify upper gastrointestinal tract injury by revealing blood in the aspirate. The route should be orogastric if a frontal base of skull fracture is suspected, to avoid passing the tube through fractures.

Similarly, a urethral catheter should be passed to measure urine output, decompress bladder and also detect haematuria. Urethral injury should be ruled out before catheterization.

Repeated clinical assessment and special investigations should be the rule in the assessment of abdominal trauma, unless there is a clear indication for early laparotomy

Finally, the patient's medical history should be ascertained using the mnemonic AMPLE:

A = allergy
M = medication
P = past history
L = last meal
E = environment or event details

5.4.3 Nursing role

The nurse in the trauma team plays an important role in comprehensive assessment of the abdomen both during primary and secondary survey. The number of nurses involved in the care of a single patient would depend on the severity of trauma.

The "nurse" initial assessment and subsequent close observation provides the trauma team with vital clues in the management of abdominal trauma

As a first hospital responder the trauma nurse often activates the trauma team and prepares the resuscitation room (lights, heaters, blankets) and the necessary equipment, e.g. monitors, blood bottles, forms. The nursing team leader may be the first person to receive details of the history and mechanism of injury, either from the paramedics or the patient, that are important for accurate triage using the Manchester system. With this information, it is then often possible to anticipate the need and prepare for steps like urinary catheterization, DPL, etc. This early contact should also be used to establish rapport with the patient.

Much of the diagnosis of abdominal trauma depends on establishing accurate vital signs and the circulation nurse needs to record these regularly on a chart and make the team members aware of the trend. During the early phase of primary survey, the nurse will also help to undress the patient and notice any external signs and wounds. This initial 'nursing' assessment is vital in gaining the patient's confidence and preserving dignity as much as practicable.

The relatives nurse is the mainstay of communication between the team members and the patient as well as the family. This is particularly important for assessment of subtle abdominal trauma as well as coordination of multidisciplinary care. Patient advocacy is a crucial role for the nurse. In abdominal trauma, this has an immediate impact on good quality care in the form of timely analgesia, informed consent for procedures and moral support in the stressful resuscitation room.

Analgesia

It is both humane and physiologically appropriate to give a conscious patient effective analgesia prior to secondary survey. This does not compromise abdominal assessment and may help to reveal clinical signs. A simple and effective method of initially providing analgesia for the patient with abdominal trauma is to give morphine titrated in small aliquots by the intravenous route. More complex techniques are discussed in Chapter 16.

5.4.4 Investigations

This section outlines the commonly available modalities that are used in the assessment of patients with abdominal trauma. Although other specialized investigations are available, local expertise and protocols must guide their use.

Blood tests

Any sample of blood taken during primary survey should be sent for a baseline full blood count, biochemistry including amylase and cross-matching. Pregnancy testing should be undertaken in all female patients of childbearing age.

Plain radiography

Early in the primary survey x-rays of the chest and pelvis are requested. They are performed in the resuscitation room.

The chest film may reveal rib fractures or evidence of diaphragmatic injury (see above). The presence of gas under the diaphragms may not be visible on supine films.

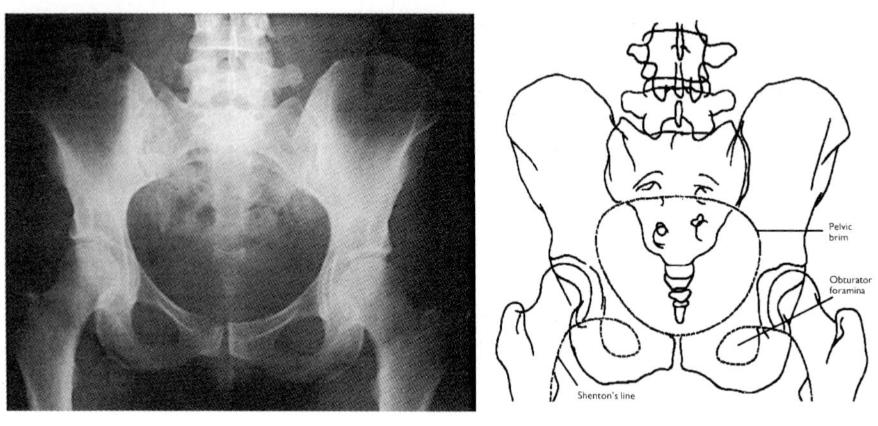

Figure 5.4 Pelvic radiograph using the 'ABCS' method. *ABC of Emergency Radiology* (1995). Nicholson DA and Driscoll PA (eds). Reproduced with permission from BMJ Publishing Group.

A plain film of abdomen is rarely useful, except to show the position of a residual bullet. Much more useful in abdominal trauma is a pelvic film. Interpretation must be undertaken in a systematic fashion to avoid missing important findings. Using a simple 'ABCS' system can allow the correct diagnosis to be made in up to 94% of cases (*Figure 5.4*).

A = accuracy, adequacy and alignment

Ensure it is the correct x-ray for the patient! An adequate pelvic x-ray should include the whole pelvis and the proximal third of femurs. The alignment of three rings is checked. The sacrum and the pelvic brim form the large one. The two small ones are the obturator foramina. If one of these circles is broken, a search should be made for fractures or joint separation.

The last check of alignment is made using a smooth curved line continuous with the obturator foramen and the inner surface of the neck of femur.

B = bones

All the bones should be traced along the cortical margin to detect a fracture, which may show up as a lucency, density or trabecular disruption.

C = cartilage

The sacroiliac joints and the symphysis pubis should be checked for widening. The acetabular margin may also reveal fractures.

S = soft tissue

A pelvic wall haematoma may be detected by bladder displacement.

Focused abdominal sonography for trauma examination (FAST)

The availability of good quality ultrasonography in the resuscitation room has led to a great increase in its use in abdominal trauma. In many centres members of the trauma team are doing this. The FAST protocol is a way of conducting such an examination, which concentrates on finding fluid within the abdomen. This examination is rapid and can detect as little as 200 ml of fluid in the subphrenic spaces, the subhepatic space, the pelvis and the pericardium. This may be repeated at frequent intervals if this is appropriate.

The FAST examination can achieve almost 90% sensitivity but is operator dependent and has low specificity, in terms of determining the source of the fluid. It has largely replaced diagnostic peritoneal lavage in many centres. Many injuries may be missed however, especially solid organ damage and retroperitoneal injuries.

Ultrasonography should never delay transfer to the operating theatre where there are clear indications for laparotomy.

Computed tomography (CT)

With modern CT scanners high-resolution images can be produced rapidly. The use of intravenous, oral or rectal contrast enhances the images. CT allows imaging of both the viscera and musculoskeletal structures, making it ideal for abdominal trauma. It has superseded many other investigations, for instance, intravenous urography for renal trauma. It has high sensitivity and specificity.

The main disadvantage of CT is the danger it poses for critically ill patients. To be safe in the CT room patients must have responded well to resuscitation and be stable. They must be accompanied by suitably trained and equipped staff. It is not reliable for injuries to the diaphragm, bowel or pancreas.

Diagnostic peritoneal lavage (DPL)

This is a highly accurate bedside test for the presence of abnormal fluid within the peritoneum – blood, bowel content or urine. It is a highly sensitive but has low specificity.

The indications for DPL are:

- suspected haemoperitoneum in a hypotensive patient;
- diagnosis of blood or hollow viscus content, where clinical assessment is unreliable (such as pelvic injury) or impossible (such as in the unconscious);
- diagnosis of haemoperitoneum in patients who are unsuitable for CT or ultrasonography.

DPL is contraindicated by a clear clinical indication for laparotomy. Previous scars, obesity, coagulopathy and pregnancy are relative contra-indications. DPL will, of course, not give any indication of injuries in the retroperitoneum, unless there is peritoneal involvement.

While the complication rate of DPL is low (1%) it is clearly invasive and must be performed by a surgeon. It cannot be repeated as part of the constant re-evaluation of the patient. It is, however, more accurate in the diagnosis of hollow visceral injury and mesenteric tears, than CT scanning. Ultrasonography and CT scanning have largely superseded DPL.

Technique of DPL

DPL is an invasive procedure that can be done closed, open or semi-open. The open method is preferred. The steps of the open method are:

(i) explain the procedure to the patient if they are conscious;

(ii) decompress the bladder and stomach by urinary catheterization and naso/orogastric tube;

(iii) Infiltrate 1% lidocaine with adrenaline (to reduce bleeding) over the midline on the middle third of the line between the umbilicus and symphysis pubis. A supra-umbilical approach is indicated where there are pelvic fractures or pregnancy;

(iv) incise vertically down to linea alba;

(v) pick up successive layers between two haemostats and incise under direct vision till the peritoneum is entered;

(vi) insert a peritoneal dialysis cannula, without the trochar, towards the most dependent point of pelvic cavity and attempt aspiration;

(vii) if nothing is aspirated, instil 1 l of warm crystalloid solution and allow the same to equilibrate;

(viii) siphon the fluid off into the bag and test contents.

DPL is considered positive if:

(i) 10 ml of frank blood, bowel content or urine is aspirated;

(ii) the red cell count in the lavage fluid is over 100 000/mm^3;

(iii) the white cell count in the lavage fluid is over 500/mm^3.

Diagnostic laparoscopy

There has been a recent increase in the use of video-laparoscopy for the assessment of abdominal trauma. Its diagnostic value is limited due to a high rate of missed injuries. It may be suitable for the confirmation of peritoneal breach in stab wounds and assessment of injuries to the diaphragm. With refinement of technique, it may help reduce the negative laparotomy rate.

Local wound exploration

A stab wound may be explored locally to determine whether there is a peritoneal breach. Penetration of the transversalis fascia or inability to find the end of the tract constitutes a positive exploration and mandates laparotomy or further diagnostic evaluation. Stab wounds in the posterior abdomen are more difficult to explore due to the thickness of the muscles.

5.4.5 Definitive care

This will be based upon the response of the patient to the treatment administered, the results of all the investigations and the extent of all the abdominal injuries identified. The trauma team leader is responsible for coordination of this process.

The disposal of the patient will depend upon the existence of associated pelvic and visceral trauma. Unstable patients with haemoperitoneum require an urgent laparotomy and surgical haemostasis. Orthopaedic surgeons may be needed to control bleeding from pelvic fractures.

Some patients with solid organ damage from blunt trauma may be managed without operation. This is only possible if close monitoring by a surgeon and serial CT/ultrasonography are available.

Penetrating abdominal trauma is mostly treated by exploratory laparotomy. In some cases of low velocity stab or gunshot wound, selective nonoperative policy may be safe.

Pelvic disruption adds to the therapeutic difficulties. External fixator or selective embolization may achieve pelvic haemostasis. The need for a laparotomy for surgical haemostasis of the abdomen has to be carefully judged.

Effective analgesia continues to be vital as the patient transfers to definitive care.

BOX 5.2 Management of injury to abdominal organs

Organ	*Haemodynamically unstable*	*Haemodynamically stable*
Diaphragm	Surgical repair	Surgical repair
Liver	Laparotomy repair/resection/ packing/conservative management	Nonoperative management/ repair
Spleen	Splenectomy or repair	Nonoperative management/ splenectomy/repair
Stomach	Repair	Repair
Duodenum and small intestine	Repair	Repair
Biliary tree	Repair and drainage	Repair and drainage
Pancreas	Debridement/excision/ drainage	Nonoperative management/ debridement/excision/ drainage
Large intestine	Repair/colostomy	Repair/colostomy
Bladder	Repair	Catheter decompression/repair
Kidney	Repair/partial excision/ nephrectomy	Nonoperative management/ drainage
Vascular injury	Repair	Repair

5.5 Summary

Injuries to the abdomen and the pelvis can vary immensely in magnitude. The presence of significant injury may not always be obvious on presentation. The clinical signs may add to the confusion. The trauma team leader must be suspicious of the existence of abdominal trauma in all patients of multiple injuries and must have a clear understanding of the mechanism of injury. It is best to assume that abdominal trauma exists unless proven otherwise.

The investigations available to establish a diagnosis all have their roles and must be used liberally according to the index of suspicion. Transfer of patients for such investigations must only be done with stable haemodynamically normal patients. Such heightened awareness and a policy of aggressive investigation will help reduce unexpected findings in the abdomen and the avoidable deaths that still occur due to abdominal trauma.

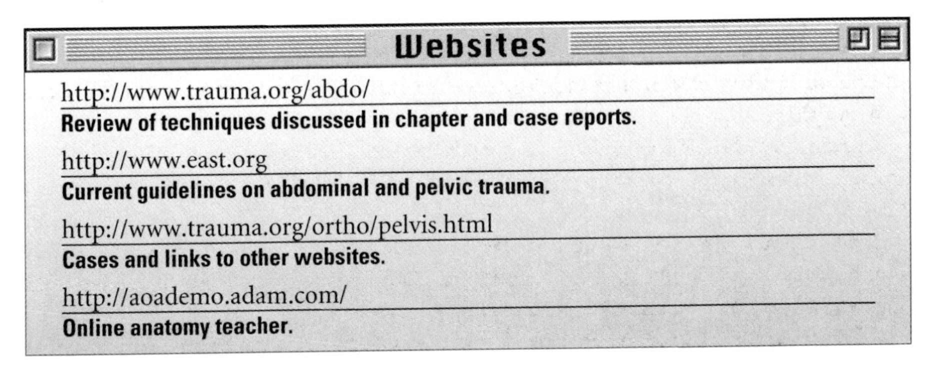

Websites

http://www.trauma.org/abdo/
Review of techniques discussed in chapter and case reports.

http://www.east.org
Current guidelines on abdominal and pelvic trauma.

http://www.trauma.org/ortho/pelvis.html
Cases and links to other websites.

http://aoademo.adam.com/
Online anatomy teacher.

Further reading

1. **American College of Surgeons Committee on Trauma** (1997) *Advanced Trauma Life Support for Physicians.* Chicago: American College of Surgeons.

6 Head trauma

D Bryden, C Gwinnutt

Objectives

In order to care for a patient with a head injury, members of the trauma team must be familiar with:

- normal anatomy and physiology;
- the anatomical and physiological changes that may occur following a head injury;
- the terms commonly used when describing the type of head injury sustained;
- how to assess the patient with a head injury;
- how safely to manage a patient with a head injury;
- when and how to communicate with a neurosurgeon;
- when to perform investigations or carry out specific treatments.

6.1 Introduction

Of all patients attending a UK ED, 11% will have sustained some form of head injury. Only 1% of patients with a head injury will be referred to a specialist neurosurgical unit, and so staff working within the ED must become familiar with managing all forms of head-injured patients, since they represent a large proportion of their workload.

As the majority of head injuries occur in younger male age groups, the economic and social consequences of delayed or inadequate treatment can be devastating. Alcohol is a contributory factor in 25% of cases of head injury.

6.2 Anatomy

A basic knowledge of neuroanatomy is important in understanding some of the clinical signs that may be seen after a head injury.

The scalp is made up of five distinct layers. The subcutaneous layer is very vascular and open scalp wounds that breach this layer can cause considerable blood loss unless the scalp injury is repaired. Scalp haematomas of a considerable size can also develop in the looser areolar layer.

The white and grey matter of the brain is contained within the rigid box-like skull and bathed in cerebrospinal fluid (CSF). The interior of the skull base has many bony projections. To prevent brain injury, two perpendicular folds of dura mater prevent excessive movement; the falx cerebri separates the two cerebral hemispheres and the tentorium cerebelli separates the cerebral hemispheres superiorly, from the cerebellum inferiorly. The dura mater is one of three layers of tissue covering the brain, the others being pia and arachnoid.

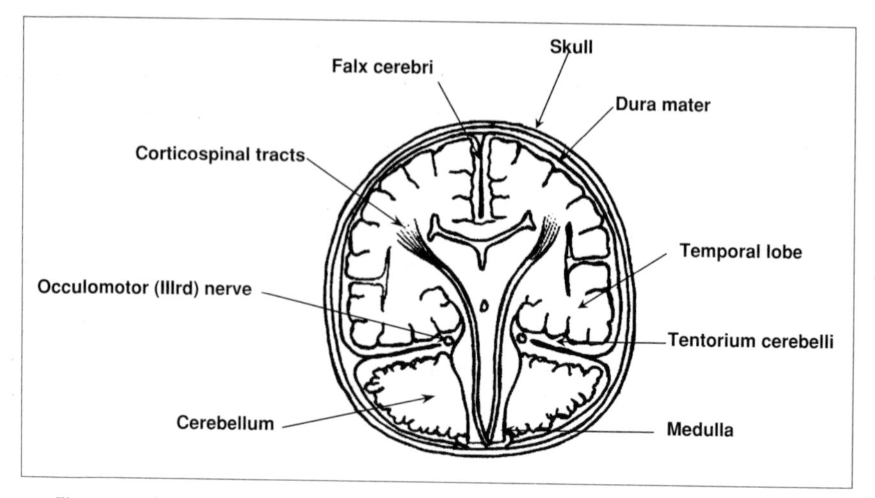

Figure 6.1 Coronal section of brain showing the folds of the dura mater and IIIrd nerve

Arteries run between the dural folds and the inner surface of the skull. The most important is the middle meningeal artery, which lies beneath the temporo-parietal area of the skull. Bridging veins also run in the subarachnoid space, which is a CSF-filled space between the pia mater covering the brain and the arachnoid mater. Bridging veins carry blood from the brain to the venous sinuses that run in the dura mater.

The midbrain consists of the pons and medulla and passes through an opening in the tentorium cerebelli and continues at the level of the foramen magnum with the spinal cord. The oculomotor (IIIrd) nerves leave the anterior aspect of the midbrain, run forward between the free and attached edges of the tentorium cerebelli and go on to supply many of the extrinsic muscles of the eye. They also contains pre-ganglionic parasympathetic fibres that cause constriction of the ipsilateral pupil (*Figure 6.1*).

The brain is not a solid structure but has spaces (ventricles) within it containing CSF. Two lateral ventricles, one in each cerebral hemisphere, are connected to the third ventricle at the junction of the midbrain and the cerebral hemispheres. The third ventricle is in turn connected to the fourth ventricle at the level of the medulla.

The CSF is secreted by the choroid plexus in the lateral ventricles of each hemisphere, and passes through foraminae or channels in the brain before draining into the subarachnoid space at the level of the midbrain. In the healthy person, CSF communicates freely within the skull before being absorbed by folds of arachnoid villi in the walls of the venous sinuses.

6.2.1 Anatomical changes following head injury

Primary brain injury

Damage that is sustained at the time of an accident as a result of either direct injury or inertial forces is termed primary brain injury. Either mechanism may result in many of the changes described below.

Direct injuries

These result from contact with a hard object. Contact at the point of impact may deform the skull producing a *linear fracture*, and considerable underlying brain injury. *Depressed fractures* occur when bone fragments enter the cranial cavity. *Compound fractures* occur when there is direct communication between an open scalp laceration and the meninges or brain substance. A *basal skull fracture* is a special form of compound fracture whose presence requires careful treatment (see later).

A *contusion* may develop in an area of brain lying under the impact point of a contact force. The bone is deformed inwards, and shock waves distribute out from the point of impact, producing haemorrhage, brain oedema and neuronal death. This may also occur when the brain contacts the inner aspect of the skull base. Patients usually lose consciousness at the scene of the accident, and focal signs have often developed by the time of arrival in the ED.

Inertial injuries

Inertial injuries can produce injuries that result in a significantly worse outcome than damage resulting from direct contact.

Diffuse axonal injury (DAI)

- Occurs after a rapid acceleration or deceleration of the head.
- Is associated with a high transfer of energy, e.g. shaking a child.
- Causes deformation of the white and grey matter of the brain.
- Leads to axonal damage, microscopic haemorrhages, tears in the brain tissue and the subsequent development of oedema.
- Severe DAI can cause immediate coma at the scene of the accident and has an overall mortality of 33–50%.

Concussion

- May occur after minor inertial forces to the head and is a less severe form of DAI.
- The patient is always amnesic of the injuring event.
- There may be amnesia for events before (antegrade amnesia) or afterwards (postgrade amnesia).
- Consciousness may have been lost for up to 5 min.
- There may be nausea, vomiting and headaches.
- The patient rarely has any localizing signs.
- Microscopic structural brain damage occurs, and so the effect of numerous episodes can be considerable.

Contra coup injuries

- These are brain injuries that occur away from the site of impact.
- The head undergoes an acceleration/deceleration force, the skull and brain move in the direction of the force producing injuries opposite the point of impact.
- Greater damage develops furthest from the impact point as the brain collides with the inner skull or skull base.

Haematomas

These can occur outside the dura (extradural) or beneath the dura (intradural).

Extradural haematoma (EDH) (*Figure 6.2*)

- Associated with a fractured skull in 90% of cases.
- Most often develops in the temporo-parietal area following a tear in the middle meningeal artery (rarely due to a tear in a venous sinus).
- As the commonest source is arterial, an EDH develops quickly (Box 6.1).
- The classical presentation of an EDH occurs in only one third of cases.
- The commonest clinical signs are a loss of consciousness and pupillary changes, although these can develop rapidly and late on.
- An EDH is a neurosurgical emergency, as early evacuation (within 2–4 h of clinical deterioration) will result in a better patient outcome by reduction of secondary injury.

BOX 6.1 The classic history of an extradural haematoma

- Transient loss of consciousness at the time of the injury from a momentary disruption of the reticular formation
- Patient then regains consciousness for several hours, the lucid period
- Localizing signs develop, with neurological deficits, headaches and eventually unconsciousness from the developing ECH, which causes the ICP to rise

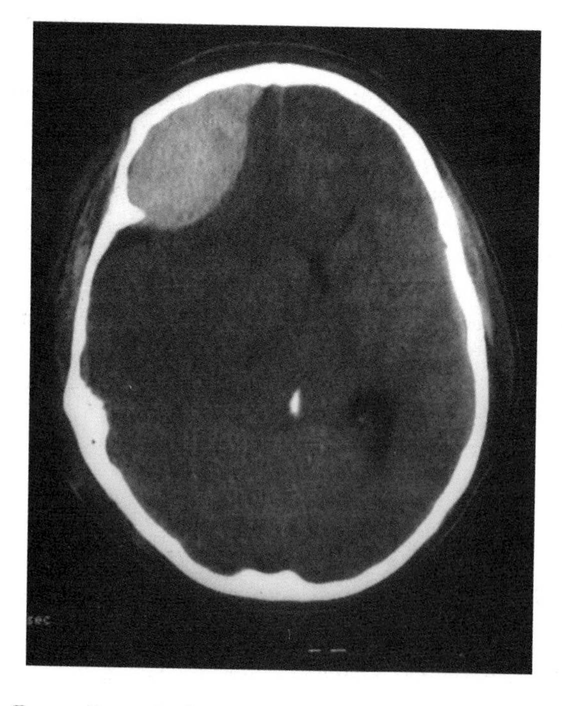

Figure 6.2 **CT scan of EDH**

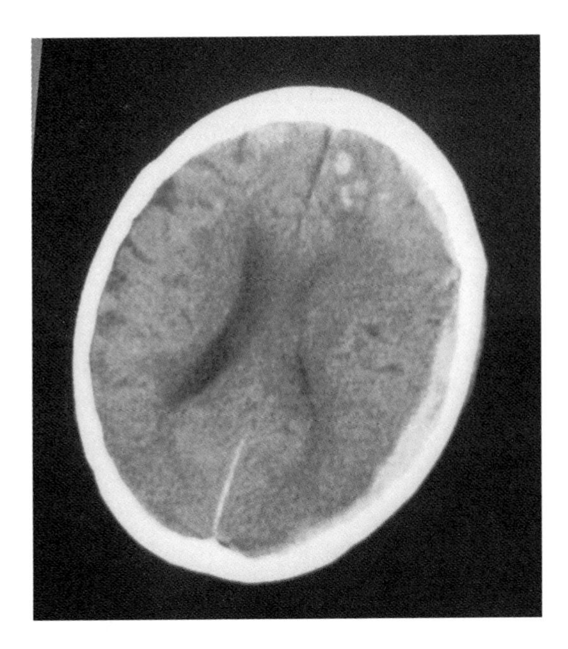

Figure 6.3 **CT scan of IDH (subdural)**

Acute intradural haematomas (IDH)

- Can be either subdural (SDH) or intracerebral (ICH).
- Both often coexist in the same patient.
- Are three to four times more common than extradural haematomas.
- Are produced by inertial or rotational forces, although considerably more force is needed to produce an ICH.

Subdural haematomas develop when the bridging veins are torn and blood collects in the subdural space, commonly over the temporal lobe (*Figure 6.3*). Clinical deterioration of the patient can be very slow (up to several days). This type of haematoma is more common where there is pre-existing cerebral atrophy, e.g. in alcoholics or the elderly, as the bridging veins are more likely to tear and a considerable blood collection can form in the space. Early evacuation within 4 h of deterioration reduces mortality and outcome so early neurosurgical referral is vital.

Intracranial haematomas are produced by much larger forces than SDH, and are rarely found in isolation. Cerebral contusions and lacerations are often present and, as a result, mortality is considerably higher than SDH. Patients frequently lose consciousness at the time of injury, or may quickly develop seizures or focal signs.

Subarachnoid haemorrhage

- May occur following head trauma.
- May be an incidental finding on CT scan following severe trauma.
- Patients may present with headaches, photophobia or other signs of meningism and with a history of head trauma.
- Treatment should be as for any other head injured patient.

Secondary brain injury

This is damage that occurs after the primary brain injury as a result of a number of factors (see Box 6.2). It is estimated that up to 30% of deaths after head injury are directly due to secondary injury, many of which are easily preventable or recognizable and treatable within the ED.

BOX 6.2 Factors important in generating secondary injury

- Delay in diagnosis
- Delay in definitive treatment
- Hypoxia ($pO_2 < 10$ kPa)
- Hypotension (systolic BP < 90 mmHg)
- Seizures
- Extremes of arterial pCO_2
- Raised ICP
- Suboptimal management of other injuries

6.3 Physiology

6.3.1 Intracranial pressure (ICP)

This is determined by the relationship between the skull, a rigid box of fixed volume and the volumes of the brain, CSF and blood. In health, small changes in the volume of CSF and blood occur in order to keep the intracranial pressure within the range of 5–13 mmHg. CSF can be displaced into the spinal CSF space or its absorption by the pia-arachnoid increased, and the volume of blood within the venous sinuses can change. The changes in blood and CSF volume are often referred to as indicative of the compliance, dV/dP (or more strictly elastance, dP/dV) of the intracranial contents. Transient rises in pressure may occur, e.g. due to changes in posture (bending over), sneezing or coughing, but these quickly return to baseline levels.

Once the capacity to make these changes has become exhausted, that is, no further CSF or blood can be displaced, or if the volume of one of the contents within the skull

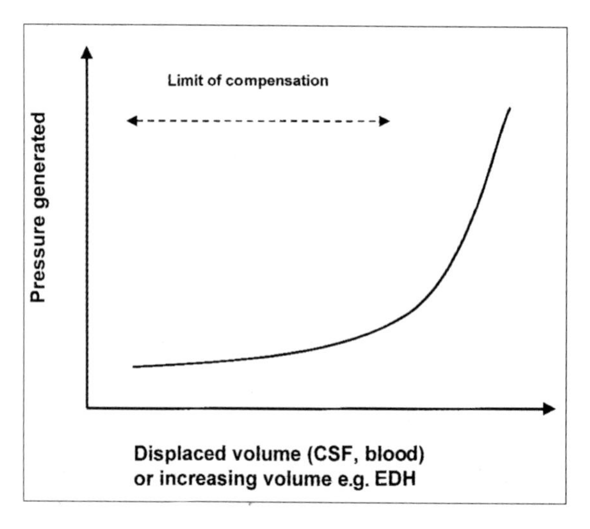

Figure 6.4 Diagram of dV/dP, Monro–Kellie principle

rises very rapidly, for example, an expanding intracranial haematoma, the compensatory mechanisms fail and intracranial pressure rises very rapidly. This is the Monro–Kellie principle (*Figure 6.4*). The rate of rise of ICP is a direct function of the rate of increase in one of the volumes within the skull.

6.3.2 Cerebral perfusion

Cerebral neurons require an almost continuous supply of oxygen and glucose. If blood flow is interrupted for as little as 4 min, neurons rapidly fail and die. Perfusion of the brain is dependent upon the pressure gradient across the vasculature and is termed the cerebral perfusion pressure (CPP). This is the difference between MAP and cerebal venous pressure (CVP). The latter is difficult to measure and in health approximates to the more easily measured ICP:

$$\text{CPP} = \text{MAP} - \text{ICP}$$

Cerebral perfusion pressure is reduced primarily by a reduction in MAP, an increase in ICP or both.

Cerebral venous pressure may also play a role in reducing CPP. When venous drainage of the brain is impaired, for example by a tight endotracheal tube tie or a patient coughing, venous pressure will be elevated above ICP and therefore reduce CPP.

Under normal circumstances, MAP and hence CPP varies, but blood flow to the brain must remain constant and this is achieved by a process termed autoregulation. The trigger to autoregulation is CPP; as CPP falls the cerebral arterioles dilate to maintain flow, as CPP rises they constrict to reduce flow, so that cerebral blood flow remains constant over a CPP range of 50–150 mmHg (*Figure 6.5*). As ICP rises, it becomes increasingly important to calculate CPP. An adequate CPP depends not only on a low ICP, but also on an adequate MAP. The threshold for developing cerebral ischaemia varies with the type of neuronal tissue, but *on average* occurs if the CPP falls to 50 mmHg or less *in a normal person.* Following a head injury the threshold for developing ischaemia is often much higher and occurs at CPPs of 60–70 mmHg.

This is due to a disruption of cerebral autoregulation in the early stages after a head injury. In the first few hours, cerebral blood flow falls although the metabolic requirements of the neurones are unchanged. Consequently, a higher cerebral perfusion

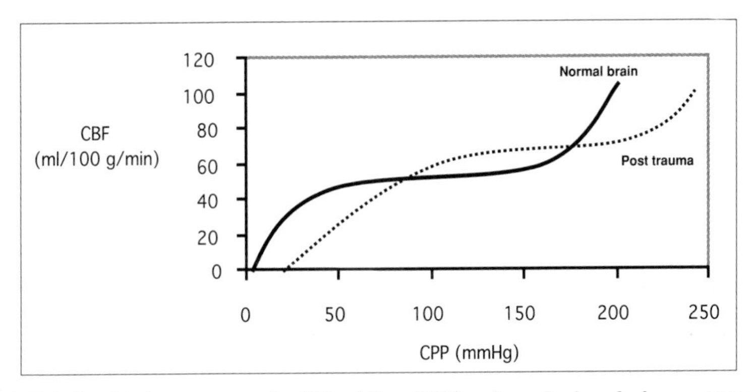

Figure 6.5 Relationship between cerebral blood flow (CBF) and cerebral perfusion pressure (CPP) in normal and traumatized brain

pressure is needed to maintain an adequate cerebral blood flow to prevent ischaemia and neuronal death.

6.3.3 Consciousness

This is determined by a number of cranial and extracranial factors. Damage to the reticular formation (a neuronal network in the midbrain and brain stem) or either of the cerebral cortices will result in a loss of consciousness. Hypercapnia from any cause will lead to drowsiness and unconsciousness, whilst hypoxia will initially result in restlessness and agitation, but if uncorrected will cause unconsciousness. Other factors which may impair a patient's level of consciousness are shown in Box 2.4.

6.4 Signs of a head injury

Signs of a head injury may be nonspecific and can develop in an atypical pattern. Practitioners must therefore always have a high degree of suspicion of injury based on the presenting history or information obtained.

Unconsciousness is an unreliable sign of the severity of injury, as it may be due to the primary injury or to treatable secondary factors such as hypoxia and hypotension. A patient with multiple injuries may possess false focal signs, e.g. pupillary dilatation due to direct eye trauma. A high degree of vigilance along with continual reassessment of the patient is therefore necessary. Early manifestations of temporal lobe problems (e.g. extradural haematoma) relate to its close proximity to the tentorium, where its medial aspect compresses the IIIrd nerve causing ipsilateral pupillary dilatation. A contralateral hemiparesis occurs due to compression of the corticospinal motor tracts crossing over at the level of the midbrain.

As intracranial pressure increases signs of a more general nature are apparent, of which Cushing's response is the most well known. If untreated, the opposite pupil enlarges, the patient becomes apnoeic, cardiovascular instability ensues as a result of brain stem herniation or 'coning' followed shortly after by death (*Figure 6.6*).

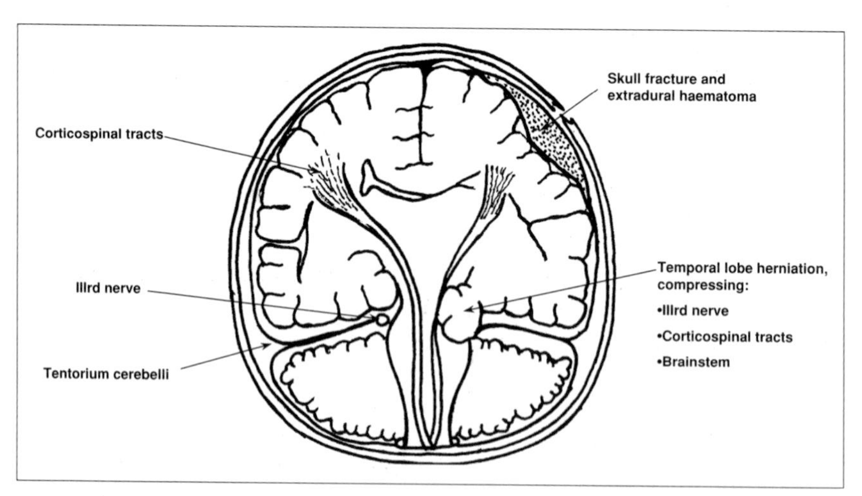

Figure 6.6 Coronal section of brain showing herniation of medial temporal lobe. Compare with Figure 6.1

Recognition of Cushing's Response is an indication of the need for urgent action to reduce ICP with control of the airway and ventilation, hyperventilation and mannitol, as progression to brain stem herniation can be extremely rapid.

Signs of a rise in intracranial pressure within the posterior fossa may be quite subtle, and often initially manifest only as changes in respiratory pattern or activity. It is important therefore to record and observe respiratory pattern in head-injured patients in addition to respiratory rate.

6.5 Assessment and management

6.5.1 Preparation

The medical team leader must:

- ascertain the mechanism of any injuries;
- establish the neurological state of the patient at the scene;
- identify any subsequent changes either with or without treatment;
- be aware of the presence of any other injuries.

If the patient was noted to have been talking at any point since the injury, the primary brain injury is unlikely to be severe, but secondary injury could still be extensive.

Resuscitation should be carried out on a trolley capable of head down and head up tilt, in order that once stabilized, the head-injured patient can be managed in a 15° head-up position to reduce ICP.

6.5.2 Primary survey and resuscitation

It is essential that the patient is managed using the approach described in Section 1.6.1. The life-threatening injury may be extracranial even if the head injury is thought to be significant.

Airway and cervical spine control

The roles of the airway doctor and nurse are:

- maintain continuous verbal communication with the patient wherever possible;
- monitor and report to the team leader any changes in the ability to communicate with the patient;
- clear and secure the airway and maintain cervical spine control;
- ensure adequate oxygenation at all times.

Indications for endotracheal intubation and mechanical control of ventilation following a head injury are listed in Box 6.3.

Attempting tracheal intubation risks aggravating any secondary brain injury as a result of hypoxia, hypertension and an increase in ICP, if not performed in a controlled manner. Furthermore, the cervical spinal cord may also be injured. It is therefore recommended that in a head-injured patient, tracheal intubation is performed by an individual experienced in the use of anaesthetic induction agents and muscle relaxants. The airway doctor must not only be capable of achieving intubation but also be confident in dealing with the problems of using anaesthetic drugs or failing to intubate.

BOX 6.3 Indications for intubation and ventilation following a head injury

- Inability to maintain an adequate airway
- Risk of aspiration, i.e. loss of laryngeal reflexes
- Inadequate ventilation:
- Hypoxia $PaO_2 < 9$ kPa breathing air
  $PaO_2 < 13$ kPa breathing oxygen
- Hypercarbia $PaCO_2 > 6$ kPa
- To assist in acute reduction of ICP by hyperventilation
- Spontaneous hyperventilation causing $PaCO_2 < 3.5$ kPa
- Rapidly deteriorating GCS regardless of initial level or absolute GCS < 9
- Continuous or recurrent seizures
- Need to transport a patient out of the department
- Development of complications, e.g. neurogenic pulmonary oedema, hyperthermia

Once intubation is achieved, it may be possible temporarily to reduce ICP by hyperventilating the patient and reducing their $PaCO_2$ to 4–4.5 kPa. This causes vasoconstriction of cerebral arterioles, thereby reducing the volume of arterial blood in the head. However, if excessive it can severely reduce blood flow to already compromised areas, and exacerbate any injury. Close monitoring of arterial blood gases is required to prevent this occurring. Hyperventilation is reserved for those patients in danger of imminent coning or after discussion with a neurosurgeon.

The risk of an associated cervical spine injury in an unconscious patient following a road traffic accident or fall is 5–10%. Manual inline stabilization is the preferred technique to maintain stability whilst intubation is being carried out, and consequently, a third person is required to maintain the neck in a neutral position whilst intubation is being performed. Leaving the semirigid collar in place limits mouth opening and makes tracheal intubation much more difficult.

Once intubation has been completed, the airway team must ensure that the collar, tape and sandbags are reapplied. It is vital to ensure the collar fits adequately and the head is maintained in a neutral position, as constriction of the neck veins from too tight a collar or tube tie, or poor positioning can elevate the ICP from venous congestion.

Breathing

In an unventilated patient, the respiratory pattern and rate gives vital information and must be continually monitored. Because of the importance of avoiding hypoxia and hypercarbia, adequacy of ventilation is best assessed by arterial blood gas analysis. Thoracic injuries should be rapidly identified and appropriate action performed to ensure adequate oxygenation.

Circulation

A closed head injury is never a cause of shock in an adult patient. Children under 18 months (with open fontanelles) or adults with massive scalp injury may lose sufficient blood to cause shock, but other life-threatening injuries must always be considered and excluded.

Assuming that the patient is *not* in a shock, then fluid administration should be confined to maintenance volumes of either normal (0.9%) saline or Hartmann's solution (compound sodium lactate). Care should be taken not to administer excessive volumes as this can aggravate cerebral oedema.

In the shocked patient, the aim should be to restore blood pressure to an appropriate level for the patient because of the deleterious effects of hypotension on CPP. An adequate volume is more important than the type of fluid used. Initially a bolus of warmed crystalloid or colloid is given, with further fluid type dictated by the patient's response.

In cases of head trauma, dextrose containing fluids (5% dextrose, 4% dextrose plus 0.18% saline) are avoided because:

- they reduce plasma sodium, thereby lowering the plasma osmolality and exacerbating cerebral oedema;
- they cause hyperglycaemia, which is associated with a worse neurological outcome.

It is vital that all fluids administered are recorded appropriately.

Dysfunction

The airway nurse must make a quick 'AVPU' assessment of the patient during the initial ABCs. Once hypoxia and hypotension have been corrected then an assessment of the patient's conscious state should be performed and any localizing signs identified using the Glasgow Coma Scale (GCS) and pupillary reactions. It is always better to record the observed response rather than the associated numerical value, as this is more useful when communicating to members outside the team, e.g. the neurosurgeon. This assessment must be repeated at regular intervals and deterioration in any one of the observed elements of the GCS must be reported to the team leaders.

Exposure and environment

Hypothermia is usually more of a problem after removal of the patient's clothes, but hyperthermia can develop in response to the head injury, and if detected should be treated by active cooling measures, e.g. ice bags, fans, and pharmacological treatments, e.g. rectal paracetamol, if possible. Brain temperature may be 0.5–1°C higher than central core temperature, and so any degree of hyperthermia may be considerably worse than predicted by increasing the metabolic demands of damaged brain tissue. There is no evidence that mild hypothermia is beneficial in the early stages of managing a head injury in the ED.

Team leaders

Upon completion of the primary survey, the team leaders should be satisfied that appropriate resuscitation is under way and all factors that contribute to secondary brain damage have been eliminated. In addition, the patient must be adequately monitored to ensure that any change in the patient's neurological status is detected early. Continual reassessment of heart rate, blood pressure, respiratory rate, blood gas analysis and GCS and pupils is mandatory. An arterial line can often be helpful, allowing continual blood pressure and heart rate monitoring and frequent arterial blood sampling.

Do not forget that extracranial injuries may be the cause of a neurological deterioration

6.5.3 Secondary survey

A detailed head-to-toe examination is carried out as described in Section 1.6.2. Features specific to patients with head trauma are described below. The medical team leader is responsible for ensuring that the examination is completed as fully as possible or if not completed that this is also recorded.

Scalp

Examine the scalp for lacerations, bruising or swelling and digitally explore all cuts for a linear or depressed skull fracture in the base. Occasionally a haematoma in the loose areolar layer can imitate a fracture. Any open fractures exposing brain tissue should not be explored, but covered with a clean dressing and left for expert assessment. Foreign matter protruding from the skull should also be left for removal by the neurosurgeons. Significant scalp bleeding should be controlled either by direct pressure on the edges or using haemostats to grip the aponeurosis and fold the scalp back on itself.

Neurological assessment

A more detailed examination needs to be performed including a repeat of the GCS, pupillary responses, and detection of any lateralizing (focal) signs that may indicate intracranial injury.

When utilized correctly, the GCS (see Box 6.4) is a very useful tool for assessment and communication, but it does not detect focal injuries. The best responses in each section should be recorded.

Common pitfalls

- Inability to open the eyes due to swelling does not automatically mean 'no eye-opening'. Record that the assessment cannot be made.

BOX 6.4 Glasgow coma scale

Eye:	
Opens spontaneously	4
Opens to speech	3
Opens to pain	2
None	1
Verbal:	
Orientated	5
Confused	4
Inappropriate words	3
Incomprehensible sounds	2
None	1
Motor:	
Obeys commands	6
Localizes to pain	5
Flexion (withdraws) to pain	4
Abnormal flexion to pain (decorticate)	3
Extension to pain (decerebrate)	2
None	1

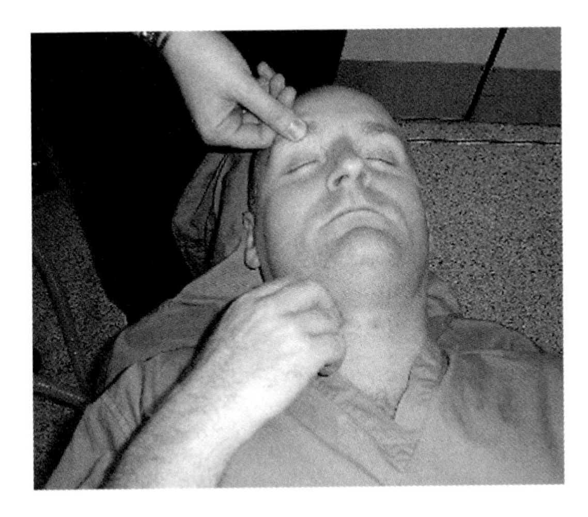

Figure 6.7 Pressure on supratrochlear nerve

- A response to pain is best elicited by applying pressure on the supratroclear nerve in the supraorbital ridge (*Figure 6.7*). A peripheral stimulus may not be sensed in the presence of a spinal cord injury.
- Localizing to pain means that a hand reaches above the clavicle following the supraorbital stimulus. Limb movements confined to below the clavicle represent 'withdraws from pain'.
- Splints and painful fractures limit limb movement. This may cause differences between sides. Record the best side and indicate there is disparity.
- A verbal response cannot be assessed in an intubated patient. Record 'patient intubated'.

As the patient's airway will be secure, regular reassessment of the GCS and pupils can be delegated to the airway nurse. The aim is to detect *any change* in neurological state that may indicate injury or worsening of the patient's condition, and so it is helpful to have the same person assessing these parameters each time.

Lateralizing signs are a strong indicator of intracranial pathology. These are most often a unilateral weakness or asymmetry of motor or pupillary responses, and strongly suggest the presence of focal injury. In a conscious patient, upper-arm drift is a sensitive test of partial hemiplegia. The patient is asked to close their eyes and hold their arms out in front of them, palms facing upwards. Rotation of the arm so the palm faces downwards is an early and sensitive sign of cause for concern. Congenital pupillary dilatation may be present in 10% of the population, but the pupils on both sides should have normal light reflexes.

Fully conscious patients with apparently mild head injuries may also need assessment of their short-term memory to aid in decision-making regarding admission and discharge. They should be able to recollect three objects shown to them 3 min beforehand.

A poor neurological response or deterioration should never be attributed solely to the presence of alcohol. The presence of intracranial pathology or secondary brain damage from hypoxia, hypotension, hypovolaemia or hypoglycaemia must always be considered.

Base of skull

Examine the patient to elicit any clinical signs of a basal skull fracture. The base of skull lies along a line joining the landmarks of the mastoid process, tympanic membrane and orbits, and a fracture is suggested by any of the findings in Box 6.5. In the acute situation, the later signs of fracture may not be present.

Blood dripping from the nose or ear can be tested for CSF by dropping some of the fluid onto an absorbent sheet, e.g. paper towel. If CSF is mixed with the blood, a double ring pattern will develop. The presence of CSF also delays clotting of any blood discharge, although this is not such a reliable sign.

Routine administration of antibiotics is not of proven value in a base of skull fracture, even if there is a CSF leak, indicating the presence of a compound fracture. Antibiotics are generally reserved for those patients with a depressed compound fracture to prevent meningitis and abscess formation. The antibiotics chosen will depend on local policy, and should be known by the team leaders.

A nasogastric tube should not be used if there is a fractured base of skull, as the tube may be pushed up into the skull vault. As a general rule, it is safer to use the orogastric route for gastric drainage in an unconscious head-injured patient.

BOX 6.5 Signs of a fracture to the base of the skull

Early:

- Haemotympanum
- Bloody CSF from the ear or nose
- Scleral haemorrhages with no posterior margin

Late (occurring up to 12–24 h after injury):

- Bruising over the mastoid (Battle's sign)
- Orbital bruising ('panda' or 'racoon' eyes)

Eyes

Penetrating injuries may occur through the orbits into the anterior cranial fossa. The eyes should always be inspected therefore for obvious trauma or haemorrhage and the pupils compared for size and reactivity.

Other injuries

Cardiovascular instability in an unconscious trauma patient must always be investigated and treated prior to moving the patient for further investigation, for example, CT scanning. Depending on local facilities, an abdominal ultrasound scan or diagnostic peritoneal lavage may need to be carried out in the Emergency Department to exclude occult abdominal injury.

6.5.4 Other relevant conditions

Agitation

This is common after head injury, and may indicate intracranial pathology, pain or hypoxia. Efforts should be made to detect and treat the cause as agitated patients are at risk of further injury to themselves. Sedative drugs should never be used as a first-line treatment for agitation, as the cause of the agitation may be missed and secondary injury worsened. If after excluding other causes, the patient remains agitated, expert anaesthetic assistance is required to administer general anaesthesia. Additional investigations, for example CT scanning may therefore be required as a result, since the ability to assess and monitor the patient is impaired.

Convulsions

These may occur spontaneously in patients with epilepsy or more seriously indicate primary or secondary brain damage. Further brain damage can occur if the fits are left untreated due to the hypoxia and hypercapnia that can develop during fitting. An initial convulsion can be treated with a slow intravenous bolus of diazepam to a maximum dose of 5–10 mg depending on age and size. If this fails or the fitting recurs, it is preferable to use a slow intravenous infusion of phenytoin at a dose of 17 mg/kg rather than give further diazepam. Phenytoin should never be given at a rate faster than 50 mg/min as it can precipitate cardiac dysrhythmias. All anticonvulsants can depress both the cardiovascular and respiratory systems so blood pressure and respiration should be closely monitored.

In cases of uncontrolled fitting unresponsive to phenytoin, an intravenous barbiturate (commonly thiopental), will be required. An expert (often an anaesthetist) should administer this, as it will also necessitate intubation and controlled ventilation of the patient. Muscle relaxants should never be given alone, as muscle paralysis does not terminate convulsions.

Completion of secondary survey

At this point, the nursing and medical team leaders should ensure the following:

- the neurological state of the patient following injury, on arrival and any subsequent changes have been recorded;
- they have identified and wherever possible, treated any factors causing secondary brain damage;
- they have assessed and treated any associated injuries;
- any cervical injuries have been detected.

6.5.5 Definitive care

Investigation

This is partly determined by the stability of the patient. If, for example, hypotension due to a ruptured viscus is detected, it is imperative the patient undergoes a laparotomy to treat this prior to undergoing cranial CT scanning. If, however, the patient is stable after completion of the secondary survey, then it is appropriate to carry out a CT scan to determine the exact nature of any cranial and associated injuries. Box 6.6 lists the indications for cranial CT scanning after head trauma.

Wherever possible, cranial CT is the investigation of choice, as it allows earlier detection and possible earlier neurosurgical treatment of intracranial complications with an improved outcome. The Canadian CT Head Rule suggests that a CT should be performed in patients with minor head trauma with any one of the following:

BOX 6.6 Indications for urgent CT scanning

- Skull fracture or after a fit
- Confusion or neurological signs present after assessment and resuscitation
- Deteriorating consciousness or coma after resuscitation
- Significant head injury, haemodynamically stable, needing anaesthesia
- Uncertain or difficult diagnosis, e.g. alcohol, drugs

- GCS < 15 at 2 h after injury;
- suspected open or depressed skull fracture;
- any signs of a base of skull fracture;
- vomiting, ≥ 2 episodes;
- age > 65 years.

Current UK recommendations are under review by the National Institute for Clinical Excellence (NICE) and new guidelines are expected in 2003.

If CT scan facilities are not available on an urgent basis, it may be necessary to transfer the patient to a hospital with these facilities. Performing skull x-rays prior to this may enable the team leaders to clarify the necessity for transfer (see Boxes 6.7 and 6.8).

6.6 Terminology applied to head injuries

Head injuries are grouped into three general categories to aid further management and assessment.

BOX 6.7 Indications for performing skull radiographs

Unconscious patient or with neurological signs:

- All patients, unless CT performed or transfer to a neurosurgical centre

Orientated patient:

- History of loss of consciousness or amnesia
- Suspected penetrating injury
- CSF or blood loss from nose or ear
- Scalp laceration (to bone or > 5 cm long), bruising or swelling
- Persistent headache or vomiting
- Violent mechanism of injury, e.g. fall, RTA, assault with weapon

BOX 6.8 Relative risk of haematoma

No skull fracture	
• Orientated	1:5983
• Not orientated	1:121
Skull fracture	
• Orientated	1:32
• Not orientated	1:4

6.6.1 Minor head injuries

These constitute the majority of attenders to the ED. Patients who meet this description have:

- minimal disturbance of conscious level (GCS 14–15);
- amnesia < 10 min duration;
- no neurological signs or symptoms at the time of examination;
- no skull fractures, clinically or radiologically;
- a responsible adult at the place to which they are discharged.

They must be given appropriate written instructions, e.g. head injury card.

6.6.2 Moderate head injuries

These patients require admission for observation and investigation. Wherever possible it is recommended they remain under the care of a local admitting team with experience of caring for head injuries. This will include patients with:

- confusion or any depression of the level of consciousness (GCS 9–13);
- a skull fracture, on x-ray or clinically;
- difficulty in assessment, e.g. alcohol, drug intoxication, epilepsy;
- patients with relevant co-existent medical disorders or treatment, e.g. blood clotting disorders, anticoagulants;
- patients without a responsible adult to monitor them.

If there is any deterioration in their condition during admission their status must be discussed with a neurosurgeon.

6.6.3 Severe head injuries

These patients need urgent neurosurgical referral. Such patients include:

- coma (GCS < 9) after full resuscitation;
- those with a skull fracture and neurological signs;
- a compound or depressed skull fracture;
- basal skull fracture;
- post-traumatic epilepsy;
- deteriorating consciousness or neurological state regardless of initial presentation;
- neurological disturbance lasting more than 6 h;
- amnesia > 10 min;
- abnormal head CT scan.

6.7 Referral to a neurosurgeon

Any patient with potential or actual need for neurosurgical intervention, or where a CT scan cannot be performed within a reasonable time should be referred to a neurosurgeon. This will include all of those patients in the category 'severe head injury' and those in whom a CT scan is indicated (see Box 6.6) but cannot be arranged within 2–4 h.

6.7.1 Communication with a neurosurgeon

Not every patient discussed with a neurosurgeon will need to be admitted under their care, but advice about investigation and treatment can often be useful. Neurosurgeons require a detailed referral as indicated in Box 6.9.

BOX 6.9 Patient information needed by neurosurgeon

- Name, age and sex
- Time and mechanism of injury
- Neurological state at the scene (description)
- Any change in neurological status during transfer to hospital
- Initial assessment (ABCDE), other injuries
- Localizing signs of neurological injury or convulsions
- Treatment administered and any response
- Results of any investigations
- Relevant past medical history and medication

6.7.2 Treatment to discuss with a neurosurgeon

The following are recognized treatments for head injuries, but should not be used routinely and ideally after neurosurgical referral.

Mannitol

This is an osmotic diuretic agent that has a dual effect in reducing ICP. Its early effect is due to an improvement in cerebral blood flow by altering red cell deformability and size. It also reduces interstitial brain water by establishing an osmotic gradient and movement of water between brain tissue and blood. In areas where the blood brain barrier is damaged it can, however, leak into the brain tissue and increase the local water content. Initially, 0.5 g/kg of 20% mannitol (175 ml in 70 kg adult), is administered and the patient reassessed, e.g. a reduction in pupil size. A urinary catheter is always required if not already in place. Repeated doses can cause hypovolaemia or electrolyte disturbance.

Frusemide

This is a potent diuretic that also reduces ICP by reducing brain water and the rate of CSF production. It can be used instead of mannitol at a dose of 0.5 mg/kg. The effect of frusemide can be extremely potent if used in conjunction with mannitol, and will cause hypovolaemia, hypotension and biochemical derangement.

Hyperventilation

This has been discussed above. Its use should be confined to cases of imminent coning in conjunction with other treatments, e.g. mannitol.

Neurosurgery

This is rarely required in the ED as it is preferable to transfer the patient to the neurosurgeon once stabilized. Burr holes should only be placed by a trained surgeon who has consulted a neurosurgeon.

6.7.3 Neurosurgical transfer

Transfer to a neurosurgical unit should only occur after adequate resuscitation and stabilization of any life-threatening injuries. The escorting team should consist of a trained nurse and a doctor experienced in dealing with any patient deterioration in transit. If the patient is intubated, the doctor should be a trained anaesthetist. Preparation and equipment for transfer should be in accordance with accepted guidelines and is described elsewhere. Adequate records including vital signs and GCS must be maintained during transfer.

6.8 Summary

Head injury management in the ED should be directed at identifying and treating the factors that cause secondary brain injury. Life-threatening injuries to other systems need to be treated prior to transfer for further neurosurgical investigation or treatment. Coordination of the resuscitation team is vital in order to detect these injuries and prioritize their treatment. The majority of head injuries seen in the ED do not require admission or neurosurgical input. The team must be able confidently to detect those that do.

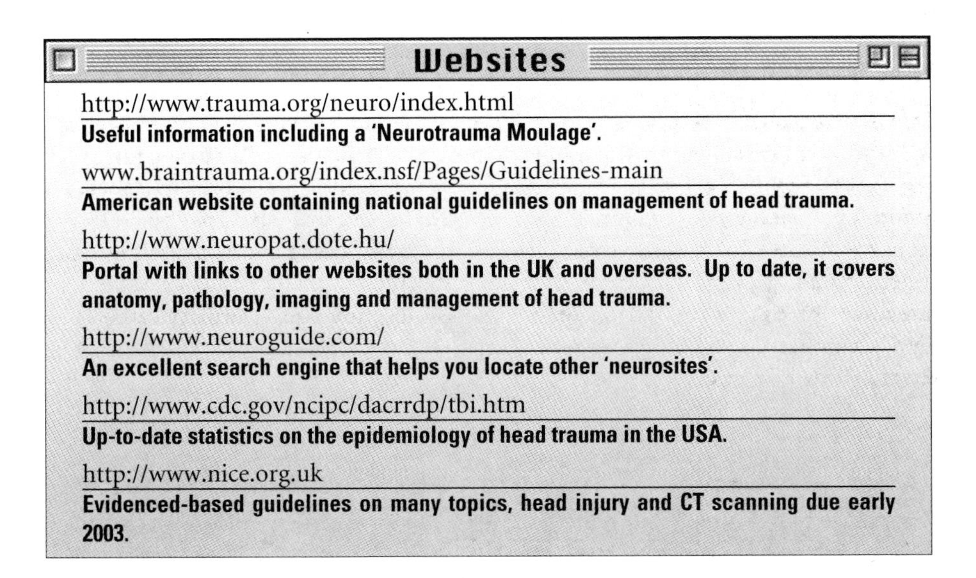
Websites

http://www.trauma.org/neuro/index.html
Useful information including a 'Neurotrauma Moulage'.

www.braintrauma.org/index.nsf/Pages/Guidelines-main
American website containing national guidelines on management of head trauma.

http://www.neuropat.dote.hu/
Portal with links to other websites both in the UK and overseas. Up to date, it covers anatomy, pathology, imaging and management of head trauma.

http://www.neuroguide.com/
An excellent search engine that helps you locate other 'neurosites'.

http://www.cdc.gov/ncipc/dacrrdp/tbi.htm
Up-to-date statistics on the epidemiology of head trauma in the USA.

http://www.nice.org.uk
Evidenced-based guidelines on many topics, head injury and CT scanning due early 2003.

Further reading

1. **Stiell IG, Wells GA, Vandemheen K, *et al.*** (2001) The Canadian CT Head Rule for patients with minor head injury. *Lancet* 357: 1391.

2. **The Royal College of Surgeons of England** (1999) *Report of the Working Party on the Management of Patients with Head Injuries.* The Royal College of Surgeons of England: London.
3. **Maas AIR, Dearden M, Teasdale GM, *et al.*** ((on behalf of The European Brain Injury Consortium) 1997) EBIC Guidelines for management of severe head injury in adults. *Acta Neurochir.* (Wein) **139:** 286.

7 Spinal injuries

P Kelly, P Johnson, C Gwinnutt

Objectives

The aims of this chapter are to:

- discuss the epidemiology of spinal injury;
- review the applied anatomy of the spinal cord and vertebral column;
- describe the common mechanisms of spinal trauma;
- review the pathophysiological changes which occur after spinal injuries;
- describe the key features of the primary and secondary survey in patients with spinal injury;
- outline the principles of interpretation of the lateral cervical spine x-ray;
- outline the principles used to rule out injury to the cervical spine.

The statistical risk of spinal injury is relatively small. Nevertheless the potential for life-long morbidity is so high that great caution must always be exercised to ensure that further neurological damage does not result from medical interventions. To this end it is essential that, initially, all trauma patients are managed as if they all have an underlying spinal injury until it has been excluded.

The initial assessment and management of the patient with a spinal injury is a challenging and difficult problem

7.1 Epidemiology of spinal injury

The aetiology of spinal injury varies worldwide, but the commonest cause is road traffic accidents, which generates approximately 50% of all spinal injuries. The exact nature of the injury varies according to the direction and speed of the vehicle at impact, the victim's position and the presence or absence of seat belts and airbags. Similarly, pedestrians struck by motorcycles or cars are at risk of sustaining virtually any form of spinal injury.

Sporting accidents are the next most common cause. Data from the Royal Society for the Prevention of Accidents (ROSPA) has identified activities including gymnastics, trampolining, horse riding, rugby, skiing and hang gliding as most likely to result in spinal injury. In any given population, the prevalence of spinal injuries is also dependent upon both the recreational facilities and the popularity and activity of the various sports clubs.

7.1.1 What are the risks?

- Spinal cord injury (SCI) affects mainly young adults in the age from 16–30 with almost 80% of them being male.
- Post-mortem studies indicate that the incidence of spinal cord injury in the UK approaches almost 50 per million population per year.
- Of those surviving a spinal injury, approximately 15–20 per million population per year will suffer a major paralysis as a result of their injury.
- In a patient with multiple injuries, approximately 3% will have sustained spinal trauma.
- Approximately 10% of patients with a significant head injury will also have damaged their cervical spine.
- If the patient is known to have a spinal fracture at one level there is an 8% risk of there being a second injury present elsewhere in the spine.

Traditionally it has been taught that the majority of spinal fractures occur in the cervical spine with the remainder being fairly evenly split between the thoracic and lumbar region. More recent figures from the Trauma Audit Research Network (TARN, personal communication) reveal a different distribution (see Box 7.1).

Further analysis of this data for 1000 patients with spinal cord injury indicates a much higher incidence of cord injury with cervical spine fractures, compared with either thoracic or lumbar injuries. In addition there are a small number of patients who present with spinal cord injury without radiological abnormalities, often referred to as SCIWORA.

BOX 7.1 Site of spinal fractures or dislocations without cord injury*

Site	%
Cervical	22%
Thoracic	28%
Lumbar	41%
Multiple	8%

(*Based on data from approximately 9000 patients presenting to Emergency Departments in England and Wales.)

7.2 Anatomy of the vertebral column and spinal cord

7.2.1 The vertebral column

The vertebral column is made up of 33 vertebra, consisting of seven cervical, 12 thoracic, five lumbar and nine fused as the sacrum and coccyx.

The typical vertebra consists of two main parts: anteriorly, the body, which is essentially a cylinder of bone, and posteriorly, a vertebral arch that encloses the spinal canal (*Figure 7.1*). From the body of the vertebra a pair of pedicles project backwards and from these pass the lamina which fuse together in the midline, thereby forming the spinal canal. From each arch a spinous process projects posteriorly and from each lateral side projects a transverse process. The superior and inferior articular processes of the facet joints are formed from the transverse processes. Each pedicle contains a notch

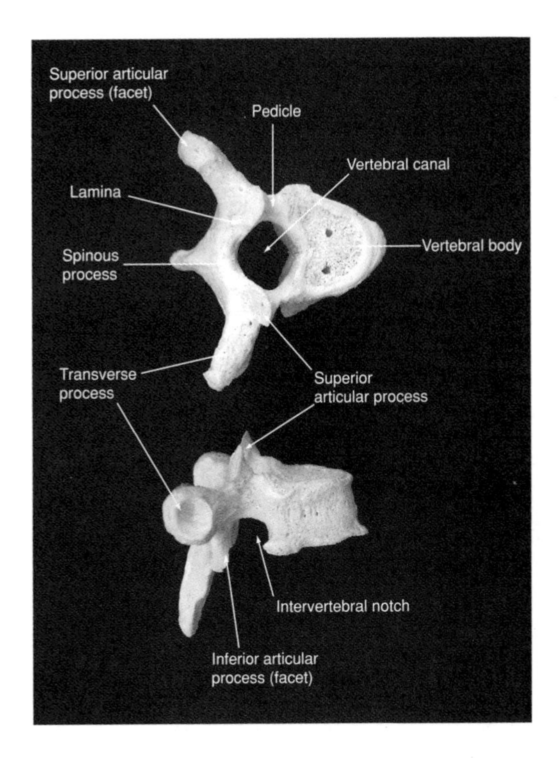

Figure 7.1 Lateral and bird's eye view of typical vertebra

both superiorly and inferiorly to align with corresponding notches on adjacent vertebra to form the intervertebral foramina, through which pass the spinal nerves.

In man, with his erect posture, the vertebral column has to support the weight of the head and the trunk and therefore must have great axial strength whilst retaining flexibility. A series of curves, produced partly by the wedge shape of the vertebral bodies and the shapes of the intervertebral discs, give rise to the characteristic cervical and lumbar lordoses. The bodies of the vertebra and the intervertebral discs provide axial support while the flexibility of the spine is facilitated partly by the natural curves, the intervertebral discs and the presence of the synovial facet joints. The strength of the spine and its stability during movement is maintained by a combination of the bony structure, the lie of the facet joints, the intervertebral discs and the muscles and ligaments that connect the vertebra (*Figure 7.2*). Clinically the most important ligaments are the anterior and posterior longitudinal ligaments, ligamentum flavum and interspinous ligaments between the spinous processes.

Cervical spine

There are seven cervical vertebra, of which the top two are structurally distinct. The 1st cervical vertebra (atlas) has no body but, instead, lateral masses that articulate by synovial joints with the occipital condyles on the base of the skull (the atlanto-occipital joints). These joints allow for a considerable degree of both flexion and extension of the head. The 2nd cervical vertebra (axis) has an upward projection like a finger called odontoid process (or dens) and articulates with the back of the anterior arch of the atlas – in other words it lies within the spinal canal itself (*Figure 7.3*). The joint between

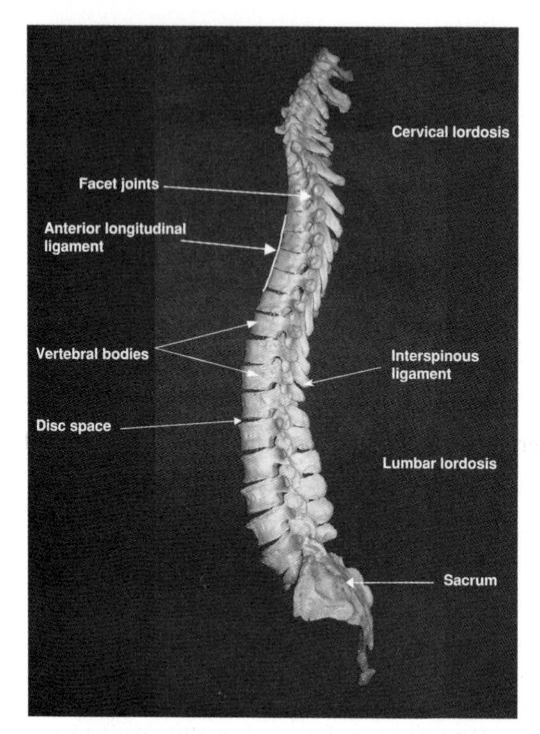

Figure 7.2 Lateral view of vertebra and ligaments

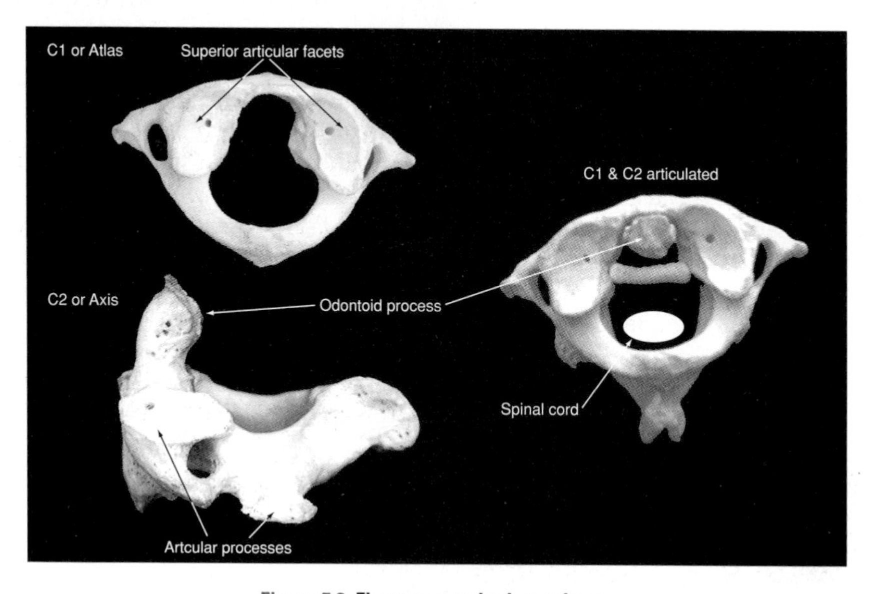

Figure 7.3 First two cervical vertebrae

the atlas and the axis (the atlanto-axial joint) allows mainly for rotation of the head in a line passing through the long axis of the odontoid peg.

The lower five cervical vertebra all have backward sloping facet joints stacked somewhat akin to a series of roof tiles. These are synovial joints and allow mainly for flexion and extension and to a lesser degree rotation.

Thoracic vertebra

There are 12 vertebra, characterized by relatively long transverse process and facet joints on the sides of the vertebral bodies allowing for articulation with the ribs. The facet joints through which adjacent vertebra articulate with each other are aligned more vertically than within the cervical spine and, whilst allowing flexion and extension, significantly restrict rotation.

Lumbar spine

The five lumbar vertebra are characterized by having the largest bodies, shorter transverse processes and retaining the vertical lie of the facet joints.

Sacrum and coccyx

The sacrum consists of five fused vertebrae and is triangular in shape. The vertebral canal is bounded by pedicles and laminae and there are very short spinous processes. Laterally there is an articular facet for articulation with the ilium. The coccyx consists of three to five fused vertebrae articulating with the sacrum.

Intervertebral joints

Movement between adjacent vertebrae is relatively slight but there is a considerable additive effect. The two regions of greatest flexibility are the junctions between the cervical and the thoracic spine and between the thoracic and lumbar spine. Combined with the fact that these are the points where the direction of curvature of the spine changes, this makes them also the two most common sites for spinal injury.

Spinal canal

The spinal canal extends from the foramen magnum in the base of the skull to the sacral hiatus. It is bounded anteriorly by the vertebral bodies, intervertebral discs and the posterior longitudinal ligament (*Figure 7.4*). Posterior are the laminae and the interspinous ligaments and laterally the pedicles of the vertebra and the vertebral foramina.

7.2.2 The spinal cord

The cord is approximately 45 cm long and is continuous above with the medulla oblongata at the level of the foramen magnum, terminating as the conus medullaris. In

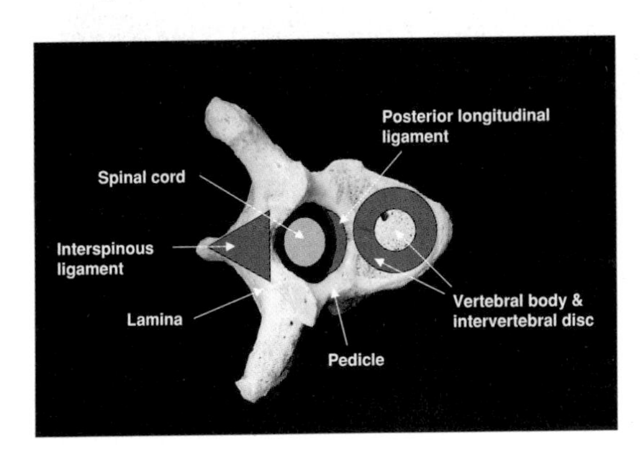

Figure 7.4 Boundaries of the spinal canal

the adult, this lies at the lower level of the 1st lumbar or the upper level of the 2nd lumbar vertebra. The cord is surrounded by the dura mater and between this and the bony canal is the extradural space, normally filled with fat and blood vessels. The size of the space varies with the different levels of the cord, being minimal in the thoracic region and maximal at C2 where there is a large space behind the odontoid process. This affords the spinal cord at this level a degree of protection and is often referred to as Steel's rule of three (see Box 7.2).

BOX 7.2 Steele's rule of three

'One third of the spinal canal within C1 is occupied by the odontoid, one third by an intervening space and one third by the spinal cord' (see *Figure 7.3*)

Structure of the spinal cord

The spinal cord consists of nerve fibres that transmit impulses from the periphery to the brain (ascending tracts) and vice versa (descending tracts). In transverse section the cord has a central canal around which is the H-shaped grey matter (*Figure 7.5*). The posterior horns of the grey matter contain the nerve cells of sensory fibres entering via the posterior nerve roots and the anterior horns contain the nerve cells of the motor nerves that give rise to the anterior nerve roots. The remainder of the cord consists of the white matter that contains the nerve fibres of the long ascending and descending tracts. The nerve fibres in some of these tracts cross (or decussate), an important factor in interpreting signs after trauma to the spinal cord.

Ascending tracts

(i) The anterior and lateral spinothalamic tracts carry pain and temperature. Having entered the spinal cord, they ascend and then cross to the opposite side within the height of two vertebral bodies before ascending to the thalamus and then the sensory cortex.

(ii) The posterior columns comprise the medial and the lateral tracts, or the fasciculus gracilis and the fasciculus cuneatus respectively. They convey sensory fibres

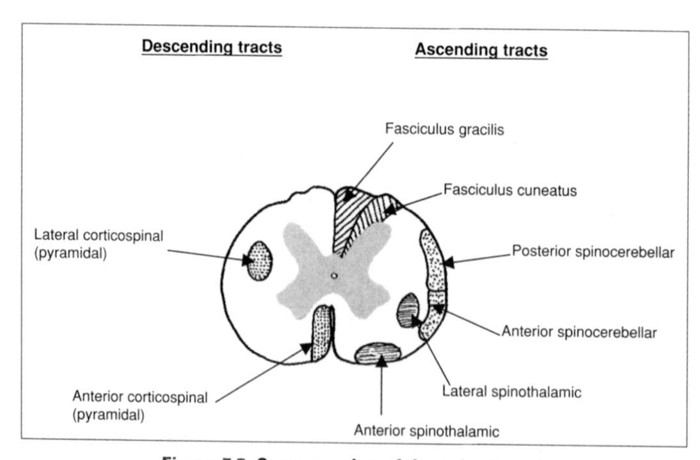

Figure 7.5 Cross-section of the spinal cord

serving fine touch, vibration and proprioception (position sense). These fibres ascend uncrossed until they reach the level of the medulla.

(iii) The anterior and posterior spinocerebellar tracts carry proprioception and ascend on the same side of the cord as they enter to the cerebellum.

Descending tracts

(i) The lateral corticospinal or pyramidal tract has its origin in the motor cortex and the fibres cross to the opposite side in the medulla, that is, before they reach the spinal cord. They then descend in the contralateral side of the cord.

(ii) The anterior corticospinal tract is a smaller motor tract and descends uncrossed from the cortex. Crosssover only occurs at the level at which these fibres leave the cord.

Spinal nerves

The anterior and posterior nerve roots pass from the spinal cord to the appropriate intervertebral foramina where they unite to form a mixed sensory and motor spinal nerve. Below the level of L1 the anterior and posterior nerve roots pass almost vertically downwards to form the corda equina.

Blood supply of the spinal cord

The main arterial supply comes from the anterior and posterior spinal arteries that descend from the foramen magnum. The anterior spinal artery supplies the whole of the cord anterior to the posterior columns, and the posterior spinal arteries supply the posterior columns. There is additional supply from radicular arteries that originate mainly from the descending aorta (*Figure 7.6*). The largest usually arises in the lower thoracic or upper lumbar region and sends branches to both anterior and posterior spinal arteries and supplies a significant part of the lower spinal cord. As there are no anastamoses between the anterior and posterior circulation, the cord is susceptible to any reduction in blood supply and may result in infarction of the cord, particularly in the watershed areas between vessels.

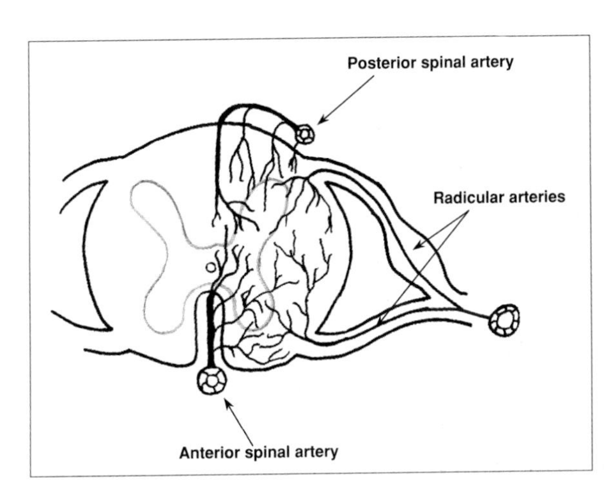

Figure 7.6 Blood supply of the cord

7.3 Mechanism of injury

7.3.1 The vertebrae

The spinal cord can be injured either:

- directly as a result of penetrating trauma;
- indirectly as a result of excessive flexion, extension, rotation, axial compression or distraction.

The latter mechanism may injure the spinal cord either as a result of a fracture dislocation or damage from displaced fractures or an intervertebral disc within the spinal canal.

Following the initial injury to the spinal cord whatever the cause there is usually some further or secondary deterioration due either to impairment of blood flow in the region of the damaged cord or as a result of traumatic oedema.

Although most injuries to the spine can be identified radiologically, spinal cord injuries occurring without any radiological abnormality (SCIWORA) are occasionally seen either in the very young children or in the elderly. In the young it occurs because there is potential for much greater mobility of the vertebral column without causing a fracture. In contrast in the elderly there are often pre-existing degenerative changes leading to significant narrowing of the spinal canal.

Stability and instability of the spine.
A spinal injury is considered stable when controlled movement will not cause neurological injury. An unstable injury exists when any movement can cause or exacerbate a neurological injury.

Hyperflexion injuries

- In adults commonly occur between T12–L2 for example as a result of flexion over a seatbelt following frontal impact. In children it tends to be higher, T4–T6.
- Often result in wedge (compression) fractures.
- May be stable or unstable depending on the severity of compression.
- May occur in the cervical spine, usually C5/6 for example following a diving injury.
- May result in a fracture of the anterior superior corner of the vertebra or *tear drop fracture*.
- Because of the associated ligamentous damage are usually considered unstable.

Hyperextension injuries

- Are usually only found in the cervical and lumbar regions due to the stabilizing effect of the ribs.
- May result in fragments of the vertebral body being pushed into the spinal canal.
- If associated with rotation may result in fractures of the laminae and pedicles.
- A special type of hyperextension with distraction in the cervical spine results in a fracture through C2 and is known as a *hangman's fracture* for obvious reasons.

Compression injuries

- Tend to affect the cervical and lumbar regions, the commonest site being L1.
- If severe may push fragments into the spinal canal.
- May be seen after diving accidents, usually at C5.
- A special type of injury occurs when axial loading compresses C1 between the occipital condyles and C2, known as a *Jefferson fracture*.
- This is often accompanied by C1 sliding forward on C2, but the cord remains uninjured thanks to Steel's rule of three.

7.3.2 The spinal cord

Injuries of the spinal cord are classified into either complete or incomplete. In a complete injury the patient has neither sensory nor motor function distal to the level of the injury. One should suspect this when there is no return of sensation or motor function within 48 h. The outlook is poor, as there is likely to be little or no further improvement. With incomplete injuries there are several well-recognized patterns of injury.

Anterior cord syndrome

- Due to the loss of function of the anterior two-thirds of the spinal cord.
- Usually the result of a flexion injury or an axial loading leading to a burst fracture and damage to the anterior spinal artery.
- May also be seen after a period of profound hypotension.
- On examination there is loss of motor function (flaccid paralysis), sharp pain and temperature sensation below the lesion.
- Proprioception, vibration and deep pressure sensation are all retained because they are transmitted in the intact posterior columns in the cord.

Central cord syndrome

- Often follows hyperextension to the neck, such as from a fall on to the face, typically in older patients who have degenerative changes in their spine, narrowing the spinal canal.
- Usually results in a vascular event, compromising blood flow to the centre of the cord.
- Results in damage to the corticospinal and spinothalamic tracts.
- On examination there is a flaccid paralysis of the arms, worse distally and spastic paralysis of the legs.
- There may be disturbance of sensation with hyperaesthesia, arms more than legs.
- There is variation in the degree of neurological presentation, usually a disproportionate loss of power in the arms with little abnormality to be found in the legs.

Brown-Séquard syndrome

- A rare injury resulting from a hemitransection of the spinal cord and associated unilateral spinal tracts.

- The neurological findings are of loss of power and proprioception, vibration and deep pressure sensation on the side of the injury at the level of the lesion.
- On the opposite side of the body there is a loss of pain and temperature sensation below the level of the lesion.
- The mechanism of injury is most commonly the result of a penetrating wound from either a gunshot or stabbing.

Neurogenic shock

- Injury to the cord above T6 results in progressive loss of sympathetic outflow.
- The higher the lesion the greater the loss of vasomotor tone and peripheral vasodilatation causing hypotension.
- A lesion at T2 or above will also result in loss of sympathetic innervation of the heart and the ability to mount a tachycardia.
- Such a patient will be hypotensive, bradycardic and vasodilated with the lack of ability to maintain temperature control.
- Because of cardiac denervation, the patient will not be able to mount a normal response to any co-existing hypovolaemia caused by any other injuries.
- The lack of any sympathetic activity may unmask profound parasympathetic reflexes, for example severe bradycardia during laryngoscopy.

Spinal shock

- This term defines the condition seen after spinal cord injury when there is a *transient* loss of tone, power and reflex activity (flaccid areflexia).
- This may last for a variable length of time (days or weeks) but there is the potential for full recovery.
- The patient's cardiovascular status and ability to respond to insults is normal.
- Areas of the cord that are permanently damaged will eventually resolve to reveal a spastic weakness.
- If there has been a complete transection of the cord, there will be a gradual return of exaggerated reflex activity, but a lack of power and sensation.

7.4 Assessment and management

7.4.1 Initial reception

The development of the ambulance paramedic service has led to an improvement in the care of patients with spinal injuries as a result of:

- recognition of the importance of the mechanism of injury;
- advance warning to the receiving hospital of a patient with either a spinal, head or multiple injuries;
- the widespread use of full immobilization, semirigid collars, head blocks and long spine boards.

Injuries are, however, still missed, particularly in either the young or the elderly. Other causes of missing a spinal injury are shown in Box 7.3. As the team leader expecting a

BOX 7.3	Common causes of missing a spinal injury
	- Unconsciousness - Distracting injuries - Lack of pain or deformity in the spine - Inadequate interpretation of x-rays - SCIWORA - Failure to consider the possibility of spinal injury

known trauma case it is worthwhile remembering the statistical chances of dealing with a spinal injury are approximately 3% in a multiply injured patient and 10% in a head-injured patient. Around 50% of patients with a spinal cord injury will also have another potentially life-threatening injury as well. The team leader must ensure that all team members are aware of the potential for spinal injury.

It is important to ensure as with all forms of resuscitation to take heed of the principle 'Do no further harm'. In the case of spinal injury nothing could be more apt. It is therefore vital for the team leader to ensure that the patient is not subjected to any undue movement of the spine and that they are lifted and moved in one, thereby protecting the cord against the possibility of secondary injury.

Who is at risk?

- The conscious patient complaining of severe neck or back pain.
- The conscious patient unable to move or feel either arms or legs.
- The patient with severe facial injuries.
- Patients involved in high-speed road traffic accidents.
- Falls from a height.
- Patients unconscious or with a head injury.
- Patients who have suffered multiple injuries.
- Distracting injury.

In all the above groups one should assume the presence of an underlying spinal injury until this can be positively excluded during resuscitation in the ED.

Transfer of the patient to a trolley

There are two ways of transferring the patient to the ED trolley when they are not appropriately immobilized on a long spine board.

- An ambulance scoop stretcher can be inserted beneath the patient, the head and neck immobilized and then the patient lifted over.
- When this device is not available a minimum of five people will be required. It is vital that the team has been fully trained in the procedure and knows only to act on the direct instructions from the person controlling the stabilization of the head and the cervical spine. Using his hands and forearms this person controls the neck and head of the patient whilst three other members position themselves for lifting, one for the thoracic spine, one for the lumbar spine and pelvis and one for the legs. On the controller's command all four gently lift the patient and the fifth member removes the trolley.

It is also useful to have an additional, sixth member, to hold IV infusions and monitors whilst the patient is being transferred. At no time during the course of this manoeuvre should the patient be subjected to a bending or twisting force.

7.4.2 Primary survey and resuscitation

Spinal injuries are frequently identified early, often before arrival in the ED. It is therefore all too easy to make the mistake of assuming that you are dealing with a patient with a spinal injury rather than a patient with potentially multiple injuries and a spinal injury. Do not be distracted from the routine of the primary survey, the team leader must ensure that the basic rules of assessment and resuscitation, as described in Section 1.6.1, are followed to prevent deterioration secondary to hypoxia or hypoperfusion.

Airway and cervical spine control

The first and most urgent priority is for the airway doctor and nurse to secure the airway as described in Section 2.4. At the same time, the neck must be stabilized in a neutral position, without any distracting force being applied. This is best achieved by the nurse applying MILS, in order not to compromise airway management. If the victim is still wearing a motorcycle crash helmet, it should be removed by two skilled operators: one expands the helmet laterally and gradually 'rocks' the helmet off the head until it can be rotated free, while the other person immobilizes the cervical spine from below. In the conscious patient whose airway is clear, a semirigid collar, blocks and tapes can replace the nurse to immobilize the cervical spine. However, some patients are likely to be anxious and at times claustrophobic from their presence and the nurse must continue to reassure, to give hope and to explain what is happening. If at any time it becomes necessary to remove the collar and blocks then it is essential that MILS must be reapplied.

Two groups of patients with spinal injuries require urgent tracheal intubation. First, the unconscious patient who rapidly develops a paralytic ileus and an incompetent gastro-oesophageal sphincter, which combined with the potential of a full stomach, puts them at a high risk of regurgitation and aspiration. The second group are those with signs of a high cervical cord injury; diaphragmatic breathing, neurogenic shock, tetraplegia, forearm flexion whose ventilation will be inadequate. Intubation in these individuals is more difficult because of reduced neck movement and is best performed by an experienced anaesthetist, who may require specialized equipment for example a fibreoptic laryngoscope.

Patients with spinal injuries who start to vomit are managed as described in Section 1.6.1.

An additional problem that occurs is the conscious patient with a suspected spinal injury but who is confused, restless and agitated, and refusing to lie down. On no account should this patient be forcibly held down but instead should be reassured, allowed freedom to move and encouraged to retain the cervical collar if possible. The muscle spasm associated with spinal injury does result in the patient instinctively holding the head and neck still and avoiding movement and it is therefore unusual for a patient to worsen a spinal injury. At the same time the team must try and identify and treat the cause of the restlessness.

Once the airway has been secured, as close to 100% oxygen as possible should be administered via a nonrebreathing mask, with reservoir. The neck is then inspected for the presence of:

- swelling, bruising and wounds;
- subcutaneous surgical emphysema;
- deviation of the trachea;
- distended neck veins;
- laryngeal crepitus.

Breathing

The chest is examined as already described looking for the immediately life threatening thoracic conditions (see Section 3.4.1). Diaphragmatic breathing may be the first clue of a significant injury to the cervical spinal cord. The finding of a fractured sternum in a road traffic accident victim should raise the suspicion of an injury to the thoracic spine. Early consideration should be given to arterial blood gas analysis to assess the adequacy of oxygenation and ventilation.

Circulation

Assessment and management are as for all trauma victims; it is important not to assume that shock is due to the spinal injury, that is, neurogenic shock (see Section 7.3.2). Even if this is the cause, resuscitation will be required and it may be exacerbated by the presence of other injuries causing blood loss that must not be overlooked. Major external haemorrhage is controlled by direct pressure, two large intravenous cannulae are inserted and blood is taken for grouping and cross-matching and any other appropriate tests. The circulation nurse should record the patient's respiratory rate, pulse and blood pressure, capillary refill time, colour and level of consciousness. The type and rate of fluid infused will need to be judged according to the circulatory status of the patient and the presence of associated injuries.

The presence of a bradycardia with hypotension in the unconscious patient may be the only indication of a significant spinal injury

Care is required to ensure optimal fluid resuscitation. Too little and the tissue ischaemia will increase; too much may precipitate pulmonary oedema. A central venous line should therefore be installed early and used to monitor the response to fluid challenges. In an isolated cord injury, a mean arterial blood pressure should be maintained near the individual's pre-injury level to ensure cord perfusion. Those patients who respond inadequately to fluid resuscitation and remain bradycardic will require the administration of vasopressors and invasive haemodynamic monitoring. Expert help should be sought early. Atropine should be used only in the emergency situation. It causes drying of the mucous membranes, thickens secretions and may cause or worsen a paralytic ileus.

Dysfunction

The team leader should assess the patient's level of consciousness either grossly, using the AVPU system and checking the papillary responses to light, or preferably with a full

GCS assessment. During this assessment it may become apparent that there is a symmetrical weakness. This should be noted, but the full definitive neurological assessment must wait until the secondary survey.

Exposure and environment

The patient should be completely divested of all remaining clothes to allow them to be examined in entirety, while at the same time not forgetting their dignity. This is usually achieved using a log roll. All patients cool rapidly once exposed, but particularly those with spinal cord injury due to the associated vasodilatation. Every effort must be made to keep them warm, using blankets, warm air blowers or overhead heaters. At the same time it is essential to ensure that there is no undue movement of the spine. During the course of the log roll, as well as removing the clothes, a rectal examination can be performed and finally the patient is removed from the spine board.

7.4.3 Secondary survey

This consists of a detailed head-to-toe examination and is usually carried out by the team leader as described in Section 1.6.2. There are some occasions when this needs to be delayed because of the need for surgery in order to stop the bleeding or transfer to the ICU. Whatever the reason, if the secondary survey is not completed in the Emergency Department, this must be clearly documented in the patient's notes and the team leader should remind the clinicians responsible for the inpatient care on handover. All too commonly for the lack of a detailed secondary survey, injuries that are eminently treatable are missed and go on to produce problems long after the immediate life-threatening conditions have been forgotten.

The remainder of this section will concentrate on those aspects of the secondary survey that relate to the management of patients with spinal injuries.

The conscious patient

A number of symptoms are associated with spinal injury:

- pain in the spine at the level of the injury worsened with movement;
- in the absence of pain ask the patient to cough or tap their heels; this may reveal a painful area;
- abnormal or absent sensation;
- ignorance of other injuries, particularly fractures;
- presence of weakness or inability to move a limb or limbs.

A full neurological examination must be performed on both sides to detect any abnormalities:

- cranial nerves;
- sensation in all dermatomes (light touch and pain, *Figure 7.7*);
- muscle power using the MRC scale (Box 7.4);
- reflexes;
- rectal examination, if not already performed during the log roll.

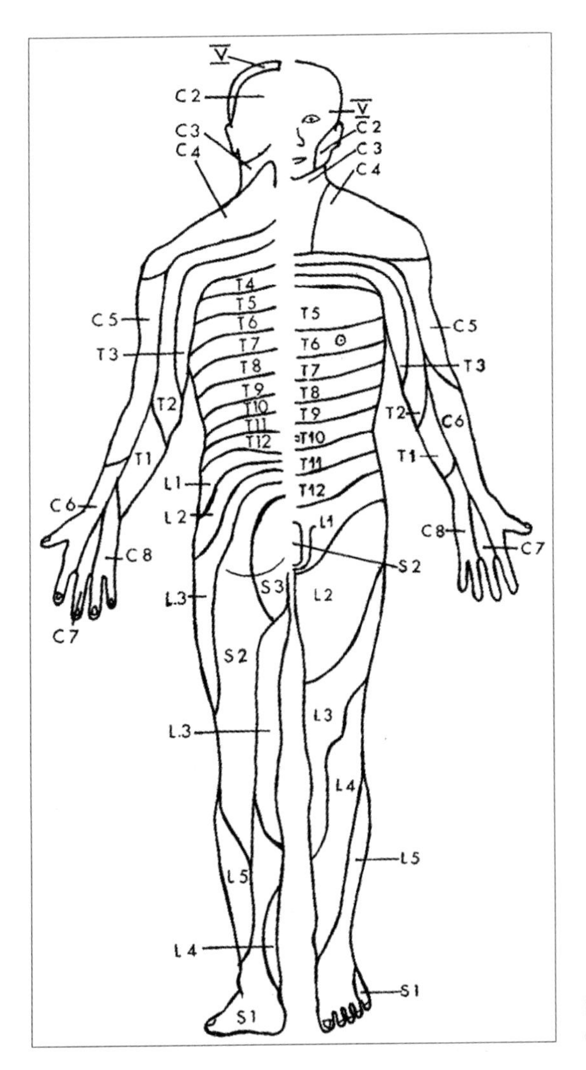

Figure 7.7 **Diagram of the dermatomes**

BOX 7.4	The MRC scale for assessing muscle power
	0 = total paralysis 1 = A flicker of contraction, but no movement 2 = Movement with gravity eliminated 3 = Movement against gravity 4 = Movement against resistance, but reduced power 5 = Normal power

Myotomes

Although strictly speaking most muscles are innervated by more than one nerve root, the following actions can be regarded as being performed predominantly by muscles as having one spinal root value:

C5 – shoulder abduction

C6 – wrist extension

C7 – elbow extension

C8 – finger flexion

T1 – finger abduction

L2 – hip flexion

L3 – knee extension

L4 – ankle dorsiflexion

L5 – great toe extension

S1 – ankle plantarflexion

Reflexes

These approximate to the root values:

S1,2 – Ankle

L3,4 – Knee

C5,6 – Supinator

C7,8 – Triceps

The unconscious patient

The key to recognizing the potential presence of a spinal injury is a continued high index of suspicion. The features listed in Box 7.5 increase the chance of there being a spinal injury. If there is any spontaneous movement it is important to note it and try to identify if it was actually spontaneous or a response to pain, and any difference between limbs.

A rectal examination is performed to assess the sphincter tone and the bulbocavernosus reflex. The latter consists of contraction of the bulbocavernosus muscle that can be detected by palpation in response to squeezing the glans penis. There will be no response if the cord is uninjured or a state of spinal shock exists. This assesses spinal roots S2, 3 and 4.

The vertebral column must be examined and this will entail log rolling the patient with an appropriate number of staff to ensure that the spinal alignment is maintained and not subject to any undue forces. The team leader should examine the whole spine from occiput to coccyx, looking and feeling for any deformity, swelling, tenderness, mal-alignment, bogginess, muscular spasm or wounds. If not done so already, a long spine board must now be removed to minimize the risk of the development of pressure sores and at the same time a note must be made of the state of the pressure areas.

BOX 7.5 Features suggesting spinal injury in an unconscious patient

- Hypotension with a bradycardia
- Flaccid areflexia
- Diaphragmatic breathing
- Loss of response to pain below an identified dermatome level
- Absence of reflexes below an identified level
- Priapism

7.4.4 Investigations

Plain x-rays

Although ultimately a number of x-rays of the spine may be required depending on the clinical indications, a lateral cervical spine film is the most common. A number of errors are made when looking at these films that can result in injuries being missed, these include:

- an inadequate x-ray;
- assuming a normal x-ray excludes the possibility of spinal injury;
  – a good quality lateral x-ray is only 85% sensitive;
- spinal cord injury due to a vascular event with no bony injury (SCIWORA);
- failure to appreciate the severity of the abnormality;
- failure to systematically examine the x-ray.

The latter is totally avoidable by having a system to examine the x-ray – the AAABCs system (see Box 7.6).

BOX 7.6	The AAABCS system of x-ray interpretation
	Accuracy Adequacy Alignment Bones Cartilages and joints Soft tissues

Accuracy?

Is this the correct film for the correct patient?

Adequacy?

Are all seven cervical vertebrae, the occipito-cervical junction and the C7–T1 junction visible?

If not, consider either repeating the film with the patient's arms pulled down to remove the shoulders from the field of view, or take a 'swimmer's view;. If these fail then a CT will be required. Do not be complacent, the C7–T1 junction is where the majority of missed lesions occur.

Alignment?

Check the contours of the four longitudinal curves (see *Figure 7.8).*

1. Anterior – along the anterior aspect of the vertebral bodies from the skull base to T1.
2. Posterior – along the posterior aspect of the vertebral bodies from the skull base to T1.
3. The spinolaminar line should be smooth except at C2 where there can be slight posterior displacement (2 mm).
4. The tips of the spinous processes – a tighter curve. The tips should also converge to a point behind the neck.

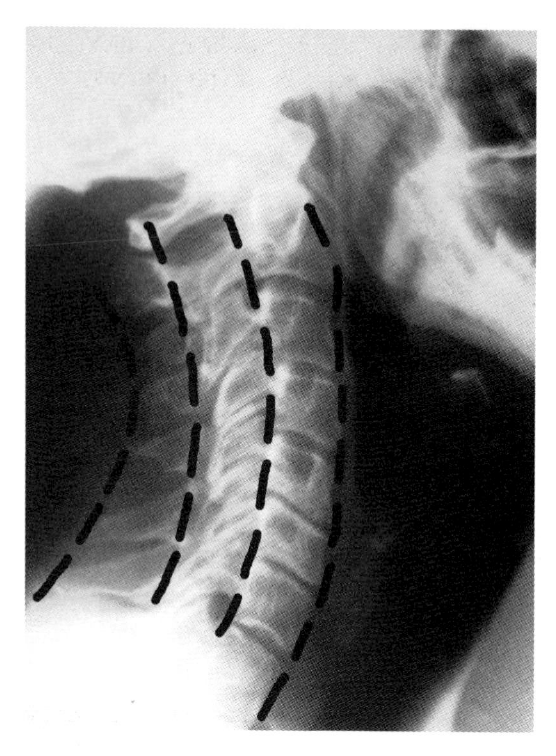

Figure 7.8 Lateral cervical spine film with curves shown

A break in any of these lines indicates a fractured vertebra or facet dislocation until proved otherwise. Divergence of the spinous processes is also abnormal.

In some patients there is a pronounced loss of the normal curve of the cervical spine (lordosis). This may be due to:

- muscle spasm;
- age;
- previous injury;
- radiographic positioning;
- the presence of a hard collar.

If identified it therefore only indicates that the patient may have sustained a cervical spine injury.

Bones

Check the cortical surfaces of all vertebrae for steps, breaks or angulation.

C1 Check the laminae and pedicles, think about a Jefferson fracture.

C2 Check the outline of the odontoid and pars interarticularis, think about a hangman's fracture.

C3–T1 Start at the anterior inferior corner of the vertebral body and proceed clockwise, checking pedicles, laminae and spinous processes. The height of the anterior and posterior bodies should be the same. More than 2 mm difference suggests a compression fracture.

Check the spinal canal – this extends from the back of the vertebral body to the spinolaminar line and is more than 13 mm wide. It may be narrowed by: dislocations, bony fragments pushed posteriorly, pre-existing degenerative disease.

Cartilages and joints

Check the disc spaces, facet joints and interspinous gaps.
Disc spaces should be of uniform height and similar in size to those between adjacent vertebrae. Facet joints have parallel articular surfaces, with a gap less than 2 mm. Widening of the gap and visibility of both facets suggests unifacetal dislocation. There will also be anterior displacement of less than half the width of the vertebral body and associated soft tissue swelling (see below). If there is displacement greater than 50%, then both facets are dislocated. There will also be narrowing of the disc space, widening (fanning) of the spinous processes and soft tissue swelling.

Check the gap between C1 and the front of the odontoid peg.
The distance between the posterior surface of the anterior arch of C1 and the anterior surface of the odontoid should be less than 3 mm in the adult; greater than this suggests rupture of the transverse ligament. This may occur without there being bony injury or cord damage (Steele's rule of three).

Soft tissues

Check the soft tissue shadow anterior to the cervical vertebrae.
Fractures of the cervical vertebrae or ligamentous injury will result in a haematoma as in any other area of the body. This will be seen as an increase in the width of the soft tissue shadow adjacent to the injury. In some subtle injuries this may be the only evidence. As a rule of thumb the soft tissue shadow between the anterior border of C1–3 and the air in the oro- and nasopharynx should be less than 7 mm wide. At the level of C5 this increases to about 21 mm, or the width of the vertebral body. Occasionally, this may be seen as anterior displacement of an endotracheal tube.

It must be remembered that the stability of the cervical spine is dependent on the ligaments that are not revealed on a plain x-ray. Therefore the lateral cervical film must be examined not only for signs of bony injury but also for clues of ligamentous injury as this may indicate the presence of an unstable injury (see Box 7.7).

In most patients who are suspected of having a significant injury to their cervical spine, further x-rays will be required, for example anteroposterior, open mouth views and, in addition, thoracic and lumbar views may also be required. These will need the patient to be transferred to the x-ray department. This should only be undertaken

BOX 7.7 X-ray features associated with an unstable cervical spine

Facet joint widening
Facet joint overriding
Widening of the spinous processes
> 25% compression of a vertebral body
> 10° angulation between vertebral bodies
> 3.5 mm vertebral body overriding with fracture
Jefferson's fracture
Hangman's fracture
Tear drop fracture

when it is safe to do so. For further details on interpretation of x-rays the interested reader should consult the references in Further Reading.

CT and MR scanning

When combined with plain x-rays, CT scanning increases the detection of fractures to over 95%. It also provides greater detail of bony injury and degree of compromise of the spinal canal and is used predominantly to allow planning of definitive care, including surgery. Its main drawbacks are that it requires a relatively stable patient and it provides limited detail about the spinal cord. It is important to remember that patients can be scanned whilst remaining immobilized on a long spine board. MR scanning is now the investigation of choice to identify soft tissue injuries, including spinal cord, ligaments and intervertebral discs. The main problem is the time taken to scan the patient and the use of MR-compatible resuscitation equipment in ill patients.

7.4.5 Definitive care

Many patients who have the potential for a spinal injury, particularly to their cervical spine, based upon the mechanism of injury, will turn out to be uninjured. A system is therefore needed to determine who needs an x-ray of the cervical spine and when it is safe to remove the devices immobilizing the cervical spine. This is commonly referred to as 'clearing the cervical spine'.

Who needs an x-ray of their cervical spine?

Any patient in whom the mechanism of injury suggests the potential for injury, and does not fulfill ALL of the following seven criteria:

1. alert and orientated;
2. not under the influence of drugs or alcohol;
3. neurologically normal;
4. no other distracting injuries;
5. age ≤ 65 years.

The cervical collar is now removed and replaced with MILS while the cervical spine is palpated:

6. no tenderness in the midline over the cervical spine.

Finally, the patient is asked to actively move their head and neck:

7. pain free, unrestricted rotation of the neck, 45° to the left and right.

If any criteria are not met, full immobilization is maintained and x-rays obtained. Conversely, if all are fulfilled, immobilization is no longer required.

The situation is more difficult in the unconscious patient. As it is impossible to carry out a neurological assessment or identify pain, it is safer to assume injury and maintain immobilization. For those patients who require care on the ITU, it may be appropriate to perform detailed CT or MR scanning to rule out the possibility of injury. This will, of course, require specialist advice.

7.5 Summary

The management of the patient with a spinal injury starts at the scene and continues through to rehabilitation in order to minimize the risk of secondary injury and maximize the potential for outcome. The basic principles of resuscitation apply at all stages, but it is equally important that the situation is not made worse by careless or uncoordinated handling of the victim at any stage.

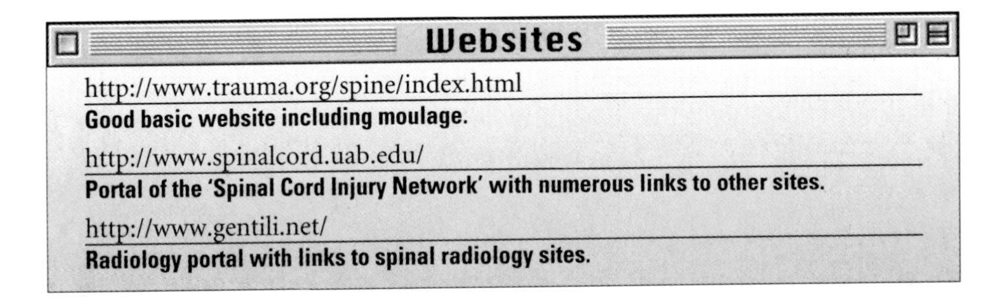

Further reading

1. **Hoffman JR, Wolfson AB, Todd K & Mower WR** (1998) Selective cervical spine radiography in blunt trauma: methodology of the National Emergency X-Radiography Utilization Study (NEXUS). *Ann. Emerg. Med.* **32:** 461.
2. **Stiell IG, Wells GA, Vandemheen KL, *et al.*** (2001) The Canadian C-Spine Rule for radiography in alert and stable trauma patients. *JAMA* **286:** 1841.

8 Maxillofacial injuries

D Patton

Objectives

At the end of this chapter, the trauma team members should understand:

- the importance of airway management in maxillofacial trauma;
- the relationship between facial injuries and injuries to the cervical spine;
- the management of severe bleeding in the head and neck region;
- the importance of the secondary survey in identifying potentially life-threatening associated injuries in the chest and abdomen.

This will allow the trauma team to assess and carry out the initial management of severe injuries to the face and jaws in the first two hours after injury.

8.1 Introduction

Following the introduction of seat belt legislation, interpersonal violence has overtaken road traffic accidents as the most common cause of facial injuries in the United Kingdom. Home Office data demonstrates that interpersonal violence more than doubled between 1974 and 1990, and continues to increase. Where facial injuries result from violent crime, 50% of the victims have raised blood alcohol levels, and this may complicate the pre-hospital and early hospital care. One study has demonstrated that in assault cases resulting in fractures, 83% involved the facial skeleton. Isolated fractures of the mandible, nose or zygoma are most common in this situation.

More extensive fractures of the midface and nasoethmoid regions are more often due to road traffic accidents or substantial falls. These are more likely to be life threatening, and also more likely to be associated with other injuries, particularly of the chest and abdomen.

8.2 Applied anatomy

For the purposes of this chapter, the head and neck region is best regarded as a closed box (the skull) below which the facial bones are suspended and attached to the inclined skull base. This is supported by the cervical spine, which is easily damaged in deceleration injuries such as road traffic accidents or falls. There is therefore a relationship between facial injuries, head injuries and injuries to the cervical spine. If a casualty with a significant facial injury is unconscious, there is a 10% chance of an associated injury to the cervical spine. The most important manifestation of maxillofacial injuries is, nonetheless, airway obstruction, and this is the most common cause of death in this type of trauma.

The middle third of the facial skeleton is a complex structure consisting of the two maxillae and nasal bones centrally, and the zygomatic bones laterally. The maxillary bones are thin, but thickened laterally to form four buttresses which pass vertically from the tooth supporting alveolar bone, up to the skull base (*Figure 8.1*). These are designed to absorb the vertical stresses of mastication, but collapse relatively easily with anterior forces. As a result of this, the bones of the central midface may function in the same way as the 'crumple zone' of a car with the application of a significant anterior force. As the middle third of the face 'crumples' it absorbs energy which would otherwise be transmitted to the skull base, increasing the chance of brain injury. As the middle third of the facial skeleton is displaced backwards it slides backwards down the inclined base of the skull, obstructing the airway, and causing a gap between the upper and lower front teeth. In this situation, dragging the upper jaw forwards with fingers behind the palate may relieve the airway. As the central facial skeleton is forced backwards it separates from the skull base at one of three levels originally described by Le Fort early in the last century.

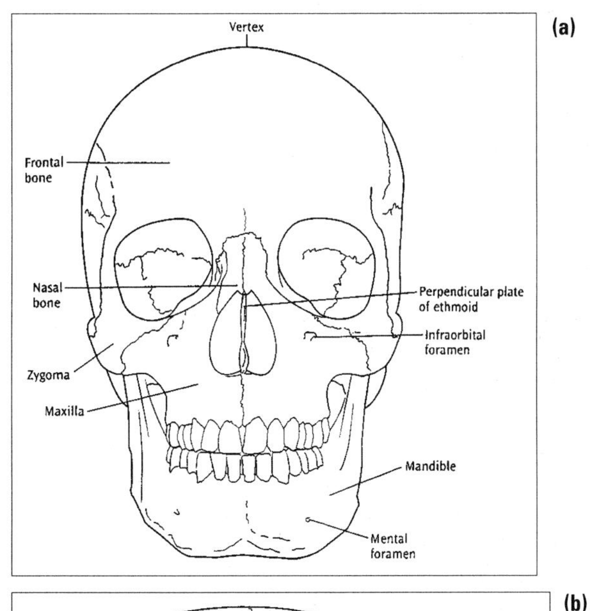

(a)

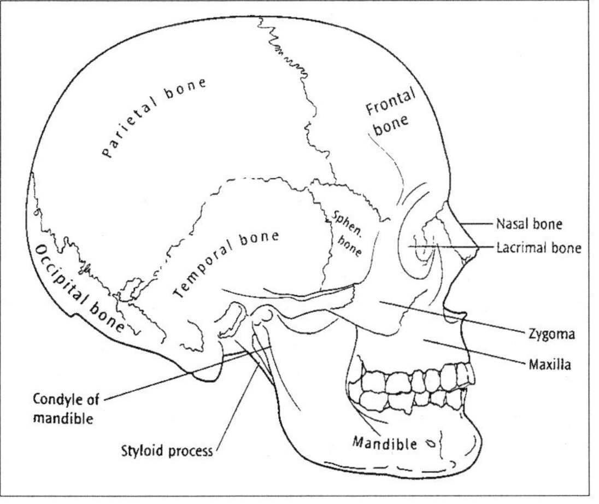

(b)

Figure 8.1 (a) Anterior view of bones and skull. (b) Lateral view of bones and skull. Greaves I, Porter K, Ryan J (eds) *Trauma Care Manual* (2001). Reproduced with permission from Hodder/Arnold.

The lateral part of the middle third is formed by the two strong zygomatic bones whose prominence is a protective mechanism for the eye. They also form part of the floor of the orbit, and so zygomatic fractures are frequently associated with eye injuries, which may be masked by the soft tissue swelling, and missed. Always 'beware the black eye'.

The mandible forms the lower third of the facial skeleton. It is a strong bone which articulates with the skull base at the temporomandibular joint. It provides the anterior support for the tongue via the muscle attachments to the genial tubercle. If there is a bilateral fracture of the mandible, or comminution of the anterior mandible, the tongue support may be lost, allowing the tongue to fall back and obstruct the airway.

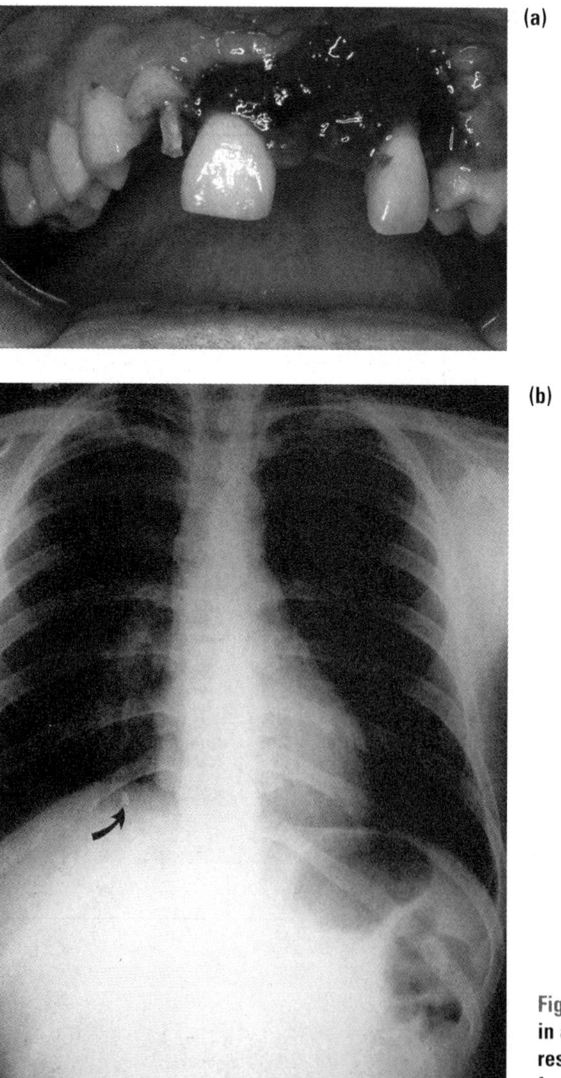

(a)

(b)

Figure 8.2 (a) Damage to teeth in a bicycle accident, resulting in inhalation of tooth fragment. (b) Chest X-ray of same case showing small fragment of tooth in right lung (arrowed).

The necks of the mandibular condyles are relatively weak and are a common fracture site. A blow to the chin such as a punch may be transmitted back through the mandible to cause a fracture of the condyle, an injury which is often missed. This injury should always be suspected if there is a laceration on the chin. The fractured condyle may also be forced back into the external auditory meatus causing a laceration of the anterior wall. This results in bleeding from the ear which may initially be misdiagnosed as a skull base fracture.

Teeth are frequently knocked out or fractured in maxillofacial trauma. Wherever possible, any missing teeth should be accounted for, as they may have been inhaled, particularly in the unconscious patient. An inhaled tooth is most likely to be found in the right main bronchus, although smaller fragments may slip further down into the more peripheral airways (*Figure 8.2*). An avulsed tooth in the right main bronchus may be overlooked on a standard chest radiograph as it may be masked by the border of the heart. In addition to teeth fragments of acrylic dentures may be inhaled or become lodged in the vocal cords. Early bronchoscopy is indicated to avoid the development of pulmonary complications. Swallowed teeth usually pass through the alimentary canal without complication.

Facial injuries, particularly those to the middle third of the face, may cause rapid soft tissue swelling, making it difficult to palpate underlying bone fractures. Gross swelling of the face should always alert the examiner to the presence of a fracture, but radiographs are often necessary to clarify the extent of the injury. The soft tissues of the face and scalp have a good blood supply. Soft tissue facial injuries bleed profusely, but the extent of blood loss is often overestimated. Where there is obvious hypovolaemic shock, it is important to search for covert bleeding elsewhere, such as in the abdomen or chest. It is easy for an examiner to be distracted by the appearance of a major facial injury, and to overlook a more life-threatening injury elsewhere. The good blood supply also means that tissue necrosis is unusual in facial injury and any debridement should be relatively conservative, preserving facial skin. Nonetheless, wounds contaminated with debris such as road grit must be thoroughly cleaned to avoid unsightly tattooing of the wound requiring later revision surgery. Extensive lacerations of the face frequently give the impression of tissue loss because muscle retraction pulls the edges of the wound apart.

8.3 Assessment and management

This section emphasizes the assessment and management of a maxillofacial injuries in the first 2 h from the time the casualty arrives in the Emergency Department (ED), until their care is taken over by the maxillofacial team. It is not the intention to deal with the definitive surgical care of hard and soft tissue facial trauma.

The initial management of the facial injury follows the procedure described in Section 1.6.1.

8.3.1 Primary survey and resuscitation

The primary survey is designed to detect and treat immediate life-threatening injuries. It is not necessary to make an accurate diagnosis of the facial injuries at this stage, only to deal with any potential life-threatening conditions, such as airway obstruction, which have arisen. Those aspects of the primary survey, which are of particular importance in injuries to the head and neck, are emphasized here.

Airway and cervical spine control

Airway obstruction is the most common cause of death in facial injury. The patency of the airway should therefore be immediately assessed. This may be rapidly determined by speaking to the casualty and assessing the response. The nature of the response will yield immediate information, not only on the patency of the airway, but also the level of consciousness. Although a large proportion of casualties with facial injuries may be under the influence of alcohol or drugs, it should not be assumed that they are the cause of confusion. Such behaviour may well be due to hypoxia, and improve once the airway is established, and other causes of hypoxia corrected. At the same time listen for stridor, snoring or gurgling, the characteristic noises of airway obstruction. If the patient is hoarse, consider an injury to the larynx, or a foreign body such as a tooth or denture impacted in the vocal cords.

Establish the airway

The conscious patient with bleeding from facial injuries is usually more comfortable sitting up with his head held forward to allow blood and secretions to drain forwards out of his mouth. Otherwise blood will gravitate to the back of his mouth causing him to cough and splutter. If he is unable to sit up, then a prone or semiprone position is preferable.

While the airway is being assessed and re-established, movement of the cervical spine must be minimized, particularly in the unconscious patient. This is achieved by an assistant holding the casualty's head in line with his body with the neck slightly extended. First, the airway must be re-established, and then safely maintained, reassessing patency at regular intervals.

Even in severe facial injuries it is usually possible to establish an airway with simple procedures, although intubation may be required to protect the airway when it is proving difficult to control bleeding within the mouth and pharynx. It is unusual in civilian practice to have to resort to a surgical airway, except where there has been a failed intubation, there is a foreign body impacted in the vocal cords, or direct damage to the larynx.

The stages to secure the airway are:

- clear debris (broken teeth/dentures) from the mouth with a careful finger sweep and suction. Keep any retrieved fragments to help the maxillofacial team account for missing or broken teeth;
- try a jaw thrust or chin lift;
- if clearing the mouth and a jaw thrust have been unsuccessful, try pulling the tongue forward. In the unconscious patient this best achieved with a towel clip, or suture passed through the dorsum of the tongue as far posteriorly as possible. Other instruments tend to crush the tongue, and increase the pain and swelling;
- if the anterior part of the mandible is comminuted, or there is a bilateral fracture, the tongue may have lost its anterior support allowing it to fall back against the posterior wall of the pharynx. In this situation, pulling the front of the mandible forward may clear the airway;
- if the maxilla has been pushed backwards down the inclined plane of the skull base, then pulling it forwards to disimpact it may also clear the airway. Backwards

displacement of the maxilla may be suggested by the lower front teeth being in front of the upper teeth, with an open bite.

In the majority of cases these manoeuvres will have established an airway, but it must then be maintained. In most cases this is achieved with a nasopharyngeal or oropharyngeal airway of the correct size, although a tongue suture may sometimes be indicated to hold the tongue forward. Note that an oropharyngeal airway is easily dislodged, and poorly tolerated in a responsive patient. A nasopharyngeal airway is much better tolerated and less likely to be dislodged, but neither will prevent the aspiration of blood or vomit. They require frequent suction to prevent them becoming blocked. Also remember that care is needed when passing a nasopharyngeal tube in a patient with fractures of the middle third of the facial skeleton, as these may be associated with fractures of the base of the skull. Nasopharyngeal tubes should be passed horizontally through the nostril, and not upwards towards the skull base. Whichever method has been used to maintain the airway, it must be checked regularly. In practice, the casualty is usually intubated with a cuffed tube, both to maintain the airway and to reduce the chances of aspiration.

When these initial attempts to establish an airway fail, the most common cause is bleeding in the pharynx or nasopharynx, which has not been controlled (see below under circulation). There may also have been direct trauma to the larynx, from, for example, a karate blow, or a foreign body impacted in the vocal cords. An attempt is made to intubate the casualty, but if the degree of bleeding is too great to see the vocal cords do not persist, but proceed to a surgical airway. If there is a foreign body impacted in the hypopharynx, this usually becomes apparent during attempted intubation and may be removed. If, however, it cannot readily be removed, do not persist but proceed quickly to a surgical airway.

The surgical airway

A cricothyroidotomy is the preferred way to establish a surgical airway in an acute emergency. It affords rapid and relatively safe access to the airway. Tracheostomy should be regarded as a semi-elective procedure to be carried out by an experienced surgeon in a controlled environment. It is usually possible to establish a surgical airway with a cricothyroidotomy within 2 min. In the presence of a fracture of the larynx, a tracheostomy rather than cricothyroidotomy will be indicated.

Surgical airways in children

Establishing and maintaining the airway in a child in the presence of severe facial injuries may be challenging. The initial methods outlined above are attempted but if a surgical airway is needed, cricothyroidotomy should be avoided in children under the age of 12. The cricoid cartilage is the only circumferential support for the upper trachea in this age group and accidental damage to it during cricothyroidotomy may have serious consequences. If an experienced surgeon is available and time permits, a formal tracheostomy may be carried out. An alternative to buy time is jet insufflation. This will generally give 30–45 min extra time to allow a tracheostomy to be performed. Oxygen at 50 psi is administered through a 14 g needle cricothyroidotomy. Remember, however, that carbon dioxide elimination is poor with needle cricothyroidotomy, and CO_2 levels will increase. The pulse oximeter may give a false sense of security as it will not detect high CO_2 levels, and tells little about the adequacy of ventilation.

Breathing

Before fitting a neck support, or prior to assessing the chest in the normal way, examine the neck. This will yield important information not only about direct injury to the neck, but also to abnormalities of the chest. There may be laryngeal crepitus or surgical emphysema associated with a fracture of the larynx.

Take particular care when examining penetrating wounds of the neck, resulting from ballistic injuries or knife wounds. If examination suggests that the wound extends deep to the platysma muscle, do not push a gloved finger in, or torrential bleeding may result if a major underlying blood vessel has been damaged. Even perforations of the internal jugular vein may have tamponaded themselves by the time the casualty arrives in the accident unit, and disturbing the wound may have dramatic consequences. Such wounds should be formally explored in theatre with the appropriate vascular instruments readily to hand.

It is always safer to assume that a penetrating wound of the lower neck or supraclavicular fossa has involved the apex of the lung until proved otherwise. A haemopneumothorax may occur even when there are no apparent injuries below the clavicle. An assessment of the breathing is therefore important even when there does not seem to have been an injury to the chest (*Figure 8.3(a) and (b)*).

Facial injuries sustained in road traffic accidents are frequently associated with abdominal injuries, and may result in a ruptured diaphragm leading to abnormal signs in the chest if the viscera have been forced upwards into the thoracic cavity. Damage to

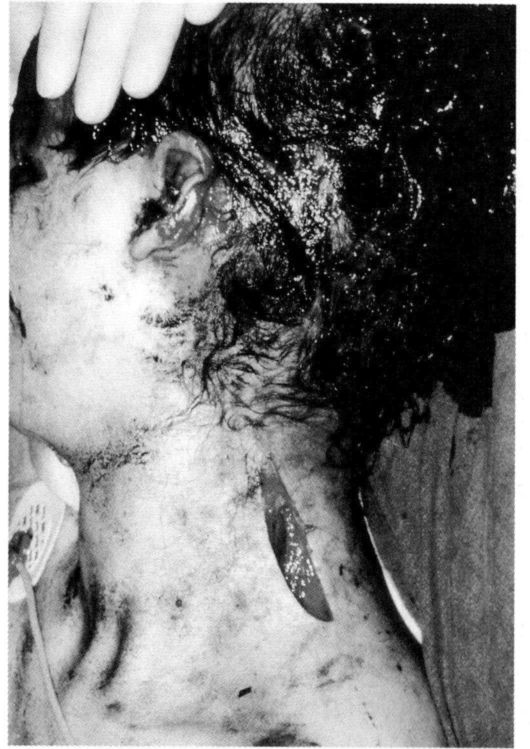

(a)

Figure 8.3 (a) Multiple stab wounds to neck and head. There were no injuries below the clavicle. Greaves I, Porter K, Ryan J (eds) *Trauma Care Manual* (2001). Reproduced with permission from Hodder/Arnold.

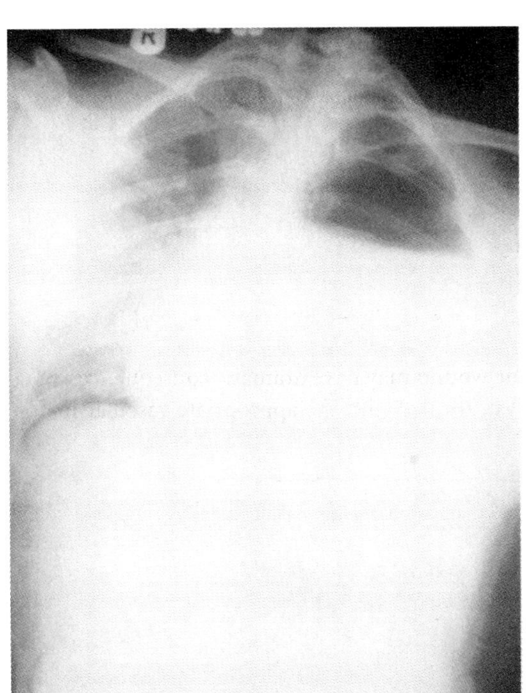

(b)

Figure 8.3 **(b) Chest X-ray of same patient as (a) showing haemothorax. Greaves I, Porter K, Ryan J (eds) *Trauma Care Manual* (2001). Reproduced with permission from Hodder/Arnold.**

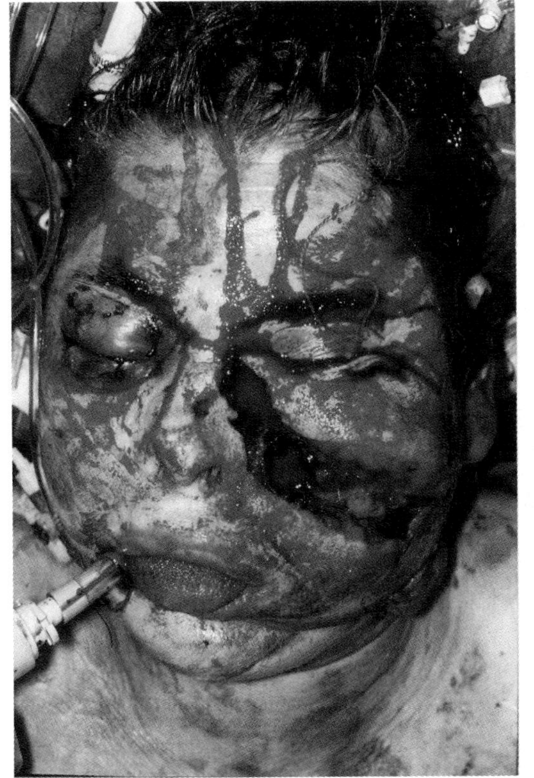

(a)

Figure 8.4 **(a) Severe facial injury (Le Fort II), car occupant, unrestrained.**

(b)

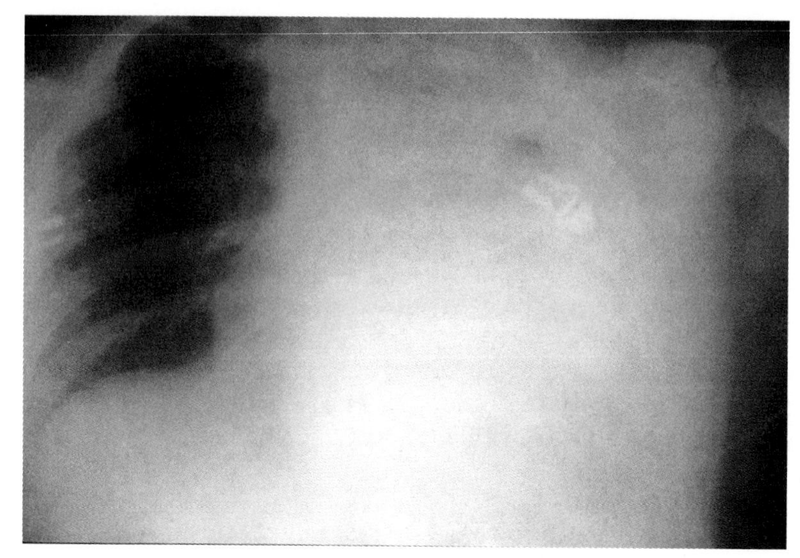

Figure 8.4 (b) Chest X-ray showing gastric air bubble in the left chest as a result of ruptured diaphragm (same patient as (a)).

the phrenic nerve in the neck following penetrating injuries will also paralyse the diaphragm on that side (*Figure 8.4(a) and (b)*).

In this section we have dealt with those aspects of breathing assessment of particular relevance in the presence of facial injuries. A full account of the chest examination is discussed in the chapter on thoracic trauma.

Circulation

The major problems relating to maxillofacial injuries in the first two hours nearly always relate to the airway or bleeding. It is the A and C of the primary survey which are therefore the most important.

It is not the intention to cover the assessment of the circulation in this section, but to emphasize the control of bleeding in the head and neck region, and to warn of the tendency to attribute hypovolaemic shock to maxillofacial injury, when covert bleeding in the abdomen, chest or pelvis is the more likely cause (*Figure 8.5*).

The tissues of the head and neck have an excellent blood supply, but this does mean that facial injuries bleed profusely. Nonetheless, in the absence of a severe middle third facial fracture or damage to a major blood vessel in the neck, the degree of bleeding is usually insufficient to cause clinical hypovolaemic shock. An exception to this are scalp injuries in children or severe fractures of the middle third of the face in adults. Scalp lacerations alone are unlikely to cause hypovolaemia in an adult, but significant scalp injuries in children may be life threatening.

Control of bleeding in the orofacial region

It is important to control bleeding in the mouth and oropharynx as quickly as possible, not only to preserve blood, but to maintain an airway. The primary survey is normally carried out with the casualty in the supine position with in-line immobilization of the neck. In this position any blood in the mouth will gravitate to the hypopharynx and obstruct the airway.

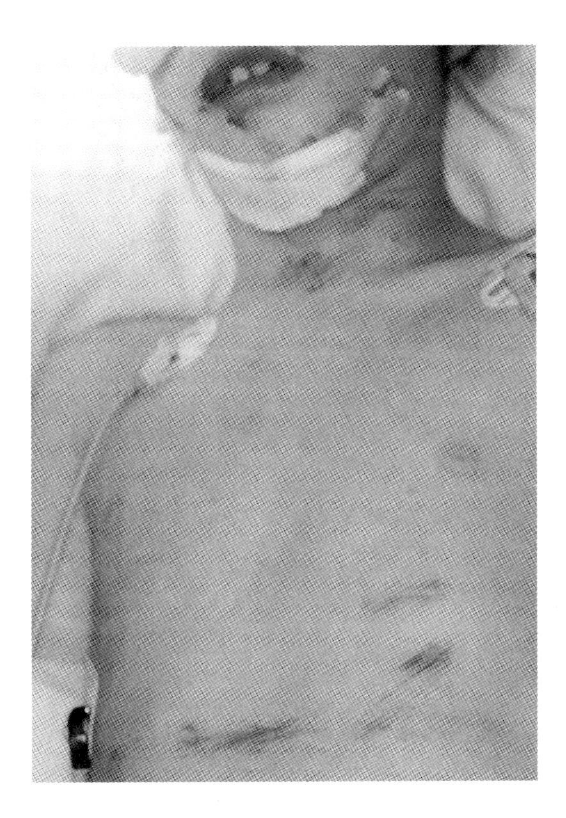

Figure 8.5 Child with fractured mandible and hypovolaemic shock after RTA. Note abrasions on abdomen. Patient also has ruptured spleen.

Most bleeding in the oral cavity is accessible and can be controlled with local pressure with a swab. The tongue is very vascular and bleeds easily. Nonetheless, bleeding from tongue lacerations is readily controlled with deep sutures to include the underlying muscle. Infiltration with local anaesthetic containing a vasoconstrictor may also help reduce bleeding from intraoral lacerations.

Mandibular fractures are often open into the mouth, and bleeding from the bone ends may be difficult to control because of restricted access. This is due to damage to the inferior alveolar vessels and will usually stop once the bone ends have been approximated and temporarily immobilized. It sometimes helps to loop a stainless steel wire or suture around the teeth on either side of the fracture site, to pull the bone ends together as a temporary measure.

A particularly difficult area is severe postnasal bleeding into the oropharynx in association with a fracture of the maxilla. The bleeding appears to be coming down from behind the soft palate and is not controlled by simple nasal packs. In this situation the bleeding is often from an associated skull base fracture. Bleeding of this type may be life threatening and many units of blood may be lost.

The following should be considered:

- secure the airway first. Intubation with a cuffed tube is often possible if the blood pooled in the oropharynx is sucked out. If unsuccessful, proceed quickly to a surgical airway. It may also help to raise the head of the trolley to reduce the venous pressure in the head;
- pass a Foley catheter back through each nostril until they can be seen behind the soft palate. Inflate the balloons and then pull them forwards to exert local pressure

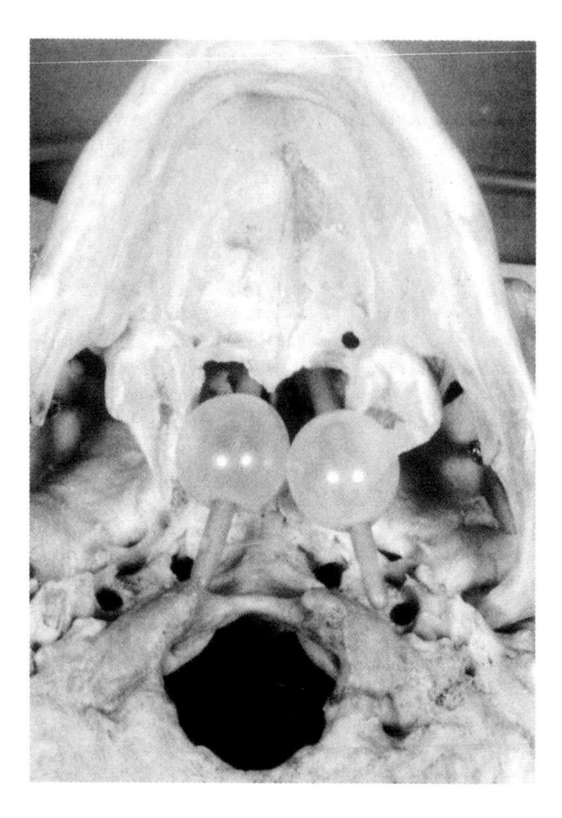

Figure 8.6 Illustration of insertion of bilateral Foley catheters inserted via the nostrils to help control bleeding from the nasopharynx.

to the mucosa in the area (*Figure 8.6*). It may then be necessary to insert anterior nasal packs. The 'Epistat™' device with anterior and posterior balloons may be used to the same end. Once the balloons are inflated, a finger may be inserted into the back of the mouth to push the back of the mobile maxilla up against the inflated bulb;

- consider hypovolaemic resuscitation maintaining the systolic pressure at 80 mmHg until control has been achieved.

External bleeding from the scalp and soft tissues of the face is generally easy to bring under control with direct pressure or sutures. Resist the temptation to use electro-cautery blindly, or to try and apply artery clips deep in wounds without adequate vision, as it is easy to damage exposed branches of the facial nerve (7th cranial nerve) leading to paralysis of some of the facial muscles. This is particularly the case in the region of the parotid salivary gland.

The management of penetrating wounds of the neck has been discussed above.

Probing wounds in the neck may precipitate bleeding. Do not probe neck wounds breaching the platysma until the casualty is in an operating theatre where unexpected severe bleeding may be controlled surgically.

Dysfunction

The assessment of the level of consciousness in the primary survey by the AVPU method is carried out in the normal way. There are some specific considerations in the presence of head and neck injuries.

Maxillofacial injuries are often associated with head and eye injuries. Many of the casualties will be under the influence of alcohol or drugs and this may complicate the AVPU assessment. It is nonetheless essential to establish a baseline level of neurological deficit. This must be reassessed at intervals so that any deterioration is detected promptly and acted on. Speech may be slurred as a result of mouth and jaw injuries, and this will alter the patient's response to questions.

Eye injuries associated with maxillofacial injuries are easy to miss. Although not life threatening, the loss of sight even in one eye is a tragedy for the individual, and early diagnosis may prevent this. Swelling may have closed the eye and made it difficult to examine. Pupil reactivity may also be changed following a blow to that part of the face. A traumatic mydriasis, for example, will cause one pupil to be larger than the other. It is essential to make at least a crude assessment of visual acuity at an early stage. This can be achieved even if the eye is too swollen to open by pushing a pen torch against the eyelid, and asking the casualty if they are aware of the light. The loss of vision in an eye may be reversible with treatment in the first few hours if it is due to a retrobulbar haemorrhage or optic nerve compression. The management of these conditions is beyond the scope of this chapter, but in this situation an urgent assessment by the ophthalmological team is required.

Exposure and environment

The casualty is completely undressed in preparation for the secondary survey. In-line immobilization of the cervical spine must be maintained as the patient's clothes are cut off. A–C are quickly reviewed.

8.3.2 Secondary survey

The secondary survey is of particular importance in the presence of maxillofacial injuries, as statistically there are often other injuries which are less evident, but which may be life threatening. This is particularly the case in road traffic accidents and fragmentation wounds from antipersonnel devices. In general, once the whole body has been exposed, the examination proceeds systematically from the head down to the feet. In this section, the important aspects of the secondary survey of the head and neck will be described. Observation and palpation are the key to examination of the head and neck.

Scalp

The scalp should be examined for lacerations and haematomas. Haematomas of the scalp may be misleading, and it is sometimes difficult to determine whether there is an underlying depressed fracture of the skull. Where there has been obvious significant blunt trauma to the scalp, regular head injury observations should be taken. Scalp lacerations should be gently probed with the gloved finger to detect fractures of the underlying skull.

Bruising and swelling

The swelling of the facial soft tissues may take some hours to develop fully. Soft tissue swelling will often mask fractures of the underlying facial skeleton, and radiographs may be the only way to make the diagnosis. For this reason, a depressed fracture of the zygoma is frequently missed. Similarly, a black eye may mask an underlying fracture of the orbitozygomatic complex, or damage to the globe of the eye. Le Fort fractures of the maxilla in particular are associated with gross facial swelling ('ballooning').

The bruises associated with skull base fractures may take 12 h or more to become apparent. The 'Panda eyes', bruising over the mastoid (Battles sign), or subconjunctival haemorrhage associated with skull base fractures or zygomatic fractures, may therefore not be obvious at an early stage.

Bruising of the neck, particularly when associated with noisy breathing and a hoarse voice should alert you to the possibility of a fracture of the larynx. Gentle palpation around the larynx may reveal crepitus.

Once the nature of the bruising has been observed, the bony margins of the facial bones should be palpated to detect step deformities.

Cerebrospinal fluid (CSF) leaks

The ear should be examined for the presence of blood and CSF in the external auditory meatus. It should be remembered that blood in the external ear may often be due to a tear in the anterior wall. This commonly occurs following a blow to chin forcing the head of the condyle of the mandible back through the tympanic plate, lacerating the lining of the anterior wall. For this reason a cut on the chin is frequently associated with blood in the external ear.

If there is a skull base fracture, CSF will not be seen if the tympanic membrane is intact. However, blood in the middle ear will cause the tympanic membrane to bulge outwards and have a blue appearance through the auroscope.

Detecting a CSF leak from the nostril may be difficult, as in the early stages it is mixed with blood or mucus. A leak of cerebrospinal fluid (CSF) down the nose is usually associated with fractures of the cribriform plate of the ethmoid, as a result of Le Fort II and III fractures of the maxilla, or fractures of the naso-orbital-ethmoid (NOE) complex. A tell-tale sign is 'tramlines' running down the cheek. These are caused by blood separating from the CSF to leave two outer lines of blood separated by CSF. They are not, however, diagnostic. After a day or two, as the bleeding stops, a more obvious watery discharge may become apparent. Where there remains doubt, further investigations such as T2 weighted MRI scans, or radio-isotope CSF studies may later be required.

Lacerations

Facial lacerations are often closed under local anaesthetic in the ED before transfer to the ward. Before closing the laceration consider the following.

- Has any branch of the facial nerve (VII cranial nerve) been divided? Microneural repair of the damaged nerve is much easier if carried out at initial wound closure in an operating theatre. Finding the fine branches as a secondary procedure after suturing can be almost impossible. The branches of the facial nerve are easily tested by asking the casualty to wrinkle the forehead, screw up the eyes and show the teeth. Particular care is needed with lacerations over the parotid salivary gland in front of the ear. Not only might the facial nerve be divided, but there may also be damage to the parotid duct.
- Is there a foreign body in the wound? Pieces of teeth or even whole incisor teeth may be concealed in a lacerated swollen lip, as may pieces of windscreen glass. If the wound is contaminated with grit, this must be thoroughly cleaned prior to closure or unpleasant tattooing may result.
- If there is a laceration of the neck, which appears on superficial examination to have perforated the platysma muscle, as in a stab wound, do not attempt to explore and

suture the wound under local anaesthesia in the ED. This may induce severe bleeding if major vessels such as the internal jugular are involved. The correct vascular instruments must be to hand before exploring such wounds. Resist the temptation blindly to try and clamp bleeding vessels in the neck. It is easy to clamp and damage important nerves such as the accessory (XIth) cranial nerve.

Examination of the eyes

Although damage to the eyes is not life threatening, detecting an eye injury with deteriorating vision within the first two hours, and seeking urgent help, may prevent permanent loss of vision. The pupil size and reactivity will have originally been noted as part of the AVPU assessment under D of the primary survey. Any change in size or reactivity should be noted over time to detect intracranial bleeding, or decreasing vision due to, for example, pressure on the optic nerve at the apex of the orbit. It is therefore important during the secondary survey to assess the eyes, and remove any contact lens. You should not be deterred by swelling around the eye. It may be necessary to delay a full ophthalmology assessment until the swelling has reduced but by shining a pen torch held against the swollen lids, it is possible at least to determine whether the visual pathway is intact. The conscious casualty will be able to tell you whether he sees the light through the eyelids. If uncooperative, the reaction of the other pupil may indicate that the visual pathway is intact.

The high incidence of missed injuries to the globe associated with cheekbone and orbital fractures has been well documented. In addition to assessing the visual acuity, if the eyelid swelling permits, look for the bloodshot eye (subconjunctival haemorrhage), examine the fundus, and test for double vision.

A subconjunctival haemorrhage may result from direct trauma to the eye, or, if the posterior limit of the bleeding is not visible, may be due to blood tracking forwards from a fracture of the orbit or cheekbone. Remember that subconjunctival haemorrhage arising from a fracture may take some hours to develop.

Double vision if present may indicate oedema in the orbit, or a blowout fracture of the orbital walls, usually the orbital floor.

Where are the teeth?

As far as possible, any missing teeth or pieces of broken denture should be accounted for. They may have been left at the scene of the accident, but consider the possibility of inhalation, particularly if the casualty was unconscious. The other possibilities to consider are:

- buried in a lip laceration, as a foreign body;
- inhaled;
- ingested.

An inhaled tooth may cause serious lung complications, and its presence must be detected as soon as possible. On the chest radiograph, a complete tooth is most likely to be seen in the right main bronchus. Here it may be obscured by the right heart shadow and easily overlooked. It is essential that inhaled teeth are removed by bronchoscopy at the earliest opportunity. Smaller pieces of tooth may work their way further down into the bronchial tree and be more difficult to remove. Swallowed teeth usually pass through the gut uneventfully.

When examining the mouth, look for any tongue lacerations, which may bleed profusely and cause airway obstruction. A step in the occlusal plane of the teeth or an obvious dental malocclusion may signify a fracture of the mandible or maxilla.

8.4 Summary

This chapter has dealt with the management of maxillofacial injuries in the first two hours after arrival in the ED, and has emphasized the management of the airway and control of bleeding. The need to stabilize the cervical spine, detect decreasing vision, and watch for neurological deterioration in this first two hours has also been stressed. The key to safe management is a seamless interface between pre-hospital and hospital care, and good communication with the surgical teams who will undertake the definitive care and reconstruction of the injuries. The exact diagnosis of the facial fractures at this initial stage has not been necessary other than to identify injuries may be potentially life threatening.

A summary of the clinical features of the most common fractures is attached in an Appendix at the end of this chapter.

Appendix

Clinical features of facial and laryngeal fractures

Injuries to the larynx and trachea

- Evidence of direct trauma to the neck (bruising and swelling).
- Noisy breathing (snoring, gurgling, croaking).
- A hoarse voice.
- Crepitus on palpation.

Fractures of the mandible

- Pain on jaw movement.
- Swelling and bruising.
- Bleeding from the mouth.
- The upper and lower teeth do not meet properly.
- Step in the occlusal plane of the teeth.
- Numbness of the chin and lower lip on that side (trauma to the inferior alveolar nerve).
- Mobility at the fracture site.

Fractures of the maxilla

- Ballooning of the soft tissues of the face.
- The upper and lower teeth do not meet properly (possible anterior open bite).
- The middle of the face may look flat before the swelling hides it.

- Numbness of the skin of the cheeks (infra-orbital nerve).
- Cerebrospinal fluid leak from the nose if associated anterior skull base fracture.
- The upper jaw can be moved:
  - In a Le Fort I fracture only the tooth bearing portion of the maxilla is mobile;
  - Le Fort II fracture – the bridge of the nose moves with the maxilla;
  - Le Fort III fracture – both cheekbones move with the maxilla.

Fracture of the zygoma

- Black eye (circumorbital ecchymosis).
- Bloodshot eye (sub-conjunctival haemorrhage).
- Numbness of the skin of the cheek and upper lip on that side.
- Loss of prominence over body of zygoma.
- Possible double vision, particularly on upwards gaze.
- Unilateral nosebleed.

Fracture of the naso-orbital ethmoid complex

- Swollen and deformed bridge of nose.
- Deepening of the angle between the nose and forehead (the depression of the root of the nose makes the nostrils more prominent from the front ('pigs snout').
- Nosebleed with possible CSF leak.
- The eyes may appear to be too far apart due to the detachment of the medial canthi (traumatic telecanthus).

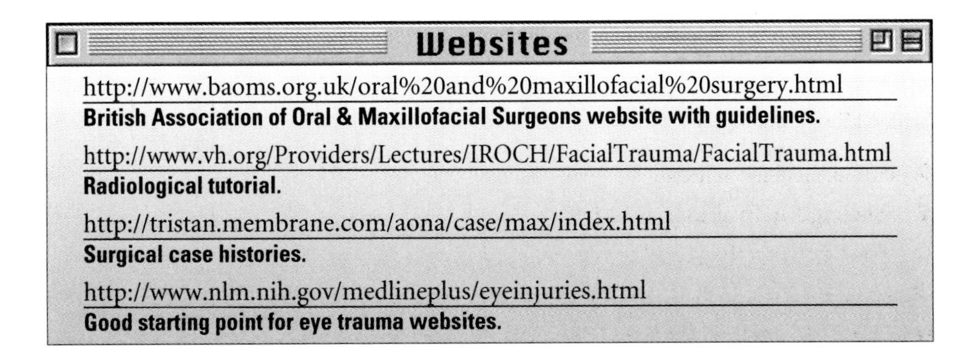

Websites

http://www.baoms.org.uk/oral%20and%20maxillofacial%20surgery.html
British Association of Oral & Maxillofacial Surgeons website with guidelines.

http://www.vh.org/Providers/Lectures/IROCH/FacialTrauma/FacialTrauma.html
Radiological tutorial.

http://tristan.membrane.com/aona/case/max/index.html
Surgical case histories.

http://www.nlm.nih.gov/medlineplus/eyeinjuries.html
Good starting point for eye trauma websites.

Further reading

1. **Al-Qurainy A, Stassen LFA, Dutton GN, *et al.*** (1991) The characteristics of midface fractures and the association with ocular injury: a prospective study. *Br J Oral Maxillofacial Surg* **29:** 291.
2. **Hutchison I, Lawlor M & Skinner D** (1992) Major maxillofacial injuries. In Skinner D, Driscoll P and Earlam R (eds). *ABC of Major Trauma*. BMJ, London, pp. 33–37.
3. **Maran AGD, Stell PM, Murray Jam, *et al.*** (1981) Early management of laryngeal injuries. *J Royal Soc Med* **74:** 656.

4. Schmelzeisen R & Gellrich NC (1999) The primary management of soft tissue trauma. In Ward Booth P, Schendel SA and Hausamen JE (eds). *Maxillofacial Surgery.* Churchill Livingstone, Edinburgh, pp. 229–244.
5. Shepherd JP, Shapland M, Scully C, *et al.* (1990) Pattern, severity and aetiology of injury in assault. *J Royal Soc Med* **83:** 75.
6. Telfer M, Jones GM, Shepherd JP (1991) Trend in the aetiology of maxillofacial fractures in the UK (1977–1987). *Br J Oral Maxillofacial Surg* **29:** 250.
7. Ward Booth RP, Brown J & Jones K (1989) Cricothyroidotomy: a useful alternative to tracheostomy in maxillofacial surgery. *Int J Oral Maxillofacial Surg* **18:** 24.

9 Soft tissue and extremity injury

G Andrew, L Light

Objectives

At the end of this chapter you should understand:

- the pathophysiology of wound healing;
- how to assess and manage soft tissue injuries;
- how to assess and manage common fractures in the emergency department (ED).

9.1 Introduction

Soft tissue and extremity trauma is rarely fatal. It is axiomatic in the early management of multiply injured patients that injuries should be dealt with in a logical and orderly fashion, in an order dictated by the threat to life and survival. This places the majority of lacerations and fractures into a category of less importance apart from a few unusual circumstances. However, it is important to consider such injuries for several reasons.

- They are very common, and relatively minor injuries of this nature compose a significant part of the workload of Emergency Departments (ED).
- Some extremity injuries can be life-threatening *per se* (for example, traumatic amputation of a limb, pelvic fractures, penetrating injuries involving major limb arteries).
- Some extremity injuries may be limb threatening (for example popliteal artery injury due to knee dislocation) (*Figure 9.1*).
- Although mortality from such injuries may be relatively low, they are a frequent cause of prolonged and sometimes severe morbidity. It is a fact that litigation is commonly a result of patient dissatisfaction with the long-term results of a relatively minor musculoskeletal injury despite exemplary management of major injuries.

Soft tissue injuries and extremity injuries may have important functional and cosmetic consequences. The cosmetic consequences may be depressingly obvious, and should not be dismissed lightly. The functional consequences include persistent pain, numbness, joint stiffness, weakness and deformity. Such problems may lead to difficulty in mobility and walking, impaired hand and upper limb function, and consequent difficulties with both work and recreation.

9.2 The pathophysiology of soft tissue and fracture healing

Skin injuries can be classified as contusions or abrasions (partial thickness damage to the skin), and lacerations (full thickness damage to the skin). Closed injuries can

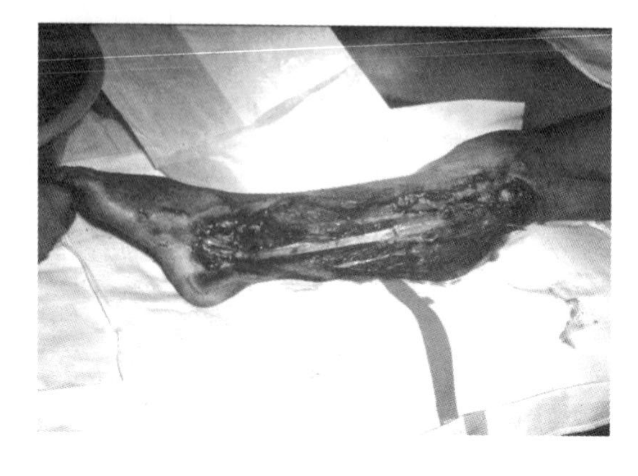

Figure 9.1 **Limb threatening injury – tissue loss, crushing and exposed, non-viable muscle. Victim run over by vehicle.**

involve full-thickness damage when the penetrating blood supply to the skin from the underlying fascia is sheared – this is known as a degloving injury and diagnosis is both difficult and important. Common causes of lacerations include knife injuries and injuries on glass. In older patients with fragile skin, lacerations can occur due to shearing of the skin, often over the front of the tibia. Skin wounds may heal by primary or by secondary intention.

9.2.1 Primary intention

A typical example of wound healing by primary intention is a surgical wound. The clean incision with a scalpel results in minimal tissue damage and contamination. The risks of infection are therefore low. The wound edges are brought together by suturing and consequently, the distance that must be traversed by the epidermis (on the skin surface) and granulation tissue (multiple capillary loops, deeper in the wound) is minimal. The wound is sealed to bacteria after one or two days, and has a functional level of wound strength (i.e. is unlikely to burst in any normal activity) within 3–4 weeks.

9.2.2 Secondary intention

Wound repair by secondary intention occurs in wounds that are left open, typically ragged or contaminated wounds. Even if contaminated material is thoroughly removed, the amount of damaged tissue and consequent necrosis will be much greater than in a clean wound. Further, the wound edges have not been brought together and the wound will initially be covered by a blood clot. This forms a protective scab over the underlying repair processes. The defect will be filled by granulation tissue, which in turn will be covered by migrating epidermis from the edges of the wound. Cicatrization (wound contracture) will reduce the size of the wound, making epithelialization faster. However, the wound contracture may give very poor cosmetic results and further may result in joint contractures if the wound crosses the flexor surface of a joint. Cicatrization typically continues for a period of approximately 6 months after the initial injury (*Figure 9.2*).

Wound healing by secondary intention is rather unreliable. The classic example is the varicose ulcer, over the distal shin. Such lesions may remain unhealed for a number of years, partly as a result of their precarious blood supply.

9.2.3 Peripheral nerve injuries

Nerve injuries occur most frequently due to lacerations, often on glass. They may also occur as a result of traction, giving rise to internal disruption of the nerve. It is commonly seen in the brachial plexus, often in motorcyclists who have fallen at high speed onto their shoulder. The shoulder is forced distally, causing massive distraction forces on the brachial plexus. Suturing techniques can be used to repair lacerations of peripheral nerves, but traction injuries are not usually amenable to operative intervention. The prognosis for nerve injuries (whether repaired or not) is relatively poor in adults.

Healing in the central nervous system occurs only by formation of scar (glial) tissue, with no attempt at nerve regeneration. In contrast, nerve regeneration does occur in the peripheral nervous system, but it is, however, rather unreliable. Nerve injuries are typically divided into three grades.

- Neurapraxia occurs due to crushing of the nerve. This is a recoverable condition where the nerve fibre remains viable. Regeneration does not need to take place, and recovery is relatively rapid;
- Axonotmesis follows a more severe crush or traction injury. The nerve sheath is not physically divided but the peripheral part of the nerve dies and regeneration is required. As the nerve sheath has not been divided, regeneration will eventually lead to reasonable recovery of function;
- Neurotmesis is the complete division of a nerve. Even after optimal repair, recovery is slow and typically proceeds, at best, at 1 mm per day. An injury proximal in the limb may therefore take over a year to reach maximum recovery.

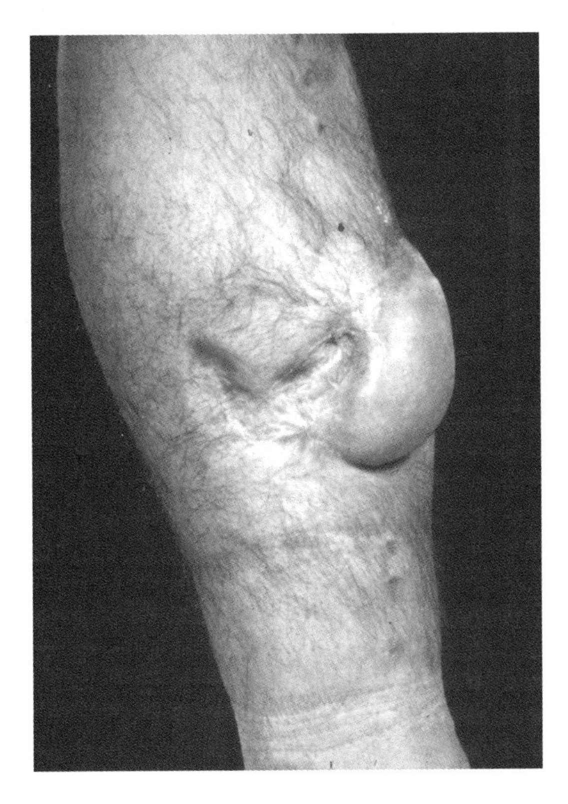

Figure 9.2 Leg wound, partially closed by reconstruction (bulging area); the remainder by secondary intention (scarring).

9.2.4 Vascular injuries

Vascular injuries can occur after lacerations or blunt trauma. A typical example is damage to the popliteal artery after a knee dislocation. Although the artery is not totally disrupted, stretching of the artery leads to damage to the intima and blocking of the arterial lumen. Such vascular injuries clearly lead to a substantial risk of severe ischaemia in the distal part of the limb. It is essential to recognize such ischaemia to avoid catastrophic damage to susceptible tissues such as muscle and nerve.

Severe vascular trauma often require repair to avoid amputation. Alternatively, if they are not recognized, gangrene may occur. Less severe injuries, or injuries in fit patients, may resolve by establishing an adequate collateral circulation – this may permit survival of the part, but not permit normal function, for example, it may cause intermittent claudication. Some vascular injuries causing occlusion will recanalize and resolve over time.

9.2.5 Tendon injuries

Tendon injuries may occur due to lacerations or to degenerative change. Surgical repairs permit healing by scarring but this may also lead to tethering of the tendon to the surrounding tissues. It is a particular problem in the hand where lacerations of the flexor tendons of the fingers may be followed by severe scarring between the tendon and tendon sheath. This may limit movement in the digits so much that the functional results are very poor (*Figure 9.3*).

Degenerative tendon injuries are common in middle-aged and elderly patients. The most frequent single tendon affected is the Achilles tendon. However, the rotator cuff, the quadriceps and patella tendons, and the biceps tendon are also frequently affected.

9.2.6 Fracture healing (Box 9.1)

Fractures are repaired by a highly organized process and in most cases, results in full functional restitution of the bone; this is termed *union* of the fracture. The phases of fracture repair seen in the shafts of bones (the callus response) are:

- haematoma;
- inflammation and granulation tissue;
- formation of woven bone matrix (intramembranous or endochondral);
- remodelling to lamellar bone.

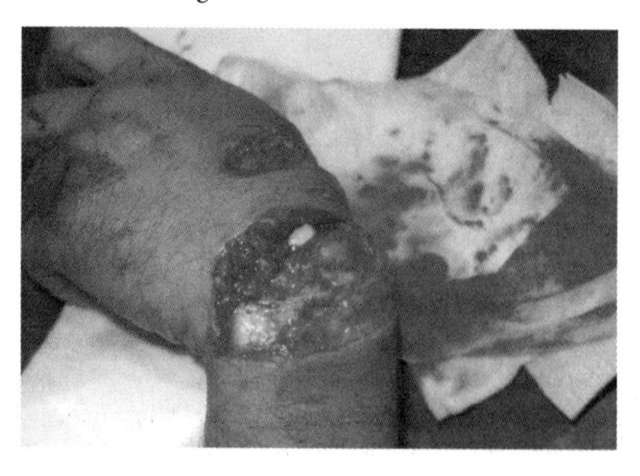

Figure 9.3 Deep laceration involving tendons of the wrist.

BOX 9.1	Three modes of fracture healing
	• External callus • Intramedullary (endosteal) callus • Primary cortical healing

These stages are the same as those seen in soft tissue wound repair, except that the matrix elaborated by the proliferating cells is bone (and not fibrous tissue), and that skin epithelium does not play a part. The matrix formed is first woven bone and then eventually the mature form of lamellar bone. The woven bone matrix becomes calcified and sufficiently strong to afford mechanical stability to the fracture (*Figure 9.4*).

Mechanical stability is much greater if the fracture callus is located circumferential to the bone (*periosteal* or external callus). If this fails to form, perhaps because of severe periosteal damage in a high-energy fracture, the fracture will be unable to heal promptly. A state of *delayed union* has occurred. Provided the fracture is adequately splinted, however, it can still heal by the formation of *intramedullary or endosteal* callus; this is a slower process. However, endosteal callus formation can also be a rapid event in an undisplaced fracture, or in metaphyseal fractures. In these cases little periosteal callus will be seen.

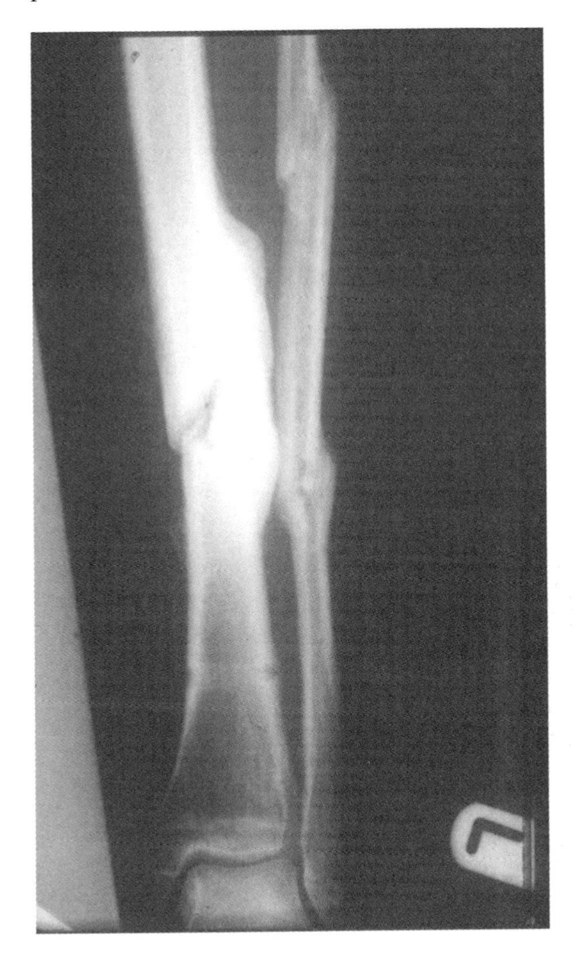

Figure 9.4 A fracture healed by external callus formation. The callus has not obliterated the fracture gap, but has 'grown' past the fracture.

The callus response described above is prevented if *all* fracture site movement is abolished. Under these circumstances, fracture union may be achieved by the process of normal bone remodelling, directly across the fracture gap. This is known as 'primary cortical healing'. It is frequently seen in fractures that are rigidly fixed with stainless steel plates attached to the bone. The disadvantages of this type of treatment are the risk of introducing infection at the time of plating, and its slowness, with the bone frequently taking over a year to return to a functional level of strength. Therefore, the use of rigid stainless steel plate fixation for fractures is now less widespread than it was 20 years ago

When fractures occur in *cancellous bone*, the method of healing is different again. There is usually a weak external callus response, but healing proceeds by 'creeping substitution'. Here the fractured cancellous bone ends join directly by establishing a bridge of woven bone. Such healing may be seen in fractures such as intertrochanteric femoral fractures, and in fractures of the condylar ends of long bones, including intra-articular fractures.

If all these possible modes of healing fail to occur, a state of established *nonunion* exists. Such a fracture will probably not heal without surgical intervention.

9.3 Clinical assessment of soft tissue injuries in the limbs

The vast majority of soft tissue wounds will be assessed and managed during the secondary survey. Management in the primary survey is usually limited to applying pressure dressings to those wounds that are bleeding heavily and covering others with sterile dressings to minimize the risk of infection.

9.3.1 History

Details of the mechanism of injury must be obtained. This allows the likely degree of contamination to be determined, but also may reveal other possible injuries. Thus, limbs run over by the wheel of a vehicle often sustain a degloving type injury, where the skin is sheared off the underlying tissues. This type of injury is often difficult to assess and may require exploration. Some elements of the history are vital. Gunshot wounds with a high-energy projectile require a different approach from an injury due to a low energy transfer. Paint injection injuries have a well-deserved reputation for bad outcomes in the fingers, but may initially appear innocuous.

- Causes of injury:
  - Sharp laceration:
    - On glass;
    - With a knife;
    - With a garden digger (with likely associated contamination).
  - Gunshot wound.
  - Blast injury.
  - Degloving injury (e.g. limb run over).
  - Injection injury (e.g. high pressure paint gun).
- Time since injury.

BOX 9.2	Nursing assessment of patient with soft tissue injury
	• History of present condition • Mechanical or medical condition precipitating injury • Last intake of fluid and diet • General health status • Medications, current and past (including use of drugs socially) • Allergies • Smoking • Antitetanus status • Family history In the elderly also consider: • Patient profile and nutritional status • Tissue viability score and prevention • Mental and emotional state • Osteoporosis and loss of function • Medical causes for falls • Social history in preparation for discharge planning • MRSA status in elderly peoples homes/nursing homes • Spiritual considerations

- Other injuries present.
- Symptoms suggestive of serious deep injury:
  - Severe pain;
  - Loss of function (e.g. inability to weight bear);
  - Numbness.

Some patients have medical problems that may compromise wound healing:

- steroid usage;
- diabetes mellitus;
- smoking;
- peripheral vascular disease;
- malnutrition.

It may not be possible to alter these, but it is often appropriate to refer these patients for specialist advice, as the risks of complications, infection or wound failure are higher.

Once the above has been completed, it is essential that a nursing member of the team performs a physical, psychological and social assessment of the patient as the foundation for planning and implementing nursing care. The key features are shown in Box 9.2.

9.3.2 Examination

It is surprisingly easy to miss soft tissue or bony injuries. To avoid this, fully expose the patient and examine the whole body in a systematic fashion. From the orthopaedic perspective:

- look – and compare with the other side;

- feel for tenderness or swelling. Feel the skin temperature and pulses and compare with the other side. Assess sensation;
- move – both actively and passively and compare with the other side.

Many patients with limb injuries will require x-rays. These and other investigations are *never* a substitute for adequate clinical examination in patients with limb injuries.

Occasionally, soft tissue injuries can be limb threatening (see Box 9.3). It is essential not to miss these injuries in patients with multiple injuries involving the torso or head. They may also present in isolation. They are rare – but must be recognized.

One important feature common to limb-threatening injuries is the risk of vascular compromise to important structures. Muscle, in particular, is vulnerable to relatively short periods of ischaemia. Once muscle cells have died, they cannot be replaced and permanent impairment or disability is likely. Vascular damage is possible even if pulses are normal, for example, with an intimal tear or with compartment syndrome, and should be assessed as described below. The signs of vascular impairment are listed in Box 9.4.

BOX 9.3 Limb-threatening injuries

- Vascular injury at or proximal to elbow or knee
- Major joint dislocation
- Crush injury
- Compartment syndrome
- Open fracture
- Fracture with neurovascular injury

BOX 9.4 Signs of vascular impairment

Pain
Pallor
Perishing cold
Pulseless – this is *not* due to vascular spasm in the patient in front of you!
Paraestheseae
Paralysis

In assessing soft tissue injuries, it is essential to have an adequate understanding of the anatomy of the area affected by the injury. A deep laceration on the dorsum of the forearm has different implications from one on the palmar surface of the wrist; the latter may typically affect arteries and nerves as well as tendons. It must also be recognized that penetrating trauma may penetrate a considerable distance. Therefore, all patients with such trauma must have an assessment of structures underlying the area of the laceration, including muscles, tendons, arteries and veins, nerves and bones. If it is not possible to exclude damage, it is wise to seek advice, as the wound should probably be formally explored to exclude significant underlying injury.

The most obvious way to describe the laceration is to quantify the size and depth of the hole that has been created. However, the state of the health of the edges of the wound is often crucial. Similarly, the degree of contamination must be assessed to judge the risk of infection. The combination of devitalized tissue and contamination is highly likely to lead to subsequent infection of the wound. This has important implications for how the wound should be managed.

When assessing the damage due to penetrating trauma, consider the patient's posture at the time of impact

Lacerations on glass require a cautious approach. An x-ray is mandatory to exclude the presence of retained fragments of glass. Most glass is radio-opaque. As glass is sharp, late injuries may occur due to retained glass fragments that move relative to the surrounding structures in normal limb movement. Substantial injuries including nerve lacerations have been described. Consequently, exploration to remove all but the tiniest fragments of glass is required. A second x-ray should be obtained subsequently to confirm that the fragments have been removed.

Clinical assessment should include examination of the following.

Nerves

Assessment of abnormal sensation early after injury may be very difficult. Patients often report the presence of sensation even when the relevant nerve supply has clearly been divided. In general, ask the patient whether sensation is normal and the same as on the other side, rather than whether sensation is present. Simple touch and moving sensation should be addressed. The examination of sharp sensation is traditionally employed, but use of hypodermic needles is not really helpful. Pressure with a somewhat blunter device (e.g. paperclip) is better. The area of abnormal sensation should be mapped out and recorded. Assessment of motor power is more reliable, but this requires accurate anatomical knowledge to ensure that 'trick' movements are not used. Motor power is usually recorded using the MRC scale outlined in Box 9.5.

BOX 9.5 MRC scale for motor power

Grade 0	No movement
Grade 1	Flicker of movement only
Grade 2	Movement not sufficient to overcome gravity
Grade 3	Movement sufficient to overcome gravity, but no additional resistance
Grade 4	Reduced power
Grade 5	Normal

If there is a suggestion of nerve injury on the basis of abnormal sensation or power, the wound should be explored and nerve repair considered. This requires good exposure, lighting, magnification, general anaesthesia and a bloodless field. This is best undertaken in the environment of the operating theatre.

Vessels

Assessment of vascular damage should include examination of skin pallor, capillary refill time, skin temperature and skin turgor. Examination of distal pulses is vital. This can be done by palpation, although the use of a Doppler device may be helpful if this is difficult. It must be recalled that vascular injuries may be present even if the distal pulses are present, and an overall assessment of vascularity should be made. If injury to a major limb artery is suspected, there is a requirement to assess this on an urgent basis, to minimize warm ischaemia time and the associated tissue damage (especially to muscle). In any event, warm ischaemia must be kept less than 5 h, so there is substantial urgency in dealing with these injuries. In patients with a probable major vascular injury an angiogram should be obtained – this may be preoperative or during the operation.

Vascular injuries are associated with a risk of substantial blood loss, particularly with penetrating injuries. Appropriate vascular access, fluids and blood cross-matching is required.

Tendons

Tendon injuries are frequent in lacerations of the limbs, with the commonest situation being injuries in the hand and wrist. Examination of these injuries should be informed by the knowledge that tendons often (usually!) retract out of the wound, and may not be evident on inspection of the wound. Sometimes an empty tendon sheath can be seen. If there is a suspicion of tendon injury, formal exploration is required with a view to tendon repair if necessary. Understanding of the anatomy of likely tendon injuries is vital; thus examination of the joint powered by the tendon is required.

It is important to understand the principles of assessment of the hand and wrist after a laceration, as these are particularly common.

- Inspection of the hand will reveal a normal arcade of finger positions, which will move in a characteristic fashion when the wrist is flexed and extended. If this does not occur after a laceration, it is likely that a tendon injury has occurred.
- The flexor digitorum profundus (FDP) powers the proximal and distal interphalangeal (DIP) joint of the fingers; while the flexor digitorum superficialis (FDS) powers the proximal interphalangeal (PIP) joint.
- Lacerations over the middle phalanx can only injure the FDP, which will cause paralysis of the DIPJ.
- Lacerations over the proximal phalanx or in the palm can injure both FDS and FDP. If both tendons are cut, then the finger will be immobile.
- If only the FDS is injured, it may nonetheless be possible to move both PIP and DIP joints with the FDP.
- To resolve whether the FDS is injured, assess the flexion of the PIP joint with the examiner holding the other fingers fully extended. This immobilizes FDP, as this is a mass action muscle where all of the tendon slips must act together. If the FDS is acting, with the FDP immobilized, the DIP joint will be flaccid despite the PIP joint movement.

9.3.3 Exploration and repair

The decision that no underlying structures are damaged can only be made if the wound has been properly explored, along with an appropriate clinical examination of the function of any underlying tendons, nerves and vessels. Failure to adequately diagnose injuries may lead to unsatisfactory results (late repairs are often less successful) and consequent litigation.

Foreign bodies in general should be removed if they are visible in the wound. If a foreign body is present but it is not visible, it is not advisable to attempt removal in the Emergency Department by probing of the wound with forceps. This is unlikely to be

The application of a tourniquet to control bleeding and permit exploration is rarely indicated in the Emergency Department. If bleeding is sufficiently severe to obscure visualization of the wound, formal exploration under optimal conditions is indicated. Exploration under inadequate anaesthesia with a restless patient, inadequate lighting and instruments, no assistance and considerable time pressure is not a recipe for success!

rewarded by success, but more likely to push the foreign body further into the wound. In particular it will obscure the track of the foreign body in the wound, making subsequent exploration in theatre more difficult. Exploring the hand or foot will frequently demand an avascular field, general anaesthetic and image intensifier screening to find the extraneous material without damaging any other structures.

9.3.4 Pain

Pain is associated with both soft tissue and bony injuries and nursing and medical staff have a responsibility to try and establish good pain control at an early stage. Initially, nonpharmacological intervention in the form of elevation of limbs, immobilization or support in slings or the application of ice should also be considered. Entonox can also be used for short-term relief. However, once a diagnosis has been made and resuscitation performed where necessary, analgesia can be given in the form of morphine, intravenously (see Section 16.3). Nerve blocks, particularly femoral nerve block, may be considered as an alternative in the elderly injured patients with femoral neck fractures, to reduce the risks of respiratory depression and sedation. Whichever technique is used, the patient's pain score should be recorded before administration of analgesia and after for evaluation of pain relief gained.

9.4 Simple wound closure

Simple lacerations, particularly if superficial (i.e. affecting only the skin and subcutaneous fat), may reasonably be treated under local anaesthesia in the Emergency Department. Prior to closing the wound it must have been thoroughly cleaned, irrigated and explored to ensure that there are no extensions that cannot be seen and assessed. In order to obtain good results from suturing, practice is essential. Deeper tissues are usually sutured using an absorbable suture, whereas the skin may be sutured using either an absorbable or nonabsorbable suture.

9.4.1 Materials used for wound closure

Suturing.	Reliable, strong, versatile, time honoured; requires some skill and equipment and anaesthesia.
Adhesive strips.	Reliable in wounds not under stress or movement, good cosmesis, spread tension on the wound; may fall off in moist wounds or if there is a lot of blood.
Adhesive.	Reliable for small wounds; no need for anaesthetic.

Some apparently simple lacerations pose particular problems:

- eyelids – scarring may be disastrous – refer to plastic or ophthalmic surgeons;
- pretibial flap lacerations – often associated with paper like skin, especially in older patients. Better to use taping techniques for closure, but risks of complication still high. Follow up carefully, and ask patient to stay off their feet if possible.

Severely contaminated wounds require adequate cleaning before closure. Material such as grease, soil, coal dust or paint must be removed to maximize the chances of healing without complications, and to give the best cosmetic result. For particulate material (grit, soil), if this is not removed primarily, it is usually not possible to get rid of this as a secondary procedure. Unpleasant tattooing of the wound may follow. The principles of adequate wound cleaning are (in order of increasing vigour):

- irrigation with clear fluid;
- use of pulsed lavage (high pressure irrigation);
- physical removal of material with forceps; and
- scrubbing with a brush.

Anaesthesia sufficient to permit the required level of activity will be required. Wounds requiring more than the first level of irrigation should be left open at initial exploration. Wounds may subsequently be closed at an interval of a few days (delayed primary closure) or longer, up to 2 weeks (secondary closure). Delayed primary closure gives results that are very similar to those of primary closure, with a dramatic decrease in the risk of wound sepsis as a result of the thorough debridement and drainage for a few days while the tissue swelling settles. Extensive lacerations should be referred for assessment by an appropriate surgical specialty.

9.4.2 Suturing a wound

You cannot learn to suture a wound from a book, but it is reasonable to indicate some of the key points. This technique can be best learnt, like most manual skills, by having it demonstrated and then practising under supervision.

To suture a simple laceration under local anaesthesia you will need the following.

Drapes

- Needle holding (suture) forceps; dissecting forceps; suture scissors.
- Antiseptic and irrigation fluid (saline), sterile drapes.
- Local anaesthetic (usually 1% lidocaine in an adult, max 3 mg/kg).
- Needles (22 g) and syringes.
- Swabs, receivers.
- Sutures: typically 4/0 nylon for the skin and 2/0 vicryl for subcutaneous tissues. Finer sutures (5/0 or 6/0) should be used on the face to minimize scarring.
- Adequate illumination.

Simple, interrupted sutures

- Expose the wound; the patient must be comfortable and warm.

- Clean the wound with irrigation and swabs so the wound edges are well defined.
- Isolate the wound with sterile drapes.
- Infiltrate the wound edges with local anaesthetic using an appropriate sized needle. Most patients get some pain from this as the local anaesthetic is a fairly strong alkali.
- The suture needle is held with the forceps, half way along the curve.
- The skin edges are held *gently* with toothed forceps and the point of the needle introduced vertically through the skin, 3–4 mm from the wound edge.
- Pass the needle through the tissues using a rotational movement of the forceps.
- The needle should exit the opposite side of the wound, equidistant from the edge and be grasped with the forceps.
- Remove the needle, again in a rotational movement, taking care not to pull the suture completely through the wound.
- Form a knot either by hand or using the forceps, using enough tension to bring the skin edges together.
- Cut the excess suture material, leaving sufficient length to allow easy removal.
- Clean once more and apply a dressing.
- Sutures may be removed at or 7–10 days from most sites or after 4–5 days on the face.

In deep lacerations, the subcutaneous tissues will need to be coapted using interrupted sutures prior to closing the skin.

Local anaesthetics

- Are toxic at excessive doses (nausea, tremor, convulsions, cardiac arrhythymias).
- Can be used with adrenaline (epinephrine) to minimize bleeding and to retain the local where it is needed (but *not* in the digits, nose, penis or on flap lacerations).
- Can be used for field blocks (infiltration), ring blocks (on digits) or regional blocks.
- Takes a few minutes to work – patience is required.
- Rarely provides complete anaesthesia to touch, but should block pain.

9.4.3 Records

It is essential to maintain adequate records. If wounds or lacerations are present, a diagram and description should be included in the documentation.

9.5 Extensive wounds

If a wound is non-closable, a variety of techniques are available:

- a small wound in an area with limited cosmetic importance, no risk of joint contracture – clean and allow to heal by secondary intention;

otherwise:

- skin grafts will take on muscle, granulation tissue or well vascularized periosteum. They will not take on bare bone or cartilage. Split thickness grafts are used most frequently and are taken with a skin graft knife;

BOX 9.6 Key points – skin wounds

- Soft tissue injuries must be assessed in the overall context of the patient – e.g. is the patient hypovolaemic due to an associated injury?
- Vital signs must be recorded and monitored other than in trivial injuries.
- Assess which structures may have been injured – is formal exploration required?
- Assess degree of tissue damage and contamination – is primary closure indicated?
  - If yes:
    - cleaning and primary closure under appropriate anaesthesia
    - consider prophylactic antibiotics
  - If no, consider:
    - cleaning/debridement and delayed primary closure?
    - cleaning/debridement and healing by secondary intention
    - referral for flap or skin graft closure.

- flaps are 'paddles' of more than one tissue (skin, fat and often muscle). They may be raised and moved with a local pedicle to support them, or moved to a remote site with microvascular anastomosis of artery and veins from the flap to appropriate local vessels.

The specialized judgement of whether to use a graft or a flap is the province of a plastic surgeon. In general, grafts are relatively rapid and simple but are prone to shrinkage and the skin graft donor sites are often painful. Flaps are much more extensively used than previously; this follows the remarkable expansion in microsurgical technology and ability, so that free flaps are now widely employed. They are often time consuming to perform, and have a variable failure rate.

9.6 Specialized wounds

9.6.1 Gunshot wounds

These injuries are relatively uncommon in the UK, but present intermittently in all countries. They may arise from low or high velocity projectiles. The clinical consequences are dependent on both the energy transfer to the surrounding tissues (see Box 9.7) and the path of the missile.

The kinetic energy (KE) is proportional to the missile's velocity and mass:

$$KE = m \times v^2/2$$

Velocity is the major determinant of KE, hence a rifle bullet will have considerably greater KE than a knife blade, despite a much smaller mass.

It is the impact velocity that determines the kinetic energy available for transfer to the tissues, not the velocity on leaving the weapon. If the missile impacts in the tissues and fails to exit, all the KE will be transferred and the maximum amount of damage will have occurred for that particular missile. When a large amount of energy is transferred, tissues are pushed away from the missile track and two cavities are formed. A permanent cavity results from the immediate destruction of tissues in the direct path of the missile, while a temporary cavity results from the energy transferred to the tissues and distorting them. This temporary cavity only lasts a few milliseconds but can reach 30–40 times the size of the missile. As the energy is dissipated the tissues then return to their normal positions.

BOX 9.7 Factors affecting energy transfer from a missile

- Kinetic energy of the missile
- Presenting area of the missile
- The missile's tendency to deform and fragment
- The tissue density
- Tissue mechanical characteristics

Cavitation has three consequences. First, there is the functional and mechanical disruption to the tissues and neighbouring structures, the extent depending on the amount of energy transferred and the tissue characteristics. Solid organs, for example, the liver, spleen and kidneys, will sustain more damage than low-density organs, such as the lungs, as a result of their greater elasticity. Secondly, any material overlying the point of entry of the missile will be carried into the wound. The higher the impact velocity, the more widely the material is spread. Further contamination can also occur as a result of debris being sucked into the wound. Finally, if a missile traverses a narrow part of the body, then the exit wound is generally larger than the entry wound. This is due to the temporary cavity extending along the wound track to the point of exit.

Low velocity projectiles (most handguns or shotguns) transfer relatively small amounts of energy and cause damage mainly to the tissues that they traverse. Accordingly, these wounds may be treated in a similar fashion to other incised wounds, with appropriate exploration and wound closure. Many gunshots may result in non-radio opaque foreign bodies being driven into the wound, including the cartridge wadding in shotgun injuries and fragments of clothing. Shooting at close range may result in powder being driven into the skin or wound and local thermal injury (*Figure 9.5*). Exploration of these wounds is mandatory. It is important not to dismiss low-energy transfer injuries as unimportant – they can be fatal if they involve vital organs, for example the heart.

Conversely, high velocity gunshot wounds pose major problems as a result of the large amounts of energy transferred to the tissues. There is often a small entrance wound, but the exit wound may be very large. There are no absolute certainties and variations in the relative sizes of exit and entry wounds are well recognized. Significant cavitation occurs with these weapons as a result of the supersonic speed of the projectile that is extremely disruptive and may cause necrosis of an extensive amount of tissue. The following lessons had to be learnt repeatedly in the armed conflicts of the 20th century:

- high velocity GSWs should be explored to remove necrotic tissue. Excision of such tissue should be thorough, including soft tissues and bone;
- primary closure should not be attempted – it is extremely difficult to assess the amount of necrosis, and the extent of marginally viable tissue, at initial exploration. If there is bony injury, this should probably be treated with external fixation initially;
- secondary exploration, reconstruction and closure should then be undertaken within a few days.

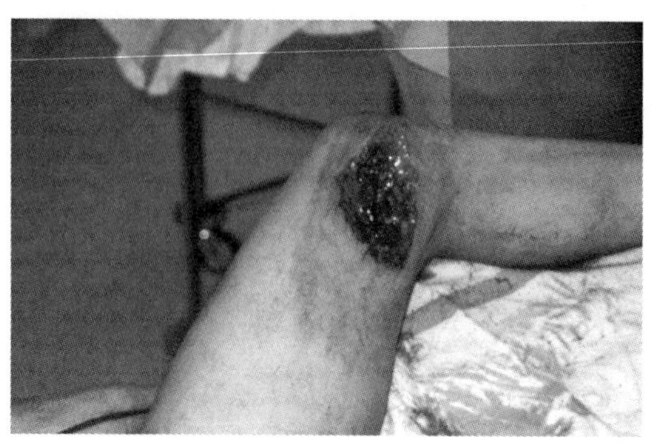

(a)

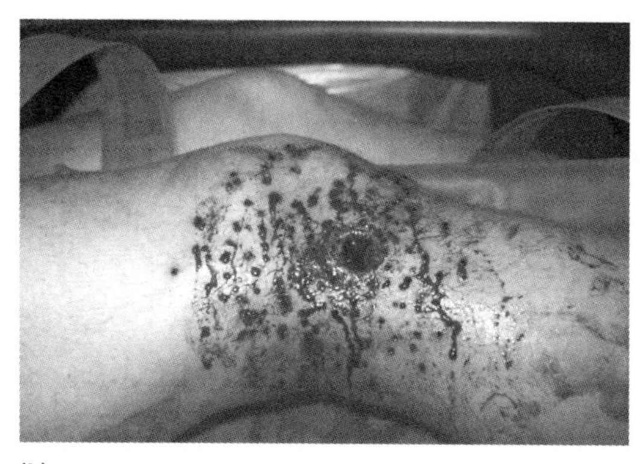

(b)

Figure 9.5 **(a) Gunshot wound to left knee. Note massive soft tissue wound. (b) Shotgun wound to right knee. Note 'peppering' effect from shot fragments.**

All GSWs must be taken seriously, but high energy GSWs, in particular, routinely require exploration. As well as considering the local effects of the projectile, attention should be paid to neurovascular and bony injuries. X-rays should be obtained to assess the presence of skeletal damage and the presence of foreign bodies including projectiles.

9.6.2 Blast injuries

Extremities may be injured by blast injuries. Such injuries may be associated with penetrating injury due to shrapnel, which may act as high or low velocity projectiles. As well as penetrating injury, the blast may lead to a closed injury arising from the shock wave. This leads, *per se*, to injury to vascular structures in soft tissues causing gross soft tissue swelling and ischaemia. Consequently, exploration may be required to decompress fascial compartments (fasciotomies) and assess the viability of tissue. Primary closure in such injuries is contraindicated.

9.7 Fractures

9.7.1 Assessment

History

The degree of violence sufficient to cause a fracture varies between patients. Older patients with osteoporosis may suffer fractures with minimal trauma, while younger patients may suffer high-energy injuries with no fractures. Such violence may be direct (assault with a blunt weapon) or indirect (twisting injury to planted foot causing a tibial fracture). Generally, a fall from greater than body height is described as a high-energy injury.

A further factor determining the degree of damage is the direction of the force. A fall to the tip of the shoulder is likely to be associated with a clavicle fracture, while a fall to the outstretched hand may lead to fractures more distally in the upper limb. Application of force to the front of the pelvis (during a RTA) may lead to an 'open book' type of fracture, whereas longitudinal force along the femur (from a head on impact during a RTA) may cause a shear fracture.

During the secondary survey, all patients must be assessed for the presence of other possible injuries on the basis of the history and mechanism of injury. Fractures of the extremities (especially open fractures) frequently look impressive but are rarely immediately life threatening.

Examination

Classic signs of a fracture include:

- pain;
- obvious deformity;
- tenderness at the fracture site; such tenderness is usually around the circumference of the bone and not just one part of it;
- swelling;
- redness;
- loss of function.

Fractured bones are often very painful in the early aftermath of injury. There is restricted use of the upper limb, and weight bearing is not usually possible in the case of lower limb injuries. Some fractures (especially pelvic and femoral fractures) are associated with considerable blood loss and will require appropriate resuscitation during the primary survey before a detailed assessment is carried out.

Gross displacement of the fracture may be associated with tenting of the overlying skin and the potential for skin breakdown. Similarly, severe displacement may lead to neurovascular compromise of the distal limb (*Figure 9.6*). For these reasons, it is sensible to correct such displacement upon completion of the ABC of the primary survey, without awaiting x-rays. In fractures at the midshaft level, establishing the presumptive diagnosis is usually easy. Conversely, injuries close to a joint may be more difficult to assess. Even with experience it may not be possible to differentiate these fractures from a fracture/dislocation or a simple dislocation. Reduction of such injuries is important to prevent skin and neurovascular consequences, but can be difficult. An x-ray prior to manipulation in these cases is usually essential. This helps to predict the direction of traction and manipulation that will be required.

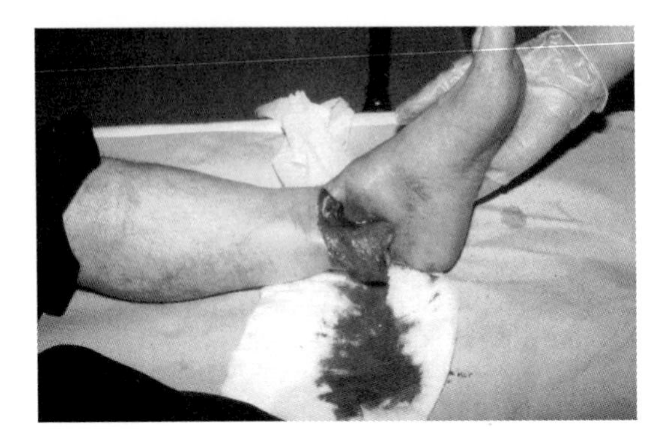

Figure 9.6 Fracture dislocation of the ankle.

Prior to obtaining x-rays, temporary splintage or support should be applied. In an upper limb fracture the use of a sling is usually sufficient at this stage, while in the lower limb a back slab or three-sided plastic splint may be used. This will minimize the pain due to both the fracture and the movement during the x-ray examination.

As a minimum, anteroposterior and lateral x-rays should be obtained and they should show the whole length of the bone. It is also important to obtain x-rays centred on the fracture adequately to understand the fracture anatomy. In frequent and typical fractures at the end of the bone (e.g. Colles fracture, malleolar fractures) it is acceptable to obtain an x-ray of the affected part only but it is essential to examine the whole of the affected bone for tenderness, mindful of possible patterns of injury, for example:

- injury of the medial malleollus may be associated with fracture of the proximal fibula (Maisoneuve fracture);
- fracture of the mid radius may be associated with a dislocation of the distal ulnar (Galeazzi fracture).

9.7.2 Interpretation of x rays

This requires practice. X-rays should always be examined on a light box. Fractures (*Figure 9.7*) are identified by:

- a break in the cortex of the bone on one or more of the views;
- a radiolucent line (in the case of a distracted fracture) or a radiodense line (in an impacted fracture) across part or all of the bone at the injury site;
- soft tissue swelling adjacent to the suspected site of the fracture (e.g. the prevertebral soft tissue shadow in neck injuries; lipohaemarthrosis in knee injuries, which suggests the presence of an intra-articular fracture).

The principal aspects of the *fracture pattern* that the x-rays should define include:

- is the fracture in the diaphysis, metaphysis or epiphysis? This predicts the healing potential and is important for planning what sort of fixation to use, if any;
- fracture pattern – is the fracture transverse, oblique or spiral? This indicates the stability of the fracture to axial loading after reduction and may determine whether operative treatment is required;
- does the fracture involve a joint surface; if so, is there displacement of the subchondral bone (and hence articular cartilage)? Is the fracture actually a fracture-

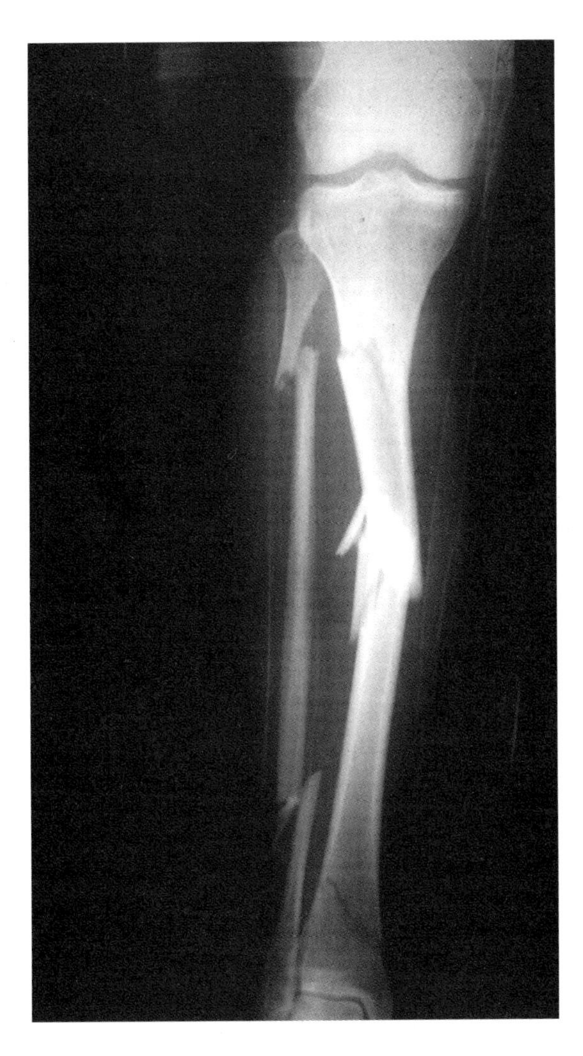

Figure 9.7 X-ray of lower leg demonstrating all the key features of a fracture.

dislocation or fracture-subluxation? These are associated with risks of secondary osteoarthritis and may indicate open reduction and internal fixation;

- does the fracture involve a growth plate (in children)? If the fracture line actually crosses it, this is associated with risk of growth disturbance.

It is frequently not possible to understand fully the fracture anatomy on the initial x-ray. Additional plain x-rays may be helpful, but a CT scan is often required to elucidate the situation and to plan fixation.

Sometimes it is not possible to identify a fracture on an initial x-ray. If careful clinical examination indicates the presence of signs of fracture (bony tenderness and swelling in the case of undisplaced fractures), there are the following possibilities:

- decide that it doesn't matter anyway (undisplaced fracture in an unimportant site) – think very carefully about this, it may be reasonable if the presence of a fracture would not really have any treatment implications (e.g. lesser toe);
- splint the limb and repeat the x-rays after a few days or a week. If the fracture is not visible on the original x-ray, it may become visible due to the healing reaction over

a few days. This approach is frequently used in scaphoid fractures, where a repeat x-ray (with repeat clinical examination) at 2 weeks is typically obtained;

- MRI scan. This is currently the most sensitive test for the presence of a fracture, as perifracture oedema is readily detected. It clearly depends on the availability of a scan, but is particularly valuable in patients with suspected but radiologically invisible proximal femoral fractures.

9.7.3 Early complications after a fracture

Impairment of circulation to the limb beyond the fracture

It is vital to check for the presence of pulses below the fracture, while keeping in mind the possibility that, even with palpable pulses, arterial damage may have occurred. Pulses may be present initially and then disappear, for instance with intimal flap tears of the arterial wall. The only adequate guard against ischaemia due to arterial injuries is repeated examination of temperature, sensation and pulses of limbs. If a vascular injury has occurred, an emergency vascular surgical assessment is needed (see above under soft tissue injuries).

Compartment syndrome

This is one of the most important complications of fractures. It is commonest after tibial fractures, but may occur in the absence of a fracture, often after a direct blow (e.g. a violent kick on the front of the quadriceps). Muscles in the limbs are invested in a fascial sheath, which only provides limited volume for expansion. When this volume change is exceeded (with swelling due to oedema or haematoma), the pressure in the sheath rises rapidly and soon exceeds capillary pressure. Tissue function including gas exchange and nutrition is then disrupted due to lack of capillary flow. *This condition may occur before there is any change in distal pulses,* because capillary pressure is so much lower than arterial pressure. The result of compartment syndrome may include muscle death, and permanent deformity with contracture (Volkmann's ischaemic contracture). The key clinical feature that should alert suspicion is the pain, which is greater than would be expected from the fracture, especially if the latter has been adequately immobilized. This occurs because muscle ischaemia is exceptionally painful. Paraesthesiae can also develop due to ischaemia affecting the nerve in the compartment. Compartment syndrome may be present very soon after a fracture, but more commonly develops in the days afterwards as swelling increases (see Box 9.8).

Box 9.8: Compartment syndrome

Common sites for compartment syndrome:

- Lower leg
- Forearm
- Hand
- Foot
- Thigh
- Buttock

Causes of compartment syndrome:

- Fractures
- Crush injury
- Reperfusion injury

Remember: severe pain after fracture, persisting after immobilization = compartment syndrome until proved otherwise

9.7.4 Management of fractures

Principles

- First-aid:
  - cover wounds with a clean (preferably sterile) dressing;
  - immobilization of the fracture using temporary external splintage The pain relief provided by adequate immobilization for a fracture has to be experienced to be believed;
  - administration of analgesia.
- Assess for neurovascular injury. Minimize gross deformity at once to minimize risk to neurovascular structures and overlying skin.

9.7.5 Assessing the severity of the fracture

The more energy dissipated in the tissues at the time of fracture, the greater the degree of tissue damage and the lower the probability of swift, problem-free fracture union. It is important to consider the likely fracture energy on the basis of the fracture history. The x-ray also contains clues as to the severity of injury. A high degree of comminution (multiple fragments), large distances between fragments, wide displacement between the main bone ends, gross overlap with shortening of the limb are all signs that a significant amount of energy was absorbed. In these cases, the deep soft tissues nourishing the bone will have been badly damaged.

One of the important clinical signs of fracture severity is damage to the soft tissues overlying the fracture. There may be an open wound, crushed or devitalized, but intact, skin. Secondary damage may continue if a grossly displaced fracture or dislocation is left to damage the skin; such an injury should be reduced without waiting for x-ray confirmation. All fractured limbs must be carefully inspected for wounds that might connect with the fracture site. As there is good evidence that many of the infections that occur in open fractures are hospital-acquired, in the Emergency Department:

(i) inspect the wound ONCE. If possible obtain a Polaroid or digital photograph;

(ii) cover the wound with a sterile dressing. A betadine soaked swab may help to minimize contamination;

(iii) do not re-expose the wound for further inspections until the patient is in theatre for wound exploration, debridement and lavage;

(iv) give antibiotics. Usually a cephalosporin (with metronidazole in the case of severe contamination).

Fractures with open wounds require emergency treatment (fracture to theatre time of 6 h or less). Wounds should be debrided, and copious wound irrigation carried out (8 l is usual for a tibial fracture). They should be managed by a combined approach by orthopaedic and plastic surgeons.

The severity of an open fracture can be graded as follows (Gustilo and Anderson, 1976):

1. wound caused by protrusion of bone (inside to out), < 1 cm, minimal contamination;
2. wound < 5 cm, minimal contamination, would be closable by suture;

3a. wound > 5 cm, minimal contamination, and probably closable by suture (all after debridement of damaged tissue);

3b. wound > 5 cm, severe contamination, or probably not closable by suture (all after debridement of damaged tissue);

3c. open wound with significant neurological or vascular injury.

Compartment syndrome requires *emergency* assessment and decompression. A relatively simple procedure to decompress the fascial compartments is needed; measurement of the compartment pressure using a pressure transducer may be helpful in decision-making.

9.7.6 Treatment of skeletal injuries

The best pain relief for most fractures is adequate immobilization. The degree of intervention needed to achieve this may vary from a sling to internal fixation. A primary reason for internal fixation in some patients (e.g. after femoral neck fractures) is to obtain adequate pain relief. It is clearly desirable to achieve adequate temporary stability to relieve pain before internal fixation is performed. Typically, plaster back slabs may be provided to give stability while awaiting definitive treatment (whether as an outpatient or inpatient). Outpatients with fractures should be reviewed in a fracture clinic within a few days.

The *principles* of fracture treatment include:

- *reduction* (i.e. reduce the deformity and replace the bone fragments in their anatomical position);
- *maintenance of reduction* for as long as it takes for the fracture to unite;
- provision of *optimum conditions for healing,* both for the fracture and other damaged structures such as ligaments and joint capsules;
- *early mobilization* of adjacent joints to prevent stiffness. This first phase of *rehabilitation* aims at achieving sufficient function to promote early return of the patient to activities of daily living and to work;
- *minimization of complications* including infection.

BOX 9.9 Treatment of skeletal injuries

Site of fracture:	Preliminary stabilization:
Clavicle, humeral neck	Sling
Humeral shaft	U slab and collar and cuff
Forearm	Full arm back slab
Distal radius, metacarpal	Short arm back slab
Femoral shaft	Traction splint
Around the knee, tibia	Full leg back slab
Ankle, foot	Short leg back slab

There are a wide variety of *methods* of fracture treatment, and none of them fulfils all of these conditions perfectly. All fracture treatment involves compromise, in order to minimize the risk of complications and the impact of any disadvantages of the particular method selected, while maximizing its benefits. Broadly, there are six methods of fracture treatment:

- immediate or early mobilization, essentially ignoring the fracture, providing minimal support (e.g. a sling for a clavicle fracture);
- support/immobilization in a plaster cast or plastic brace (e.g. humeral fractures);
- traction, which immobilizes the fracture by applying a longitudinal force along the limb (e.g. femoral fractures in children);
- external fixation using a fixator applied with screws to the bone (e.g. open tibial fractures);
- flexible internal fixation, usually with an intramedullary nail (e.g. femoral shaft fractures in adults);
- rigid internal fixation, usually with a stainless steel plate (e.g. forearm shaft fractures).

The essential logical step in planning treatment is to balance the risks of a given line of treatment against what is required to achieve a good functional result. It is vital that early management of fractures aids this, and does not compromise possible outcomes.

How to apply a backslab

These are often applied poorly – too long (this immobilizes other joints unnecessarily), too short, joint in the wrong position, inadequate immobilization.

Wear a disposable apron and gloves.

1. Get the patient in a comfortable position:
   (a) in an upper limb injury, have the patient with the forearm vertically in the air, with the elbow resting on a couch and the wrist in a neutral position;
   (b) for a lower limb injury, have the knee supported so it is flexed. It is important to have the ankle roughly in neutral; it may be necessary to push the ankle upwards from a plantar flexed position.
2. Prepare the slab:
   (a) for an upper limb slab measure from a couple of inches distal to the elbow to the metacarpal heads. The upper limb slab will typically use 8 layers of 6-inch plaster bandage;
   (b) for a short leg slab, measure from a couple of inches distal to the popliteal fossa to the tips of the toes; the lower limb slab will use 3 × 8 thicknesses of 8-inch bandage.
3. Apply a stockinette from above the proximal joint to the end of the limb.
4. Apply a plaster wool bandage evenly over the intended extent of the slab. Start with two turns proximally and end with two turns distally.
5. Wet the bandage thoroughly in lukewarm water.
6. Apply the slab:
   (a) In the upper limb, to the dorsum of the wrist, starting just (1 cm) proximal to the metacarpophalangeal joints, and finishing distal to the elbow. Apply a cling bandage;

(b) in the lower limb, apply one slab to each side of the ankle, and one slab along the sole of the foot and dorsum of the calf. This gives a slab that has a U-shape in section, and is sufficiently strong to resist ankle plantar flexion. Start by applying the slabs distally, so the slab on the sole of the foot reaches the toes. Apply a cling bandage and press the ankle up into a neutral position on your chest. Make sure that all of the toes are visible so that the circulation can be checked.

How to apply a Thomas traction splint (*Figure 9.8*)

Two people are required to do this. Before commencing the patient should have received adequate analgesia, for example, intravenous morphine, femoral nerve block or both.

- Use a splint of the appropriate size – at least 2.5 cm greater in diameter than the thigh.
- Fit the splint with fabric to support the leg (calico or stockinette).
- Apply the skin traction device to the leg – this is a rubber device with a footpiece to take the traction string and held in place with a bandage. One person applies longitudinal traction to the foot while the other applies the device. It should *not* be used in patients with poor skin, for example, patients with steroid damaged skin or rheumatoid arthritis.
- While the assistant controls the leg with the traction, the foot is passed through the splint ring. Lift and support the fracture, advancing the ring until it reaches the groin. The fracture should now be supported by the fabric.
- Support the fracture site with more fabric (usually gamgee).
- Attach the strings from the foot part of the traction device to the end of the splint, and construct a 'Spanish windlass' with a pair of tongue depressors to apply traction.
- Traction has now been applied to the fracture; counter traction is supplied by pressure between the ring and the groin. If possible the ring should be pulled out of the groin by immediate application of a weight (usually 2.5 kg) applied to the foot of the splint via a pulley over the end of the bed. In any event, a splint without counter traction should not be left for more than 24 h due to the risk of perineal pressure sores.

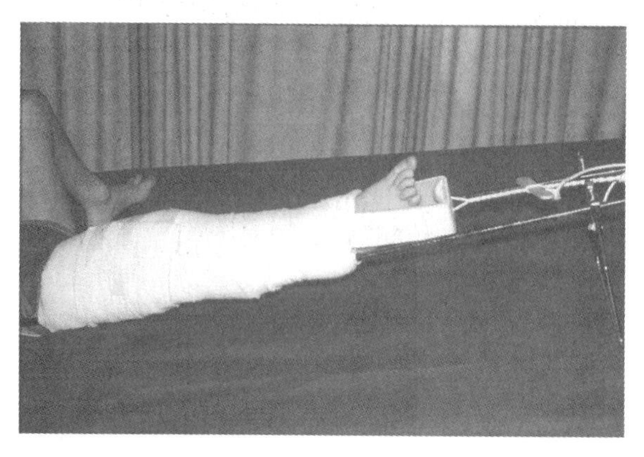

Figure 9.8 Thomas splint applied to a child for a femoral fracture.

9.8 Dislocations

Dislocations are joint injuries where the two joint surfaces are no longer in contact. Partial dislocations also occur (subluxation). These are often difficult to distinguish from periarticular fractures and it is important to obtain adequate imaging. However, if there is gross deformity, neurovascular compromise or a problem with overlying skin, it is proper to reduce the deformity prior to obtaining x-rays. Experience will help, as there are a limited number of characteristic deformities with dislocations.

A typical dislocation is the anterior dislocation of the shoulder (*Figure 9.9*). It usually follows a fall to an outstretched hand. This is frequently recurrent, and is associated with a typical deformity of the shoulder (empty glenoid). Neurovascular injuries may occur (axillary nerve) but are uncommon. X-ray appearances are as shown. Reduction may be achieved by a number of methods, including longitudinal traction (Hippocratic method) or by rotation (Kochers manoeuvre). Recurrent dislocation is common.

9.8.1 Methods of reducing anterior shoulder dislocations

Hippocratic method

Adequate pain control and relaxation is required. This can usually be attained with sedation and analgesia, but generally anaesthesia may be required. Longitudinal traction is applied to the patient's arm, with counter traction applied either by placing the (unshod) foot in the armpit, or getting an assistant to pull longitudinally in the same place with a towel. Pull along the line of the limb and use the foot or towel to press the humeral head laterally. This will press the humeral head back into the glenoid with a 'clunk'.

Kochers manoeuvre

As before, adequate pain control is required. With the patient supine or semirecumbent, externally rotate the arm – this may not be easy. Without traction, adduct the arm across the patient's chest and internally rotate it. The manoeuvre is associated with a small risk of humeral neck/head fracture so excessive force should not be used.

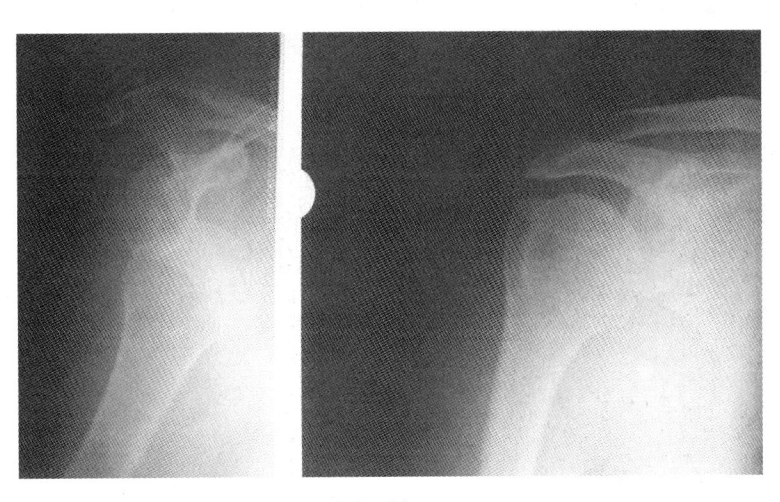

Figure 9.9 X-rays of dislocated and reduced shoulder.

9.8.2 Treatment of other dislocations

Other dislocations are associated with a much higher risk of neurovascular injury, e.g. elbow and (particularly) knee dislocations. The latter has a high risk of injury to the popliteal artery, and angiography should be considered after such an injury. If the patient presents with the knee still dislocated then it must be reduced. Careful clinical examination is required to assess the presence of a vascular injury.

Hip dislocations are typically seen after road traffic accidents and may be difficult to differentiate from the (much commoner) proximal femoral fractures. The hip is usually dislocated posterior, which will give the limb a posture of shortening, flexion and internal rotation. Dislocations usually occur in young patients and are often associated with a posterior lip fracture of the acetabulum, or a sciatic nerve injury. Careful clinical examination is required to exclude this. A major risk with this injury is of avascular necrosis of the femoral head. Urgent reduction is vital, as there is clear evidence that the risk of avascular necrosis increases with the length of time that the hip is dislocated. Reduction requires general anaesthesia with muscle relaxation.

Ankle and hindfoot dislocations may tent the overlying skin dangerously, and are injuries that require treatment before x-rays are obtained. Following adequate analgesia, longitudinal force is usually sufficient to reduce the deformity, reduce the tension on the overlying skin and allow x-rays to be taken.

9.9 Ligament injuries

Soft tissue injuries around joints are common and there are several potential pitfalls. These include the following.

- Wrist sprains. Be sure to examine the anatomical snuffbox and exclude a scaphoid fracture. Longitudinal compression along the thumb metacarpal will typically cause pain if there is a fracture in the scaphoid, and there will be pain dorsally or over the scaphoid tubercle in most fractures.
- Beware of the possibility of an injury to the scapholunate ligament. Check for dorsal tenderness over the wrist. In such patients consider obtaining a clenched fist PA view of the wrist as well as the standard scaphoid views. An increase in the gap between scaphoid and lunate denotes scapholunate instability and the patient must be referred to the appropriate specialist.
- Haemarthroses of the knee (early onset of severe swelling after injury) should be referred for assessment. This usually requires examination under anaesthetic and sometimes arthroscopy. Adequate examination of the knee ligaments after severe injury is rarely possible in an awake patient. Examination of the knee must include the medial and lateral collaterals and the cruciate ligaments.
- The best sign of meniscal injury is joint line tenderness. Remember to look for a block to full knee extension by comparing the knee with the other side. Many meniscal injuries are now repairable, so it is important to try to establish the diagnosis. Assessment may require MRI or arthroscopy.
- Ankle ligament injuries can usually be accurately diagnosed by clinical examination. Tenderness is present over the ligament, and minor or absent over the malleoli. The usual pattern is that the anterior talo fibular ligament is injured, giving tenderness just anterior to the lateral malleolus. Under this circumstance, diagnosis is provided

by accurate clinical examination; the Ottowa rules indicate that x-ray is not necessary if there is no posterior bony tenderness. Ankle ligament injuries are best treated by early physiotherapy and mobilization, often with a supportive splint, rather than a cast.

9.10 Summary

Soft tissue injuries and fractures are frequently challenging, potentially disabling and occasionally life threatening. Careful assessment of the anatomical extent of these injuries and appropriate treatment can make an enormous difference to the initial symptoms and the degree of long-term disability experienced by patients after trauma.

Appendix

Minor trauma 'checklist'

Pain relief should be administered and nonpharmacological intervention considered as previously stated.

Nursing assessment continues and local specific injuries treated.

- Conservative treatment of fractures:
  - cast application;
  - splintage;
  - slings;
  - strapping.
- Surgical intervention of fractures:
  - admission;
  - bed management;
  - immobilization;
  - neurovascular status;
  - intravenous fluids.
- Wound management:
  - wound closure with sutures;
  - wound closure with steristrip or glue;
  - environmental dressings;
  - admission for wound closure;
  - admission for debridement;
  - admission for incision and drainage;
  - admission for cellulitus and mark area to determine extent of involvement.

In the case of either soft tissue injury or fracture to upper limbs remove jewellery to avoid complications. Nail varnish should be removed to be able to assess and establish the neurovascular status of digits.

Discharge planning checklist

If the patient is to be discharged from the ED discharge planning is vitally important especially in the elderly. Arrangements and referrals to the following areas should be considered:

- social worker;
- community nurse;
- general practitioner;
- home from hospital agencies – Age Concern / Red Cross;
- meals on wheels.

Family support and needs must be explored and appropriate arrangements made. Nursing staff must ensure that patients are discharged with specific information related to their injuries:

- head injury card;
- PoP instructions;
- discharge summary;
- discharge medication, especially pain relief;
- follow-up instructions, to:
  - general practitioner;
  - nurse practitioner;
  - fracture clinic;
  - dressing clinic;
  - A&E follow-up.

Wound management instructions:

- physiotherapy clinics.

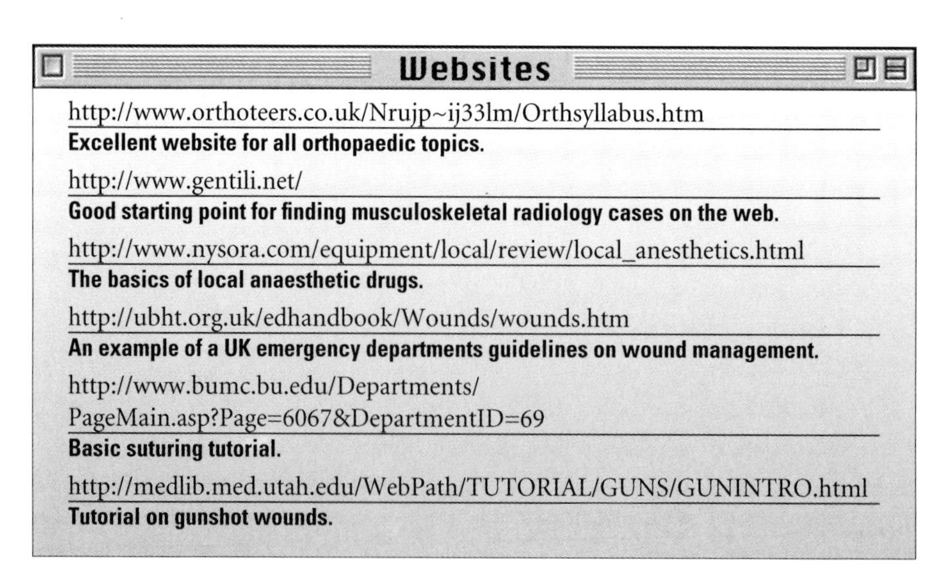

Websites

http://www.orthoteers.co.uk/Nrujp~ij33lm/Orthsyllabus.htm
Excellent website for all orthopaedic topics.

http://www.gentili.net/
Good starting point for finding musculoskeletal radiology cases on the web.

http://www.nysora.com/equipment/local/review/local_anesthetics.html
The basics of local anaesthetic drugs.

http://ubht.org.uk/edhandbook/Wounds/wounds.htm
An example of a UK emergency departments guidelines on wound management.

http://www.bumc.bu.edu/Departments/PageMain.asp?Page=6067&DepartmentID=69
Basic suturing tutorial.

http://medlib.med.utah.edu/WebPath/TUTORIAL/GUNS/GUNINTRO.html
Tutorial on gunshot wounds.

Further reading

1. Charnley J (1968) *The Closed Treatment of Common Fractures.* Churchill Livingstone, Edinburgh. (Recently reprinted by the John Charnley Trust.)

2. Gustilo RB, Gruninger RP & Davis T (1987) Classification of type III (severe) open fractures relative to treatment and results. *Orthopedics* **10:** 1781.

3. Macrae R & Esser M (2002) *Practical Fracture Treatment*, 4th edition. Churchill Livingstone, Edinburgh.

10 Psychological and psychiatric issues in the resuscitation room

D Alexander, S Klein

Objectives

The aims of the chapter are to help the trauma team to:

- describe the presentation and management of
  - normal reactions to highly stressful and traumatic events;
  - common acute psychiatric conditions;
  - grief reactions;
- provide guidelines for the breaking of bad news;
- highlight issues concerning the presence of relatives in the resuscitation room;
- describe the impact of patient care on staff;
- identify measures to help staff cope with the demands of their work.

10.1 Introduction

If the contemporary media were to be believed the resuscitation room would represent a high-profile crucible in which the dramatic issues of life and death, romance, heroism, scientific inspiration and awesome clinical judgement were uniquely blended. The reality is different. Undeniably, of course, this setting is frequently dramatic and professionally challenging, but its demands can also take its toll of staff who work in it, and it poses major challenges in terms of patient management and staff welfare.

10.2 Normal reactions to highly stressful and traumatic events

For patients and relatives, the resuscitation room is likely to provoke anxiety and concerns about privacy, unfamiliar procedures and faces, and intimidating equipment. Our own familiarity with these matters should not prevent us from realizing how alien these may be to our patients and their relatives. Also, we need to remember that accidents and medical emergencies can cause marked reactions with which the layman may not be familiar.

The following are some of the reactions commonly observed.

- Numbness and shock. This is probably Nature's way of shielding us from otherwise overwhelming experiences.
- Fear. In particular it is helpful to reassure the 'stiff upper-lipped' male that fear is a normal biological reaction.

- Depression, apathy, and helplessness. Such reactions are commonly associated with sudden and unexpected 'loss', and medical emergencies are nearly always associated with real or anticipated loss. *All suicidal talk should be taken seriously, and therefore recorded and reported. Do not be reliant on the old adage, 'If they talk about it, they won't do it'.*
- Irritation and anger. These reactions may compromise safety and the stability of catheters, iv lines, and our own composure. It is important, however, not to take such reactions personally.
- Guilt. If patients express guilt about their contribution to a tragic event it is important not to offer superficial reassurance as it is unlikely we will know all the facts.
- Cognitive and perceptual distortions. Following intensely emotional events, individuals' memories may be distorted either in terms of the order of events or the speed at which they are perceived to have happened.
- Autonomic hyperarousal and hypervigilance. Heightened autonomic reactions and an increased sensitivity to risk represent Nature's way of preparing us for the next threatening event. From a medical point of view, it is important to be aware of these changes as they may lead in the longer term to self-medication, that is, the use of alcohol and other psychoactive substances as patients try to 'calm down'.
- Intrusive experiences. 'Flashbacks' are commonly experienced following some traumatic event. These may involve any modality but are characteristically distressing and beyond conscious control. Nightmares are a related phenomenon. They represent an inability of the brain to process deeply disturbing memories and experiences.

10.3 Psychological first aid

This approach was first described in the 1980s and subsequently developed by Alexander in 1990. Described below are some basic ways we can help victims of tragic events in the early stage to ensure matters do not become worse.

- Comfort and protect: A traumatic event leaves people feeling bewildered and shocked. Sometimes, they lose sight of further risk to themselves and of the need to protect themselves against further risk. As a consequence, they may even fail to recognize the need for urgent medical care.
- Counteract helplessness: One of the hallmarks of trauma is that dreadful moment when the individual feels totally helpless and hopeless in the face of some distressing event. That feeling may carry itself over into the resuscitation room. Whenever possible, therefore, counteract that sense of hopelessness and helplessness by involving individuals in their own care or in the care of others, for example, by providing information, comfort and reassurance or by contacting other relevant persons in the family.
- Reunion with friends or relations: Family networks are an essential ingredient in trauma care. It is very important that professionals do not usurp the role of the family who are in a better position to provide a degree of care and support for their loved ones. Thus, we should allow time and provide the facilities for victims to contact their loved ones.

- Expression of feelings: It is not helpful to attempt to dredge up deep felt and painful feelings. It is better to reassure patients and their relatives that it is alright to express their feelings, however unpleasant.
- Provision of accurate information: Information is a powerful antidote to uncertainty and anxiety. Giving people accurate information helps them to feel more in charge of their circumstances and welfare. It is, however, important to remember two things. First, the information must be accurate. (If we do not know the answer to a question, we should be honest about this and confirm we will do our best to find out the appropriate information.) Secondly, stressed individuals can only take in so much information at a time. We need, therefore, to *titrate* the dose of information.
- Re-establish order: Many of the above steps will contribute to this. A characteristic feature of trauma is that victims feel their world has been turned upside down and they are out of control and helpless. The composure of staff, conveyed by word and by behaviour, can do much to indicate that they are in safe and competent hands.
- Triage: Identify individuals who may need additional support or expert help. Certain circumstances may make it particularly difficult for patients and their relatives (see below). Beware also of the individuals who are particularly quiet; they may be more at risk than those expressing openly their distress.

10.4 Acute psychiatric conditions

The resuscitation room is not normally the domain of mental health professionals; their contribution is usually made once the patient is physically stable. Occasionally, however, acute psychiatric conditions may require expert help.

Below are a number of such conditions, which may confront clinical staff in the resuscitation room. For those interested, details about such conditions and their management can be found in the Further Reading section.

10.4.1 Panic attacks

The dominant symptoms are likely to be:

- sudden onset of palpitations and chest pain;
- choking sensations;
- dizziness;
- sense of unreality;
- a fear of dying or going mad;
- waves of intense fear, provoking flight.

10.4.2 Delirium

Delirium is characterized by impaired consciousness and attention, and is commonly associated with hallucinations, delusions, disorientation, social withdrawal, impaired memory for recent events, impaired sleep, and either underactivity or overactivity. In addition to these physical and intellectual symptoms, there may be emotional disturbances such as depression (or, sometimes, euphoria), anxiety, irritability, apathy and perplexity. The onset is usually rapid, and the symptoms show diurnal variation (commonly worse at night).

The causes are varied and include:

- hypoxaemia;
- hypotension;
- cerebral haemorrhage;
- hypoglycaemia;
- meningitis;
- renal or hepatic failure;
- extended sleep deprivation;
- drugs (including steroids) and drug withdrawal;
- heavy and extended alcohol misuse or withdrawal ('delirium tremens' – see below).

10.4.3 Acute stress reaction

This transient disorder is caused in otherwise emotionally stable individuals by an exceptionally stressful or traumatic event. The symptoms usually resolve within 3–4 days or sometimes even within a few hours after the individual is removed from the source of stress or threat.

The symptoms include a mixture of autonomic, mental and psychological ones.

Autonomic	**Mental**	**Psychological**
tachycardia	confusion	flushing
disorientation	depression	amnesia
dazed		anxiety
sweating		overactivity
		anger
		despair

10.4.4 Dissociation

In dissociative conditions individuals commonly display marked denial of problems or events which are obvious to others (even the death of a loved one). These symptoms may be triggered by traumatic events, and they may help the victims to cope with otherwise intolerable stress.

There may also be otherwise inexplicable physical symptoms, such as deafness, paralysis, 'pseudoseizures', or an amnesia for events relating to the trauma. Such amnesias are usually selective and partial. They may show a curious lack of concern about such symptoms.

10.4.5 Alcohol-related problems

Resuscitation room staff will be all too familiar with the problems of alcohol (in their professional lives!). About a quarter of emergency admissions to hospitals in England and Wales are due to excessive alcohol consumption, and alcohol is implicated in over three-quarters of fatal road traffic accidents.

- Patients who are acutely intoxicated may display problems of violence (see below), but, fortunately, such behaviour tends to be short-lived and dose-related.
- Those who have an extended history of alcohol misuse may present with the characteristic 'alcohol withdrawal symptoms' outlined in Box 10.1.

BOX 10.1 Alcohol withdrawal symptoms

- Tremor (fine and rapid)
- Nausea
- Excessive sweating (especially in the morning)
- Tinnitus
- Hyperacusis
- Muscle cramps
- Impaired sleep (particularly with early morning wakening and nightmares)
- Variable mood (including irritability and anxiety)
- Perceptual disturbances (including visual hallucinations)
- Convulsions (which characteristically appear about 24 hours after alcohol withdrawal)

Delirium tremens (DT)

About 5% of physically addicted drinkers experience delirium tremens (the DTs) following withdrawal, and, if untreated, may result in cerebral obtundity, convulsions and death. It tends to occur between one and four days following withdrawal.

BOX 10.2 Delirium tremens

- Vivid visual hallucinations
- Delusions
- Ataxia
- Hyperarousal
- Insomnia
- Agitation
- Impaired concentration
- Profound confusion and disorientation
- Low-grade pyrexia
- Fear

Management of alcohol withdrawal

- The acute management comprises rehydration, restoration of electrolyte imbalance, and thiamine injections when there is a risk of acute encephalopathy.
- If there is also evidence of hypoglycaemia, oral or parenteral glucose replacement is essential, supplemented by thiamine to avoid Wernicke's encephalopathy.
- Since there is a risk of fitting, long half-life benzodiazepines (e.g. diazepam or chlordiazepoxide) are recommended. In the cases of head injury and respiratory disorder, care must be taken with the use of such medication.
- As a general principle the administration of a vitamin supplement is advisable.

10.5 Post-traumatic stress disorder (PTSD)

This condition is associated with very distressing re-experiencing of the traumatic event in the fashion of flashbacks and nightmares (see case example), avoidance of any reminders of the event (e.g. talking about it, going back to the scene, or even meeting people associated with it), and hyperarousal and hypervigilance (see above).

This condition is not diagnosed until about a month after the trauma, therefore, it is rarely a condition which will confront staff of the resuscitation room. However, since it has obtained such a high profile (thanks, in large, part to the media and to the legal profession) the features are described in Box 10.3.

BOX 10.3 Case example of post-traumatic stress disorder

- The senior author was asked to examine a badly burned patient who would not use his PCA despite being in obvious pain. This puzzled the nursing and surgical staff.
- The explanation demonstrates how distressing can be such intrusive phenomena.
- The patient explained that if he used his analgesic he had no pain; if he had no pain he became sleepy; if he became sleepy he experienced flashbacks and nightmares in which he was burned and his son died.
- He preferred pain.

10.6 Grief reactions

Grief is not an illness. Most individuals will deal successfully over time with tragic loss, but grief reactions are varied, occasionally dramatic and may interfere with clinical management.

Because most deaths now occur in hospital and not at home most laymen have little personal experience of death and dying. Also, because of impressive technological advances in medical care, society now has become 'death defying', in that they feel that no patient should ever die once in expert medical care. (Staff may themselves see death as a 'failure' – see 'Impact on staff'.) Some deaths are particularly difficult to cope with (see Box 10.4).

BOX 10.4 'Difficult' deaths

- Sudden, unexpected
- Painful, horrifying, mutilating
- Where medical mismanagement is suspected
- Where there is no body (a body helps to confirm the reality of death and provides the opportunity for the bereaved to say their 'goodbyes'

It is also worth bearing in mind that, although the death of a loved one is the most obvious source of grief, in medicine there are many 'mini deaths'. These include, the loss of a limb, the loss of function or the loss of looks (e.g. through traumatic disfigurement).

There is some overlap between the normal reactions to other stressful and traumatic events (see above) and those to loss. However, the following acute reactions should be noted in particular:

- shock and denial: patients and relatives often cannot take in the reality of the loss. This may be Nature's way of shielding them from overwhelming stress. Thus, it is best not to be confrontational with regard to the 'truth';
- apathy: patients may show a lack of interest in their physical welfare (and, as a consequence, may not contribute to medical examination and treatment);
- acute distress: there are commonly paroxysms of anxiety, depression, pining, agitation and crying. (With regard to the last, the archetypical 'stiff upper-lipped' male needs to be reassured that crying is a universal human response);

- guilt: this is commonly seen in events which have resulted in a fatality. It is important not to reassure the individual idly that he/she is 'not guilty' because, at the early stages, all the relevant facts will not be known;
- anger: relatives and patients may be extremely angry about an accident or medical emergency. They may not always know with whom to be angry; thus, staff may become the target. (See 'Dealing with the bereaved').

BOX 10.5 Features of acute grief reactions

- Shock and denial
- Apathy
- Acute distress
- Guilt
- Anger

10.7 Dealing with the bereaved

It is likely that how we deal with the bereaved in the early stages will have a marked bearing on how well they cope subsequently. It may also determine how they react to staff in the future. Thus, however uncomfortable dealing with grief may make us feel, we must do our best for those who suffer a major loss. Below are some guidelines.

- Consider the setting: try to find a quiet room, which guarantees a degree of privacy. We can be sure our pager will go off at the most intimate and inappropriate moment! Leave it with a colleague or switch it off.
- Listen (when in doubt about what to say, say nothing!): the acutely bereaved rarely welcome being talked at. It is usually best, therefore, to confine ourselves to providing an opportunity for individuals to express their feelings and to ask questions.
- Tolerate their reactions: the bereaved are commonly angry ('*What did I do to deserve this?*'), bewildered, impatient and irritable (as described above). As caregivers, we may become the target of their feelings but it is important not to defend ourselves. ('*There is no point in being angry with me, I'm just doing my best.*') It is far better to show empathy and to 'normalize' their reactions. ('*I can understand why you feel so upset and angry just now. I think anybody would feel like that*').
- Ban the cliché: dealing with those in grief can make us feel uncomfortable, insecure and anxious. Thus, we commonly are not sure what to say, and we may fall back on clichés. ('*It could have been worse, you know, your son might also have been killed*' – said to a mother whose daughter died in a road traffic accident.) Such comments can be hurtful.
- Identify sources of help: it is useful to give people information about what they should do if their difficulties continue. There is of course the family doctor but, in almost any community, there are local voluntary agencies, for example, CRUSE (see Websites) which are available to the bereaved. A brief (and accurate) leaflet listing such agencies and how they can be contacted is particularly helpful to the bereaved.

BOX 10.6 Dealing with the bereaved

- Consider the setting
- Listen
- Tolerate reactions
- Ban the cliché
- Identify sources of help

10.8 Breaking bad news

How the bereaved react to news of a tragic death (or other loss) is likely to be determined in part by how we tell them what has happened. However, it is never easy to do this, and there is no blueprint for success. There are, however, some extended guidelines provided in the Further Reading section.

Nobody wants to be the bearer of bad tidings and, therefore, there is a strong temptation to avoid being in this position. (*'I'll leave it to Sister, she's had more experience'!*). It is the responsibility of the team, therefore, to consider who is in the best position (for whatever reason, e.g. age, seniority, gender or knowledge of the incident) to speak to the patient or relative. However difficult, it is a challenge that can not be avoided.

Below are three key questions you might like to consider if you are charged with this difficult responsibility.

1. Am I properly prepared in relation to:
   - whom I will meet?
   - what information I might need?
   - where we can speak in privacy?
   - how I look (clothing stained with bodily fluids may distress relatives)?
2. Have I thought about how I am going to share the bad news?
   - It is usually helpful to provide our name, status and involvement in the proceedings.
   - Find out what they already know and what they want to know – bear in mind, they may already have gleaned false information from bystanders, the emergency services or others.
   - It is usually best to speak slowly and with pauses, and, every now and again, confirm that they have taken in what has been said. Do not forget that when we are anxious we tend to speak too quickly. Also, those in a distressed state may be confused, and their attention and memory will certainly not be at their best. Diagrams and notes can be particularly helpful.
   - In an effort to protect people, we may be tempted to deceive or, to put it more bluntly, 'lie'. Well intended this may be, but it carries the strong risk of backfiring. If they find out we have been dishonest we are likely to lose their trust. Also, it is worth remembering, that contemporary society is now very much better informed about medical matters than it used to be.
3. What will I do once I have told them the bad news?

   Sharing bad news with somebody is not just an event but the start of the process of helping them to deal with a tragic circumstance. Below are some points we should bear in mind.

   - Allow the individual time to digest what they have been told.
   - Ask them if they would like a member of staff to be with them or if they would prefer to be alone.
   - Ensure that they know what will happen next (e.g. legal proceedings, post-mortem and recovery of possessions).

- Establish how they will get home and to whom and to what they are going home. Individuals' ability to cope with a tragedy may be strengthened by the support they have at home or in the community but weakened by other pressures in their lives.

10.9 Relatives in the resuscitation room

This is an emotive and contentious issue about which much has been written recently (Mitchell & Lynch, 1997). Resistance to the presence of relatives in the resuscitation room is often based on the anxiety it creates in staff, the threat of litigation and the suspicion that relatives would not cope with what they see. More recent evidence confirms that relatives may gain considerably from their presence in the resuscitation room. The advantages of relatives being present could include:

- they can see that everything is being done to help their loved one;
- it may remove some of the 'mystery' of what happens in the resuscitation room;
- it may help to develop a constructive bond between staff and relatives which may be very helpful in the aftermath and follow-up.

However, these gains are unlikely to be achieved unless we take the following steps.

1. Relatives need to be briefed as to what they will see, hear and, possibly, smell, otherwise, they are likely to find the proceedings in the resuscitation room very disturbing and bewildering.
2. We need to ensure that there is a competent member of staff with them who can advise what is happening and offer support and reassurance as the proceedings unfold.
3. Ideally, the same member of staff should be able to spend some time with them after the proceedings have been completed to discuss their reactions and to answer any questions.

10.9.1 Impact on staff

Staff are the most valuable resource in the National Health Service; we need to take steps to protect their welfare, physical and emotional. However, there is now evidence to confirm that, whilst healthcare staff gain much job satisfaction, what they achieve may be at some cost to their health and welfare. 'Burnout' and 'compassion fatigue' are recognized risks. The authors have also described recently how the adverse effect of work may spill over into the personal and family lives of healthcare staff.

- Sources of stress*:* There are two primary sources of stress for staff. The first relates to specific demands of their work, including dealing with death, dying, pain and suffering, and insufficient time to recover between incidents. The second relates to poor management and organizational practices. These include a lack of appreciation, work overload, underfunding, and poor communication and relationships. Thus, the institution has no right to assume that the responsibility for staff welfare rests solely with individual members of staff.

- Staff reactions*:* Inexperienced and younger staff may be vulnerable to work-related pressures. However, it must not be assumed that senior and experienced staff have some special immunity to the pressures of their work. Alexander and Atcheson

(1998) found that the senior trauma surgeons and nurses were more likely than their less senior and experienced colleagues to admit to the adverse emotional impact of their work.

> **'Burnout'** ***is a professional occupational disease manifest in the many specialities of healthcare and will be a disorder as long as human values and worth are disregarded by inept policy makers and managers of human resources*** **(Felton, 1998)**

10.9.2 Violence against staff

A regrettable and increasingly prevalent source of distress and, sometimes, injury to staff is violence by patients and relatives. Obviously, the institution has a 'duty of care' to ensure that every reasonable step is taken to protect staff. However, we can take some steps to protect our safety. First, we should be aware of early warning signs, and, secondly, we should conduct ourselves in a way which reduces the risk of violence and confrontation.

1. Early warning signs:
   - a history of violence;
   - overtly aggressive, abusive attitudes and/or behaviour;
   - an identifiable serious psychiatric condition* (e.g. a paranoid illness [i.e. one in which the person feels that he/she is being persecuted], alcohol/substance misuse, organic cerebral damage [including epilepsy and damage to the frontal lobes], and severe personality disorder).
2. Preventative steps:
   - whenever possible do not deal alone with volatile situations;
   - violence is commonly provoked by anxiety and uncertainty. We can reduce this by explaining in advance what we are going to do (particularly if we are behind the patient) by way of, for example, removing clothing, examining, injecting and suturing;
   - bear in mind that what is done in the resuscitation room may be regarded by the layman as intrusive and invasive not only to the person's body but also to their 'psychological space'. A courteous acknowledgement of this will make this 'invasion' more acceptable to those who might otherwise react adversely;
   - if there is a risk of violence, it is wise to keep doors and screens open whenever it is reasonable to do so. This may not only help the individual to stop feeling trapped (and, therefore, violently anxious) but it also provides a ready exit;
   - a confrontational and aggressive (or 'macho') approach by staff is more likely to be inflammatory rather than defusing and reassuring. A calm, courteous and confident (even if we don't feel it!) approach is more likely to help;
   - beware of persistent eye contact; this may be perceived as confrontational;
   - never underestimate the strength of a disturbed individual, whatever the age, gender or physical stature.

**N.B.* This does not mean that anybody who has a mental illness is likely to be violent. However, there is an increased risk of violent behaviour in certain conditions.

If physical restraints are to be used:

- ensure they are administered safely (for patients and staff);
- they should be removed only slowly and when the risk of violence has significantly lessened;
- ensure the airway is maintained;
- they should be introduced in accordance with well practised procedures. (A chaotic rugby scrum of flailing, unidentifiable limbs is certainly unprofessional and, more importantly, potentially hazardous to patients and to staff).

If sedation is required:

- injections should be administered only once immobilization has been achieved;
- avoid the prolonged use of heavy doses of antipsychotics because of the risk of sudden death.

Important signs that staff may need help

We need to be alert to signs in our colleagues (and also in ourselves) which might indicate that there are problems of coping. These include:

- excessive and unusual use of alcohol, food, cigarettes and other substances;
- unusual level of carelessness and accident proneness;
- unusual irritability and moodiness;
- reduced work competence and poorer time-keeping;
- underworking (or, sometimes, overworking since some individuals seek to over-compensate when they feel they are not coping);
- pre-occupation with a specific event;
- social withdrawal;
- excessive denial about emotional difficulties or impact of an event.

What can we do to help staff?

Staff in the resuscitation room are usually resilient and emotionally robust individuals who are self-selected for this important and demanding form of work. They will develop their own ways of coping, including 'black humour' and viewing incidents as 'challenges' or 'problems' to be solved rather than overwhelming 'crises'. Others may neutralize what would otherwise be disturbing to them (see Box 10.7).

In addition, good training and selection will reduce the risks of work-related problems. On the other hand, there are other steps which should be considered.

BOX 10.7 Case example

During a major exercise to retrieve human remains after a major disaster, one police body handler reported to the senior author:

> *Sir, when I go in there* [a large badly damaged structure] *as far as I am concerned I'm going into a spaceship looking for Martians.*

Peer support

Talking openly with colleagues is a well-recognized source of mutual support. However, it is important that time and a suitable facility are available for this to take place. (We should also consider the wisdom of sending members of staff home following a particularly distressing event. They could miss out on the discussion among and support from their colleagues.)

Support groups

There is an implicit assumption that getting together a number of staff on a regular basis will necessarily be helpful. This has been challenged (Alexander, 1993) because commonly insufficient attention is paid to the aims of the group, the methods by which it will be run, and the choice of the group leader.

Although support from colleagues may indeed be a powerful antidote to work-related stress sometimes such support is not available because:

- colleagues do not wish to be seen as intrusive by asking personal questions;
- colleagues may find it difficult to deal with the distress and personal problems of other staff (particularly if they are more senior and experienced staff);
- those who may need help may fear that by admitting this they may compromise their career prospects and run the risk of breaches of confidentiality.

Organizational and managerial practices

How the 'system' is run appears to be a powerful antidote to the adverse effects of stressful duties. Effective ingredients include:

- good team spirit;
- a clear definition of duties and responsibilities;
- good communication within the team;
- explicit appreciation and recognition of 'work well done' (rather than the common practice of identifying colleagues only when they have made a mistake);
- adequate training (training can help to establish realistic expectations of what staff can do, and also it should include opportunities to rehearse how individuals will cope with things when they do not go to plan, e.g. in a failed CPR).

10.9.3 Psychological debriefing

In the 1980s and early 1990s, there was a strong move towards setting up debriefing sessions following 'critical incidents' (i.e. those events which threaten to overwhelm the ability of staff to cope).

The aims of debriefing were to:

- confirm that the individuals' reactions are normal;
- enable them to describe their reactions to the incident;
- identify what has been learned and what gains have been made from the incident;
- reinforce the mutual supportiveness among the group;
- help individuals to disengage from (i.e. leave behind) the incident.

Strong claims were initially made for debriefing as a means of preventing the onset of post-traumatic reactions such as PTSD. More recently, however, a more conservative approach has been advocated because there has been some evidence that certain individuals, under some circumstances, may feel worse after debriefing. This is a contentious issue, and there are many important questions to be answered. For those who wish to introduce debriefing, they are advised to consult the relevant literature on the principles, practices and evaluation of debriefing to be found in the Further Reading section.

If it is decided to introduce debriefing sessions after critical incidents, the following guiding principles should be considered.

Debriefers should be:

- properly trained;
- familiar with normal and pathological reactions to critical incidents;
- familiar with group dynamics (a group is more than the sum of the individuals);
- familiar with the nature of the incident;
- familiar with the 'culture' of the resuscitation room (in terms of what goes on in that environment, who does what, and what are the prevailing values, fears and needs among the staff).

10.10 Summary

The profile of contemporary medicine is usually cast in terms of technological advances. Whilst these are certainly impressive, we will not attain the highest levels of medical care unless we address with equal commitment the psychological needs of patients and their families. Moreover, however well trained and carefully selected, staff of the resuscitation room have a right to have their emotional needs and welfare considered in order that they are able to fulfil their important and demanding duties.

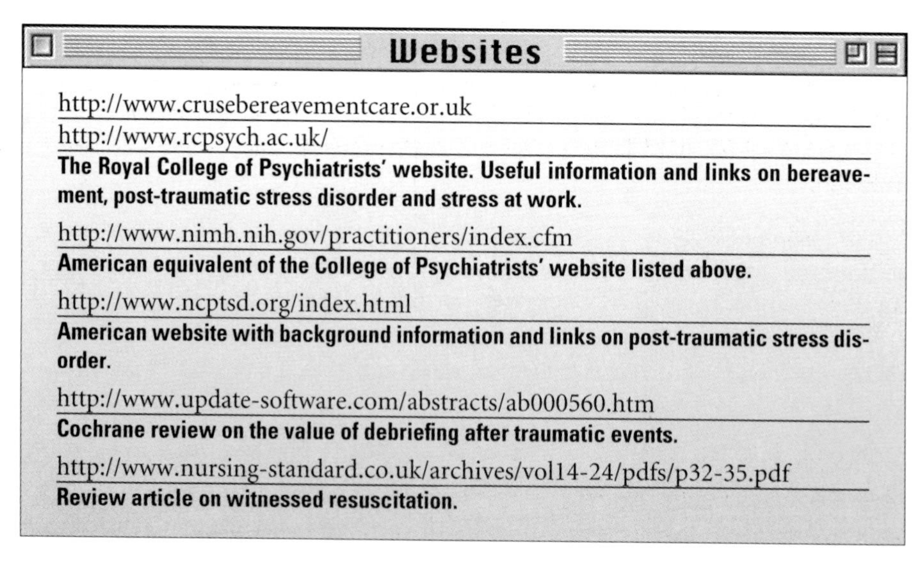

Websites

http://www.crusebereavementcare.or.uk

http://www.rcpsych.ac.uk/

The Royal College of Psychiatrists' website. Useful information and links on bereavement, post-traumatic stress disorder and stress at work.

http://www.nimh.nih.gov/practitioners/index.cfm

American equivalent of the College of Psychiatrists' website listed above.

http://www.ncptsd.org/index.html

American website with background information and links on post-traumatic stress disorder.

http://www.update-software.com/abstracts/ab000560.htm

Cochrane review on the value of debriefing after traumatic events.

http://www.nursing-standard.co.uk/archives/vol14-24/pdfs/p32-35.pdf

Review article on witnessed resuscitation.

Further reading

1. Alexander DA (1990) Psychological intervention for victims and helpers after disasters. *Br J Gen Prac* **40:** 345.
2. Alexander DA (1993) Staff support groups: do they support and are they even groups? *Palliative Med.* **7:** 127.
3. Alexander DA & Atcheson SF (1998) Psychiatric aspects of trauma care: a survey of nurses and doctors. *Psych. Bull.* **20:** 132.
4. Alexander DA & Klein S (2000) Bad news is bad news: let's not make it worse. *Trauma* **2:** 11.
5. Alexander DA & Klein S (2001) Caring for others can seriously damage your health. *Hospital Med.* **62:** 264.
6. Barratt F & Wallis DN (1998) Relatives in the resuscitation room: their point of view. *J Accident Emerg Med* **15:** 109.
7. Brewin T & Sparshott M (1996) *Relating to the Relatives. Breaking Bad News, Communication and Support.* Radcliffe Medical Press, Oxford.
8. Felton JS (1998) Burnout as a clinical entity – its importance in health care workers. *Occupational Med.* **48:** 237.
9. Figley CR (1995) *Compassion Fatigue: Coping with Secondary Traumatic Stress Disorder in Those who Treat the Traumatized.* Brunner/Mazel, New York.
10. Hardy GE, Shapiro DA & Barrill CS (1997) Fatigue in the workplace of national health service trusts: levels of symptomatology and links with minor psychiatric disorder, demographic, occupational and work role factors. *J Psychosomatic Res* **43:** 83.
11. Merson S & Baldwin D (1995) *Psychiatric Emergencies.* Oxford University Press, Oxford.
12. Meyers TA, Eichhorn DJ & Guzzetta CE (1998) Do families want to be present during CPR? A retrospective survey. *J Emergency Nursing* **24:** 400.
13. Mitchell JT & Everly GS (1995) *Critical Incident Stress Debriefing: CISD.* Chevron Publishing, Ellicott City.
14. Mitchell MH & Lynch MB (1997) Should relatives be allowed in the resuscitation room? *J Accident Emerg Med* **14:** 366.
15. O'Brien LS (1998) *Traumatic Events and Mental Health.* Cambridge University Press, Cambridge.
17. Parkes CM (1985) Bereavement. *Br J Psychiatry* **146:** 11.
18. Raphael B (1986) *When Disaster Strikes: How Individuals and Communities Cope with Catastrophe.* Basic Books, New York.
19. Raphael B & Wilson JP (2000) *Psychological Debriefing. Theory, Practice and Evidence.* Cambridge University Press, Cambridge.
20. Royal College of Physicians and Psychiatrists (1995) *The Psychological Care of Medical Patients.* Council Report CR35. Royal College of Physicians and Psychiatrists, London.
21. Smith C, Sell L & Sudbury P (eds) (1996) *Key Topics in Psychiatry.* BIOS Scientific Publishers Ltd., Oxford.

11 Trauma in the elderly

R Protheroe

Objectives

The objectives of this chapter are to inform the trauma team members of the special aspects of management in the elderly, in particular to:

- appreciate the epidemiology of injury;
- understand the differences in anatomy and pathophysiology;
- appreciate the response of the elderly to injury;
- appropriately assess and manage trauma in the elderly population.

11.1 Introduction

The elderly form an increasing proportion of the population, especially in developed countries, and their increasingly active lifestyle exposes them to events likely to result in trauma. The pattern of injury is often different from that seen in their younger counterparts and coupled with a reduced physiological reserve and increase in co-morbidities, it is not surprising they have worse outcomes, with increased complications, increased length of stay in care and the inevitable increase in costs. Despite these differences, the management of trauma is based upon the same principles already described, supplemented by an increased level of support and rehabilitation during the recovery phase. There is evidence that coordinated, aggressive management of the injuries and any concomitant diseases will improve outcome. This has been recognized in orthopaedics with the frequent close liaison between the orthopaedic and the care of the elderly teams.

Ethical issues may arise over the decision to treat the elderly, particularly in the presence of co-morbidities, although it must be stressed that age alone should not be allowed to dictate management. In the United States, triage to a trauma centre may well be considered for a lower injury severity score, purely on the grounds of age.

11.2 Epidemiology of injury

In the developed world the population is getting older and the percentage of the population living into old age is expanding rapidly. In the United States, during the last 30 years, the population increased by 39% but the number over 65 years increased by 89% while those over 85 years increased by 232%. Consequently, trauma in the elderly population is an ever-increasing problem.

Loss of sensory afferents: eyesight, hearing, joint proprioception and touch combine to make the normal environment, especially the home, somewhat hazardous, in particular the stairs. Coupled with this are age-related changes in postural stability that when combined with loss of motor strength to correct posture, increase the risk of falling. Co-morbid events, such as syncope, may add to the postural instability (see Box 11.1). Not surprisingly, falls predominate with 70% of all deaths due to falls occurring in the elderly population. This is followed by motor vehicle accidents and pedestrian accidents. As drivers, the incidence of accidents amongst the elderly is second only to novice drivers. The number of crash-related injuries and deaths per million miles increases after the age of 60 years despite the elderly driving fewer miles in total. The elderly are more likely to crash in good conditions, but the relative absence of other significant causative factors (i.e. speed and alcohol impairment) suggest that age-related impairment of driving skills may be the root cause. Medical conditions such as diabetes can have an affect as well as the catastrophic incident such as the acute dysrhythmia or myocardial infarct whilst driving.

BOX 11.1 Co-morbid causes of syncope in the elderly

- Dysrhythmias
- Autonomic insufficiency
- Hypoglycaemia
- Acute/chronic gastro-intestinal blood loss
- Medications:
  - Antihypertensives
  - Antidepressants
  - Sedatives
  - Hypoglycaemics

Pedestrian injuries form the other significant group of injuries seen in the older trauma victim, since they form the major group at risk of being struck by a vehicle. The elderly have the highest fatality effect of any age group of injured pedestrians. Again decreased mobility, impaired cognitive ability (safe to cross) and a decreased sensory input are all thought to contribute. It appears that nearly 50% of all pedestrian fatalities in the elderly occur at designated crossing points.

11.3 Anatomical and physiological changes

Ageing is a complex process of nonreversible deteriorative changes that ultimately lead to death. A progressive loss of functional reserve occurs, separate from any pathological loss of function as a consequence of states such as hypertension, diabetes, cardiovascular, pulmonary or renal disease.

11.3.1 Respiratory system

With increasing age there is a loss of lung volume, the elasticity of both the lungs and the chest wall falls, along with a decrease in pulmonary compliance. The closing volume of the lungs increases with age, allowing airway closure during normal respiration in the awake elderly. This, coupled with alveolar loss (resulting in loss of gas exchanging surface area), leads to a decrease in the normal PaO_2. These changes along with atrophy of the pseudociliated mucosa and a decrease in the ability and stimulus to cough lead to reduced clearance of sputum and thereby predispose to the development of atelectasis and hypoxia. There is also a decrease in the response to $PaCO_2$ that may cause a susceptibility to opiates and their associated side effects. Furthermore, a loss of protective reflexes increases the risk of aspiration. A gradual change of the bacterial flora in the oral cavity occurs, with an increasing incidence of Gram-negative organisms. This all contributes to a loss of reserve, and it is little wonder that there is a high incidence of orthostatic pneumonia in this population.

Pathologically, there is a greater incidence of co-existing chronic pulmonary disease in these patients that may easily lead to a marked and rapid deterioration in their condition following a traumatic insult.

11.3.2 Cardiovascular system

Over time the myocardium becomes stiffer, with a decrease in pump function, and loss of cardiac reserve and a progressive decrease in both the level of and response to catecholamines. There is an increase in the systemic vascular resistance and a decrease in the cardiac output that consequently leads to a decreased response in the vascular system to hypovolaemic shock

Pathologically, elderly patients have an increased incidence of hypertension, ischaemic heart disease, peripheral vascular disease and arrhythmias. Therapeutic medications and mechanisms (i.e. beta-adrenoreceptor antagonists, cardiac pacemakers) may mask or alter the response to hypovolaemia. It is well recognized that central venous pressure monitoring in the face of established heart disease may not be as helpful as in ordinary circumstances and a pulmonary artery catheter may be of more use.

11.3.3 Thermoregulation

The elderly have a decreased ability to thermoregulate. This may be associated with co-morbid thyroid dysfunction, loss of vascular reserve with impaired vasoconstriction, neurological impairment, or an age-related reduction in shivering and nonshivering thermogenesis. A lack of sensitivity to environmental changes, with both inappropriate behaviour and clothing, immobility and loss of exercise-induced metabolic heat production all combine to put the elderly trauma victim at greater risk of hypothermia. Following injury, the increase in the systemic vascular resistance and associated metabolic acidosis may reduce the cardiac output, thereby worsening their ability to compensate.

Hypothermia can have drastic effects. Shivering leads to an increase in oxygen demand in a patient who may not have the pulmonary or cardiovascular reserve to cope. There is also a reduction in all organ function that leads to a decrease in renal blood flow and excretion of waste metabolites and drugs, reduced hepatic metabolism of drugs (prolonged effects) and haematological consequences. Not only do we see a disturbance of platelet function and the coagulation cascade, the immune system is depressed leading to an increased risk of infection. Control of bleeding, secondary to hypothermia, is extremely difficult to resolve. There is no doubt that prevention of hypothermia (and, thereby, maintaining normal haemostasis) is much easier than treating the haemorrhagic state in the presence of hypothermia.

11.3.4 Gastro-intestinal system

Elderly patients often seem to mask the symptoms and signs of abdominal trauma. Although well recognized, it is difficult to quantify loss of gastro-intestinal tract function, resulting in an increased reliance on imaging techniques with the need for radiographic contrast and the potential for renal and other organ damage. There is also increased glucose intolerance, less muscle mass and, hence, less nutritional reserve.

11.3.5 Renal system

As people age there is an ongoing and progressive loss of glomeruli with consequent loss of function. They are less effective at retaining water in the presence of hypovolaemia. These changes are secondary to both decreased antidiuretic hormone (ADH) secretion and decreased renin–angiotensin activity. There is also a worse outcome with acute renal failure in the elderly. In addition this population is more likely to be taking diuretics for co-morbidities, with consequent relative dehydration.

11.3.6 Neurological system

As we age there is progressive atrophy of brain tissue, with consequent increase in the space available in the cranium, allowing greater movement of the tissues in the event of mechanical trauma and greater risk of subdural haematoma after relatively minor trauma. Coupled with this is the presence of amyloid plaques and a decrease in the levels of neurotransmitters. This may well lead to a progressive loss of cognitive function, memory loss and possibly dementia. Other associated co-morbidities include a higher incidence of Parkinsonism, atherosclerosis of the carotid arteries, stroke and transient ischaemic attacks. There has often been a progressive decrease in the senses with poor vision and hearing, with a greater dependence on glasses and hearing aids.

The elderly are often confused just by changes in their environment and this situation can often be worsened by the interaction of drugs. It is also important to think about intracranial haemorrhage in the elderly, as both the cause and consequence of trauma.

11.3.7 Locomotor system and cutaneous disorders

As well as the decreased muscle mass, there are degenerative changes within the bone and joints, as well as ligamentous ossification. This may well lead to a loss of flexibility of the skeleton, that can contribute to or worsen any potential injury. Over the years narrowing of the vertebral canal occurs, increasing the potential for a significant cord injury.

With increasing age, there is loss of subcutaneous fat, connective tissue and a decrease in the elasticity of skin. Reduced vascular supply, coupled with ischaemic disease leads to an increased incidence of decubitus ulcers and poor healing of both trivial skin trauma and major wounds. Previous treatment with corticosteroids may have caused a degree of localized atrophy.

11.3.8 Haematological system

The most frequent haematological disorder encountered in the elderly is anaemia. Although there are many different causes, iron deficiency predominates. There is decreased immunity predisposing these patients to a much greater incidence of infection.

11.3.9 Endocrine

There is a high incidence of diabetes mellitus with all its associated problems. The incidence of thyroid disease is greater, particularly hypothyroidism, which often goes undiagnosed in this group of patients.

11.3.10 Pharmacology

Pharmacodynamics and pharmacokinetics are frequently altered in the elderly and may lead to exaggerated effects with many drugs. This is particularly true of anaesthetic, sedative and analgesic drugs and care must be taken. With many elderly taking medicines for multiple other conditions, that is, cardiovascular agents, there is much potential for interactions.

11.3.11 Co-morbid diseases

As seen above the impact of co-morbid conditions can lead to profound problems in the assessment and management of any trauma victim, but is much more likely to be found in the elderly. With ageing, there is a gradual increase in the prevalence of co-morbid diseases, rising from 17% in the fourth decade to 70% by the age of 75 years.

11.4 Assessment and management

Resuscitation of the elderly trauma victim should progress using the principles already described in Section 1.6.1. Optimization of resuscitation assumes a greater importance in the elderly, as over-resuscitation may result in problems just as severe as under-resuscitation (see Section 4.6.1).

11.4.1 Primary survey and resuscitation

Airway and cervical-spine control

Elderly patients are often edentulous, but may occasionally have loose, inconveniently placed or very carious teeth. Along with resorption of the mandible and lax cheek muscles this may make maintenance of the airway more difficult. If intubation is required, arthritis of the temporo-mandibular joint may limit mouth opening. Soft tissues are more prone to injury, particularly the turbinates, which may bleed profusely. The airway nurse must take great care to provide cervical spine immobilization, even when the spine is clinically and radiologically intact, so that iatrogenic injury is avoided. Degenerative cervical spondylolisthesis, narrowing of the cervical spinal canal, and ligamentous instability in diseases such as rheumatoid arthritis, are more frequent than with younger trauma victims. Central cord syndrome occurs much more frequently in the elderly.

Breathing

In the elderly, it is often difficult to support ventilation using a facemask for the reasons already stated and a reduced respiratory reserve means that hypoxia ensues rapidly.

Therefore mechanical ventilation with 100% oxygen should be started early remembering that the chances of causing a pneumothorax are significantly higher in this group of patients. Repeated assessment of breath sounds and observation of the patient's chest for equality of movement and the development of surgical emphysema are important to ensure early recognition of this complication should it occur. As soon as possible, serial arterial blood gases must be performed to ensure adequate oxygenation and ventilation. Because of the potential problems, the assistance of an anaesthetist should be sought early in the management of these patients.

Circulation

Warmed fluids must be used, and the patient's response continuously and accurately monitored by the circulation nurse. The reduced fluid tolerance associated with ageing means that both hypovolaemia and overload must be avoided. In addition to the vital signs and urinary output, invasive monitoring should be established early, using expert help if necessary, in order to optimize cardiovascular function. The insertion of a urinary catheter must be carried out in a strictly aseptic manner as these patients have an increased risk of developing infection.

Dysfunction

Anxiety, disorientation and confusion in the elderly trauma patient must be treated initially by ensuring adequate cerebral perfusion with oxygenated blood rather than assuming this is the patient's normal mental state. In the conscious patient a nurse should be allocated to establish a rapport with the patient to provide reassurance and allay any anxieties. Impaired sensory function, particularly deafness, may produce inappropriate responses and make assessment difficult.

Exposure and environment

The susceptibility of the elderly to greater injuries from a given force means that they must always be completely undressed to ensure that injuries are not missed. However, they are also very prone to hypothermia (see above), so appropriate measures must be taken to prevent this being worsened or added to the patient's list of problems. Generally, doctors tend to leave patients exposed, and it generally falls to the nursing members of the team to ensure that all appropriate measures are taken to prevent hypothermia! Early consideration should be given to the use of forced air-warming devices.

11.4.2 Secondary survey

A full head-to-toe examination is warranted as a result of the inability of the elderly to withstand trauma. In view of the patient's intrinsic immobility due to degenerative diseases and the possible frailty of the skeleton from osteoporosis, care should be taken to maintain the anatomical position that is normal for each patient. Extra care must be taken during log-rolling. Padding of bony prominences during transportation is essential to prevent skin breakdown. It is the responsibility of the nursing team leader to anticipate such complications and avoid them: patients will often not notice contact pressure because of decreased pain perception.

AMPLE history

This is particularly important in the elderly. One of the nursing members of the team must be detailed to gather as much history as possible. Polypharmacy is common and it is important that the medical team leader is advised as soon as possible what medications are being taken as these may have a direct bearing on either the patient's response to injury or resuscitation. As patients get older they are more likely to have other diseases and information must be sought on site from the attending family, friends, ambulance personnel or previous hospital records. Occasionally it may be possible to obtain information directly from the patient. However, because hearing may be less acute, members of the team must remember to speak clearly to the patient, preferably looking directly at him as they speak, without shouting, allowing the patient to lip-read. They should watch the reaction during the conversation to ensure that the patient comprehends what is being said; the response to such communication will also provide further information on the patient's sensory and cognitive abilities. Further useful information may be gained directly from the patient's GP or other local hospitals, over the telephone if necessary.

Sensory overload, short-term memory impairment and senile dementia are common in the elderly. They must be allowed an appropriate amount of time to process information and formulate answers to questions, particularly about the recent events rather than assuming they are incompetent or demented. Sensitivity to these concerns can greatly assist the patient in accepting many of the intrusive procedures associated with resuscitation and subsequent hospitalization, thereby helping to maintain self-esteem.

Ethical and social implications

The patient's dignity must always be respected throughout the resuscitation period (whether conscious or not) and during admission procedures. This contributes significantly to the trauma victim's emotional outcome, as fear of becoming dependent is a serious problem for the elderly patient. The interaction of injury, advanced age and pre-existing medical conditions creates a myriad of challenging issues beyond clinical problems. Determining the survivability of injury in the elderly may not be immediately apparent, except in cases of overwhelming injury or cardiac arrest. The sudden nature of injury usually precludes any prior relation between the trauma surgeon and patient. Early frank communication with the injured patient, family and physicians about pre-injury advance directives, pre-injury quality of life and the impact of trauma on their lifestyle are required, so clearly determined goals of treatment can be established and extraordinary supportive measures are not mistakenly undertaken. Withdrawal of support at the request of the patient, family or physician may reflect humane medical care and occurs as often as in 12.5% of trauma deaths in the elderly. On the other hand, therapeutic nihilism based on age alone becomes a self-fulfilling prophecy, so early aggressive, directed care is required until such time as a comprehensive picture can be drawn and appropriate decisions made. At the same time these goals must be communicated to the entire care-giving team, and the effect of pre-existing conditions or disease must be considered through all phases of trauma care.

11.5 Summary

The elderly comprise an increasing proportion of the general population with an increasing likelihood of being involved in trauma. The anatomical and physiological changes with age result in a different response to injury. Injury severity, age and co-morbid disease all contribute to the outcome in the elderly injured patient and consequently for similar injury severity scores, their outcome is worse. Early recognition and rigorous management of all pre-existing disease, along with the injury sustained, are mandatory to maximize the outcome in this group of patients. Age must not be used as an excuse for inadequate or inappropriate treatment.

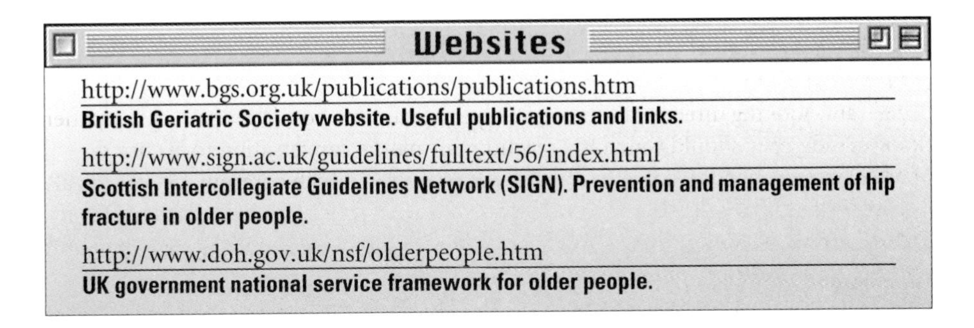

Further reading

1. **Skinner D, Driscoll P & Earlam R (eds)** (1996) *ABC of Major Trauma*, 2nd edn. British Medical Association, London.
2. **Allen JE & Schwab CW** (1985) Blunt chest trauma in the elderly. *Am Surg* 51: 697.
3. **American College of Surgeons Committee on Trauma** (1997) *Advanced Trauma Life Support for Doctors.* American College of Surgeons, Chicago, IL.
4. **Champion HR, Copes WS, Buyer D, *et al.*** (1999) Major trauma in geriatric patients. *Am J Public Health* 79: 1278.
5. **McMahon DJ, Schwab CW & Kauder D** (1996) Comorbidity and the elderly trauma patient. *World J. Surg.* 20: 1113.
6. **Milzman DP, Boulanger BR, Rodriguez A, *et al.*** (1992) Pre-existing disease in trauma patients: a predictor of fate independent of age and ISS. *J. Trauma* 32: 236.
7. **Robinson A** (1995) Age, physical trauma and care. *Can. Med. Assoc. J.* 152: 1453.
8. **Schwab CW & Kauder DR** (1992) Trauma in the geriatric patient. *Arch. Surg.* 127: 701.
9. **Waldmann C** (1992) Anaesthesia for the elderly. In: Kaufman L (ed.) *Anaesthesia Review 9*, pp 194–211.
10. **Watters JM, Moulton SB, Clancey SM, *et al.*** (1994) Ageing exaggerates glucose intolerance following injury. *J. Trauma* 37: 786.
11. **Yates D (ed.)** (1999) Trauma. *British Medical Bulletin* 55: 4.

12 Trauma in children

S Robinson, N Hewer

Objectives

The aims of this chapter are to teach staff caring for the severely injured child:

- the specific anatomical and physiological features in children relevant to the management of trauma;
- how the management of traumatic injuries in children differs to that in adults;
- an approach to the assessment and treatment of the injured child;
- the features that may help in offering a prognosis following severe injury.

12.1 Introduction

In 1999, 416 children under the age of 15 years died because of injury. Trauma is the commonest cause of death in children over the age of one year and the majority of children who die from injury do so before they reach hospital. The pattern of injury seen in the paediatric population differs from that in adults. Haemorrhagic shock and severe life-threatening chest injuries are uncommon and mortality is primarily related to head injury. It has been estimated the average ED can expect to see at most two to four severely injured children a year, therefore exposure to children with this degree of injury is an uncommon event for most doctors and nurses. Consequently, a methodical approach to the assessment and treatment of the injured child is crucial. This chapter will describe how such children can be assessed and their injuries treated.

12.2 Injury patterns in children

12.2.1 Head injuries

- Head injury is the commonest single cause of death in children over the age one year.
- The occurrence of severe cerebral oedema is between three to four times more common in children than adults.
- Cerebral oedema often occurs in the absence of contusion, ischaemic brain damage or intracranial haematoma (*Figure 12.1*).

12.2.2 Cervical spine injury

The specific anatomy of the paediatric cervical spine accounts for the different pattern of injury observed in children (see Box 12.1).

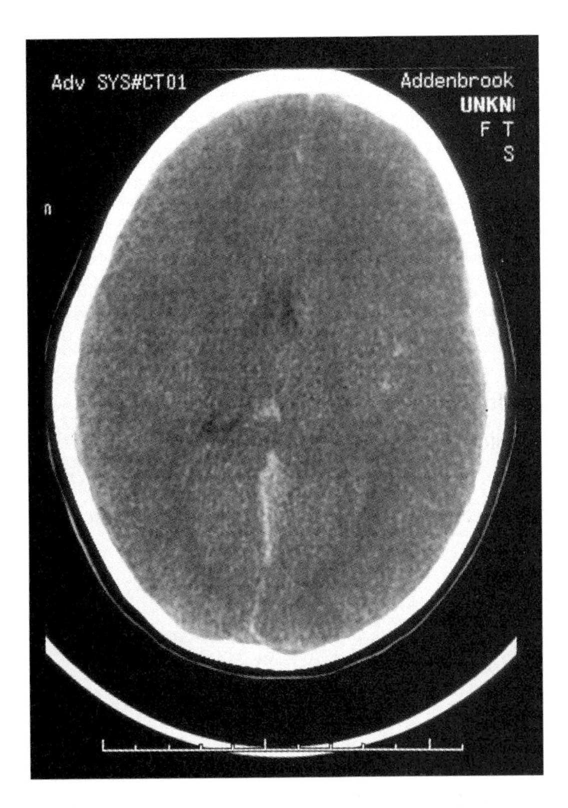

Figure 12.1 CT showing cerebral oedema

BOX 12.1 Structural characteristics of the paediatric cervical spine

Anatomical feature	Effect
• Interspinous ligament and cartilaginous structures have greater laxity and elasticity	• Greater mobility and less stability
• Horizontal angulation of the articulating facets and undeveloped uncinate processes	• Greater mobility and less stability
• Anterior surface of vertebrae wedge shaped	• Facilitates forward vertebral movement resulting in anterior dislocation
• Underdeveloped neck musculature	• More susceptible to flexion and extension injuries
• Head disproportionately large	• Causes torque and acceleration stress to occur higher in C spine and more susceptible to flexion and extension injuries

- The incidence of spinal cord injury amongst paediatric trauma patients is low (1.5%).
- 60–80% of paediatric spinal injuries are in the cervical spine (compared with 30–40% in adults).
- The frequency of upper cervical spine injury (52% C1–4) is nearly twice that of lower cervical spine injury (28% C5–C7).

- Lower cervical spine injuries predominate in older children (age > 8 years).
- Up to 50% of children with neurological deficit due to a cervical cord injury may have no radiological abnormality, 'spinal cord injury without radiological abnormality' (SCIWORA). Transient vertebral displacement with subsequent realignment to a normal configuration results in spinal cord injury with an apparently normal vertebral column.
- Mortality rates have been shown to be higher in younger children (< 10 years) than in older children (30% vs. 7%).
- Major neurological sequelae are uncommon in children who survive.

12.2.3 Thoracic injury

- Chest injuries represent between 0.7–4.5% of all paediatric trauma and are predominantly due to blunt trauma.
- Thoracic trauma is a marker of significant injury and is associated with extra-thoracic injury in 70% of cases, with mortality related to the presence of these other injuries.
- As the child's skeleton is incompletely calcified and is more compliant, serious underlying lung injury may occur without fracture of the ribs.
- Rib fractures are generally rare in paediatric trauma; children with rib fractures are significantly more severely injured than those without. Mortality increases in proportion to the number of ribs fractured.
- Isolated simple pneumothorax is relatively rare in children but tension pneumothorax develops more readily (*Figure 12.2*).

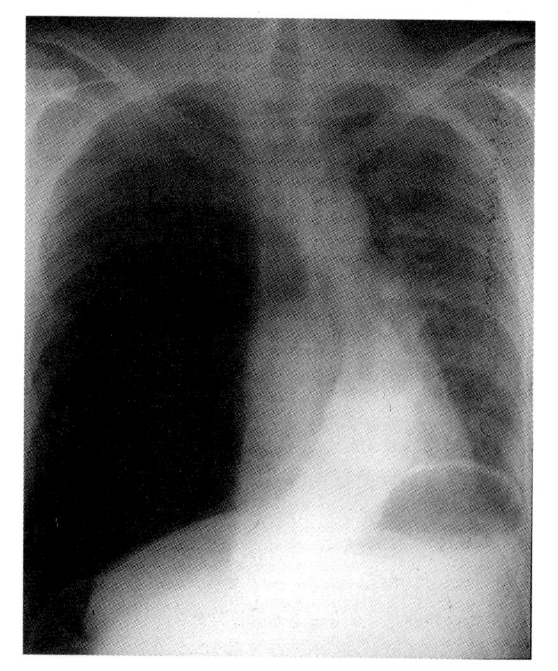

Figure 12.2 Tension pneumothorax, right lung. Note marked displacement of the mediastinum

- Pulmonary contusion is the most common injury seen after blunt chest trauma and may occur in association with pneumothorax, haemothorax or post-traumatic serosanguinous effusion. Massive haemothorax is rare in children because blunt trauma rarely results in haemorrhage from major intrathoracic arteries.

12.2.4 Abdominal injury

- Children have proportionally larger solid organs that are more vulnerable to penetrating injury.
- The spleen is the most common solid organ injured in blunt abdominal trauma.
- Liver injuries are the second most common and occur in 3% of children with blunt abdominal trauma.
- Nonoperative management is the preferred method of treatment for solid organ injury as haemorrhage is generally self-limiting and responds well to fluid or blood transfusion. Figures from one paediatric trauma centre report only 4% of blunt liver injuries and 21% of blunt splenic injuries required operative management.

The young child's predilection to air swallowing, aerophagy, can lead to painful abdominal distension, making examination difficult and increasing the risk of regurgitation and aspiration. Repeated examination, observation and monitoring of the vital signs are essential in the child with a possible abdominal injury.

12.2.5 Musculoskeletal injury

- The paediatric skeleton contains growth plates and a thick, osteogenic periosteum whilst the bones are more porous and elastic.
- Fractures are consequently less likely to cross both cortices or be comminuted.
- Bone healing is very rapid, primarily because of the osteogenic periosteum. The younger the child, the more rapid the healing. Delayed or nonunion rarely occurs.
- Growth plate injuries and epiphyseal injuries can lead to growth disturbance that may be significant (*Figure 12.3*).
- Dislocations and ligamentous injuries are uncommon in children compared with adults.
- Children with multiple injuries can have occult axial fractures and epiphyseal injuries, which are difficult to diagnose even with a good examination.

12.2.6 Nonaccidental injury (NAI)

- The possibility of NAI should always be considered when assessing a child with traumatic injuries and may account for up to 10.6% of all blunt trauma in those under 5 years.
- Children injured as a result of child abuse tend to be younger, more likely to have a pre-injury medical history and retinal haemorrhages when compared with children with unintentional injuries.

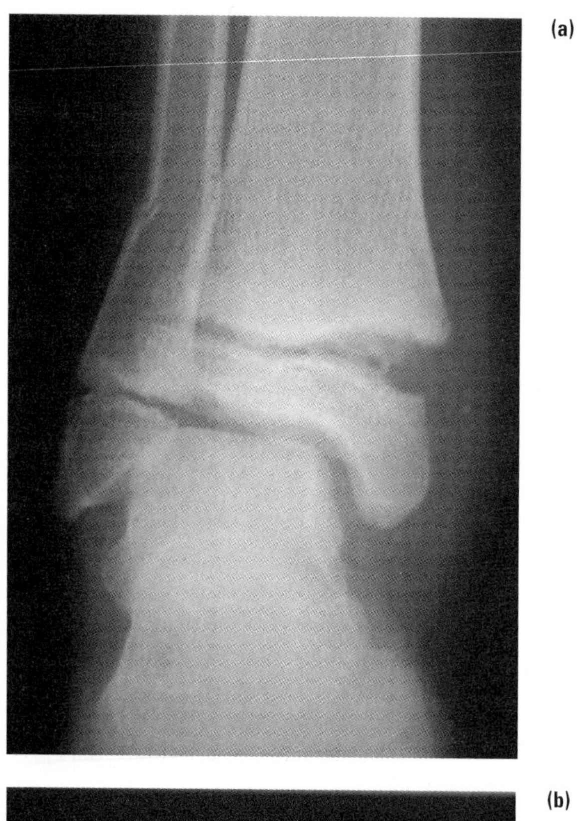

(a)

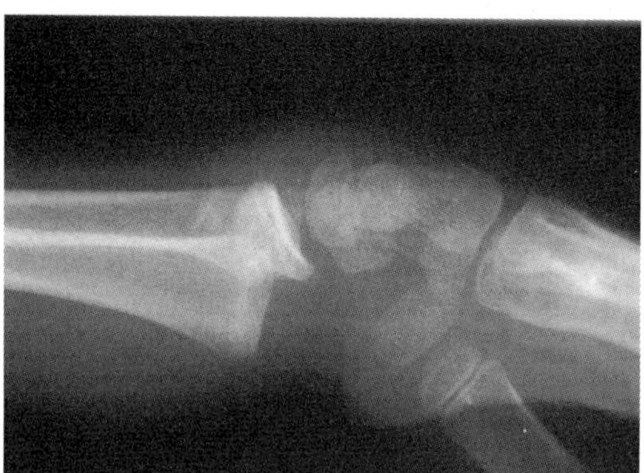

(b)

Figure 12.3 (a) Tibial fracture – Salter Harris type I. (b) Distal radial fracture – Salter Harris type II

Children suspected of being abused need to be referred to the appropriate authorities, according to local policy. Child protection procedures should be instituted in every case of suspected child abuse.

12.3 Preparation and equipment

Warning that a child with trauma is en route to the ED allows the necessary members of staff required to care for the child to be contacted, appropriate roles assigned and preparation of the relevant equipment. Paediatric staff can provide support to staff in the ED and may be able to offer additional support to the child's family during the resuscitation. This shared responsibility aids continuity should the child be transferred to Paediatric Intensive Care Unit (PICU). Most parents wish to be given the opportunity to remain with their child even if invasive procedures are required. There is little evidence to support the routine exclusion of parents from the resuscitation room; indeed most published work supports their presence. Useful guidance for caring for relatives in the resuscitation room is provided by the UK Resuscitation Council.

12.4 Assessment and management

It is essential to have a methodical approach to the assessment of an injured child to avoid missing injuries. Traumatic injury and resuscitation are dynamic processes that require assessment and reassessment. The simplest approach is that described by the Advanced Trauma Life Support (ATLS) and Advanced Paediatric Life Support (APLS) programmes.

12.4.1 Primary survey

During the primary survey a member of the team must be assigned to obtain details from the pre-hospital staff, witnesses (if present) and parents. This includes mechanism of injury, treatment administered at scene or en route, the child's past medical history, medications, allergies, immunization status and an estimate of when food or fluid was last ingested (AMPLE). An estimate of the child's weight needs to be made as soon as possible as most drugs are given on a dose/kg basis. At birth a child weighs approximately 3 kg, this increases to about 10 kg at the age of one year. As a guide the weight can be calculated by the formula:

$$\text{weight (kg)} = 2 \times (\text{age} + 4)$$

The doses of medications likely to be required can thus be calculated and prepared.

Airway and cervical spine control

Airway obstruction from the tongue, foreign material, aspiration and apnoea are particular hazards to the injured child with a decreased level of consciousness. Assessment and management of the airway follows the same principles as for adults (see Section 1.5.1). At the same time the child's head should be immobilized, initially by the airway nurse or paramedic, using manual in line stabilization, unless the child is already immobilized. Ideally, an appropriately sized collar, lateral head supports and straps are required to immobilize the head but, in practice, this cannot always be achieved in very young children or infants. In the unconscious child, care must be taken to ensure that the application of strapping and a tight fitting collar does not impair ventilation or obstruct the jugular veins and raise ICP. Any movement of the child must be performed in a controlled manner, ensuring the spine is immobilized until a spinal injury is excluded.

Potential difficulties in managing the paediatric airway can be minimized by an awareness of the anatomical differences between the adult and child airway (see Box 12.2). Indications for intubation and ventilation are outlined in Box 12.3.

Practical problems when caring for the child's airway:

- to optimize the airway in small infants, a small pillow between the upper shoulders will correct for the large occiput and help prevent excessive caudal displacement of the endotracheal tube due to neck flexion;

BOX 12.2 Structural characteristics of the paediatric airway

Anatomical feature	Effect
Large occiput (< 3 years), short neck	Neck flexes
Infants (< 6 months) breath via the nose	Complete airway obstruction may occur if blocked by blood, oedema
Relatively large tongue, floppy epiglottis	Obscures view of glottis

BOX 12.3 Indications for intubation and ventilation

- Inability to oxygenate and ventilate with a bag-valve-mask technique
- Obvious need for prolonged control of the airway, e.g. multiple injuries
- Decrease in the level of consciousness, e.g. head injury
- Inadequate ventilation, e.g. flail chest, exhaustion
- Persisting hypotension despite adequate fluid resuscitation

- avoid over-extension of the neck as this may cause tracheal compression;
- children are at greater risk of regurgitation and aspiration because of a shorter oesophagus, a lower pressure gradient between the larynx and stomach, lower oesophageal sphincter tone and gastric distension from swallowing air (a naso- or oro-gastric tube should be used to decompress the stomach if this is excessive);
- the procedure for rapid sequence induction is essentially the same as for an adult, however, intubation in injured children can be difficult and should be performed by those well practised in the technique;
- a straight laryngoscope blade can be used in the very young child to 'lift' the epiglottis and facilitate the view of the glottis;
- uncuffed, appropriately sized tubes are used in children under the age of 8–10 years to avoid subglottic oedema and ulceration;
- the oro-tracheal route is the preferred approach in the resuscitation room although a naso-tracheal tube is more easily secured and therefore often used in more controlled situations;
- cricoid pressure must be applied to reduce the risk of aspiration during induction and will decrease the volume of air forced into the stomach of small children during bag-valve-mask ventilation;
- cricoid pressure should not be released until correct placement of the tube is confirmed by a normal end-tidal carbon dioxide waveform and bilateral breath sounds;
- major complications have been reported in 25% of children who required intubation, 80% of which were life threatening.

The appropriate sizes of a tracheal tube for a child can be calculated as follows:

Oral endotracheal tube	Nasal endotracheal tube
Internal diameter (mm) = (age/4) + 4	Internal diameter (mm) = (age/4) + 4
Length (cm) = (age/2) + 12	Length (cm) = (age/2) + 15

If a surgical airway is required, needle cricothyroidotomy is the recommended technique in children under the age of 12 years. This is described in Section 2.5.7. Surgical cricothyroidotomy may result in damage to the cricoid cartilage, the only complete ring of cartilage in the airway, causing collapse of the upper airway. Healing results in tracheal stenosis and long-term airway problems.

Breathing

The adequacy of ventilation in children is assessed by the nurse and doctor simultaneously by:

- observing chest wall movement;
- counting the respiratory rate;
- examining percussion note;
- listening for air entry.

Recession of the intercostal and subcostal muscles, flaring of the nostrils and grunting is indicative of respiratory distress. A depressed level of consciousness or agitation are signs of hypoxia, cyanosis is a late sign of hypoxia; children more commonly appear pale

The treatment of life-threatening chest injuries is similar to that in adults.

Circulation

Although the blood volume/kg is higher in children than adults (100 ml/kg in a neonate, 80 ml/kg in a child, 70 ml/kg adult) the absolute circulating blood volume is small. The loss of relatively small volumes can result in significant haemodynamic compromise. Children are, however, extremely efficient in compensating for the loss of blood as a result of a relatively greater ability to increase systemic vascular resistance and heart rate. The signs of early haemorrhagic shock are subtle in children and the onset of decompensation is abrupt. Hypotension is therefore a late and pre-terminal sign. Isolated intracranial haemorrhage in infants may result in hypovolaemic shock.

Assessment

The team member allocated to deal with 'circulation' should assess skin colour, pulse rate, pulse pressure and capillary refilling time (normal < 2 s), and apply a pulse oximeter. Pulse oximetry may prove difficult in the presence of shock, hypothermia, peripheral vasoconstriction or a restless child. This is followed by attaching the ECG to allow continuous monitoring of the heart rate and rhythm, using lead II. The blood

BOX 12.4 Normal vital signs in children

Age	Weight (kg)	PR (beats/min)	RR (breaths/min)	Systolic BP (mmHg)
3–6 months	5–7	100–160	30–40	70–90
1 year	10	100–160	30–40	70–90
2 years	12	95–140	25–30	80–100
3–4 years	14–16	95–140	25–30	80–100
5–8 years	18–24	80–120	20–25	90–110
10 years	30	80–100	15–20	90–110
12 years	40	60–100	12–20	100–120

pressure (BP) is then measured by indirect techniques using appropriately sized cuffs. In the presence of massive or continuing haemorrhage, this technique is not always reliable. In such instances the BP should be monitored via an indwelling arterial catheter. This provides an accurate measurement of the BP and allows regular arterial blood gas sampling. In the initial stages, evaluation of the vital signs should be performed every 5 min.

Venous access is a high priority in the child with severe injury and should be delegated to the most appropriate person, usually a doctor or technician as the nurse performs the above tasks. The optimal sites for peripheral venous access are the veins on the dorsum of the hand or foot and the saphenous vein anterior to the medial malleolus. The antecubital vein is often easy to cannulate but the catheter is readily kinked by flexion of the elbow. The elbow should be splinted if used. Two intravenous cannulae are the ideal, the size dictated by the size of the child.

If intravascular access is not achieved within 90 s via the percutaneous route in children up to 6 years of age, the intraosseous route should be used. The most common site used for intraosseous access is 2–3 cm below the tibial tuberosity on the flattened medial aspect of the tibia. The anterolateral surface of the femur, 3 cm above the lateral condyle is another site. Fractured bones should be avoided, as should limbs with fractures proximal to the site of entry.

Alternatives to the above are percutaneous cannulation of either the femoral or central veins or venous cutdown. The latter can be difficult in the shocked child, particularly when the physician is inexperienced.

Initially, boluses of warmed crystalloid (20 ml/kg) are administered. In small children the most effective and accurate method of administration is via a syringe. The circulation nurse should make a careful record of the volumes administered, particularly in very small children. The child should be reassessed after each bolus; improvement will be evident by a fall in heart rate, an improvement in capillary refill and an increase in blood pressure. Failure to respond to fluid should prompt a search for other causes of shock whilst further fluid is administered. Any child presenting with profound haemorrhagic shock or who fails to respond to approximately 60–80 ml/kg of crystalloid and/or colloid should receive warmed, packed red blood cells, and urgent surgical referral.

Technique for insertion of intraosseous needle

- The knee and proximal lower leg should be supported by a pillow. The skin should be cleaned.
- A 16–18 g intraosseous needle is inserted 90° to the skin and advanced until a 'give' is felt as the cortex is penetrated (*Figure 12.4*). Making a small skin incision at the point of entry and a 'twisting and boring' motion of the needle facilitates insertion and entry through the cortex by the trocar and needle.
- Remove the trocar and attach a syringe. Infusion of saline can, if necessary clear the needle of any clot.
- Correct placement is confirmed by aspiration of marrow content, easy infusion of fluid with no evidence of soft tissue swelling. The aspirated sample can be sent to the laboratory for routine bloods and used for bedside glucose estimation.
- Fluids need to be administered in boluses. The flow rates are high enough for volume resuscitation. Intraosseous lines need to be replaced by venous cannulation as soon as possible.

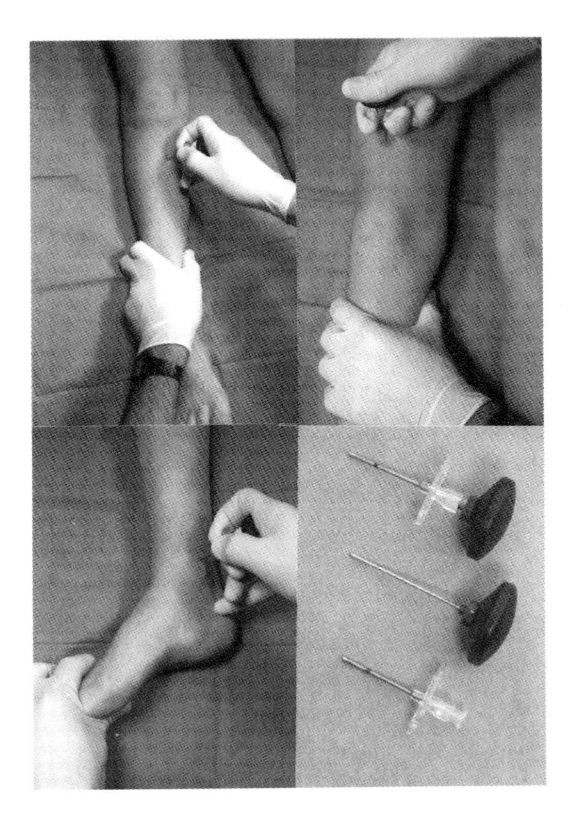

Figure 12.4 Site for insertion of intraosseous needle. Greaves I, Porter K (eds) *Pre-hospital medicine: The principles and practice of immediate care* (1999). Reproduced with permission from Hodder/Arnold.

- Complications are rare but include extravasation, subperiosteal infusion, fat and bone marrow embolism, osteomyelitis, damage to the growth plate and cortex, pain and subcutaneous oedema.

Although CT examination facilitates grading of intra-abdominal solid injury severity, it is current practice to use physiological rather than anatomical criteria to decide on the need for laparotomy. Haemodynamic instability as defined by the need for blood transfusion in excess of 25 ml/kg within the first two hours has been identified as a strong indicator of a major hepatic vascular injury. Treatment algorithms have been proposed to aid decisions regarding operative management in children with severe hepatic and splenic injury.

Dysfunction

The initial evaluation of the central nervous system in an injured child incorporates assessment of the level of consciousness by either AVPU or the GCS (see Box 12.5) and examination of the pupil size and reactivity. This can be performed by a member of the nursing or medical team and should be recorded appropriately. The assessment of GCS is not very precise in children under the age of 5 years. The presence of abnormal posturing, limb movement and tone should be noted.

Exposure and environment

On arrival, the child needs to be undressed and covered to prevent a drop in temperature. Small children have a high body surface area to weight ratio, which is at its highest

BOX 12.5	Glasgow coma scale – age < 4 years
Eye opening:	
Spontaneously	4
To verbal stimuli	3
To pain	2
No response	1
Verbal response:	
Alert, babbles, words to usual ability	5
Less than usual words, spontaneous irritable cry	4
Cries only to pain	3
Moans to pain	2
No response to pain	1
Motor response:	
Obeys verbal command	6
Localizes to pain	5
Withdraws from pain	4
Abnormal flexion to pain (decorticate)	3
Abnormal extension to pain (decerebrate)	2
No response	1

when the child is newborn. Consequently, children lose heat much more rapidly than adults do; for example, newborn children will lose 1°C every 4 min if left uncovered. Any part of the body covered by splints or collar should be examined. The back should be examined during the log roll. Wounds should be photographed and then covered in Betadine (unless allergic to iodine) soaked dressings. A member of the nursing team should have the role of monitoring the child's temperature and minimizing heat loss by ensuring that all fluids are warmed, exposure is minimal and external heating devices are used appropriately.

12.4.2 Secondary survey

If not already available, the nurse assigned to the relatives must obtain details of the child's past medical history, medications, allergies, immunization status and an estimate of when food or fluid was last ingested (AMPLE). Once the initial primary survey and resuscitative efforts has been completed, a secondary survey is performed. This consists of a detailed 'head-to-toe' examination of:

- the head, face and neck, including eyes and ears;
- the extremities;
- repeat examination of the chest and abdomen;
- log roll and, if appropriate, a rectal examination.

Appropriate radiological investigations are performed. The high incidence of spinal cord injury without radiological abnormality in children should reinforce the importance of a detailed neurological examination as the best method of identifying cord injury.

If not already done, a naso-gastric tube should be inserted. The stomach should be decompressed via the oral route if there is the possibility of a base of skull fracture. Urinary catheterization is not necessary in conscious children able to pass urine spontaneously. Urethral or suprapubic catheterization will be necessary in those children unable to pass urine spontaneously or in those where continuous monitoring of urine output is essential. A urine bag should be used to monitor the urine output of infants.

Occasionally, it is necessary for the child to be transferred urgently for surgery to control haemorrhage and it will not be possible to complete a secondary survey. If so, the physician transferring the child to theatre must be informed of this and the need for further examination recorded in the notes.

Analgesia

Analgesia must always be administered if required. An intravenous opiate is the most appropriate method in severe pain. Morphine should be diluted and the dose checked by a member of the nursing staff to ensure accurate and safe administration. The child's pain should be re-assessed at regular intervals by a nurse or doctor and further doses administered if necessary. Psychological support by parents/guardians is vital, along with other methods such as distraction techniques, regional nerve blocks, splintage and immobilization, where applicable.

Investigations

Routine laboratory investigations include FBC, blood group and cross-match and amylase. Additional biochemistry such as urea and electrolytes (U&E) or toxicology may be required but are not routinely performed in all children. Coagulation studies should be performed on patients with severe trauma. Hypotension, a GCS < 13, compound or multiple fractures and extensive soft tissue injuries are all associated with disturbances in coagulation. Arterial blood gas analysis is mandatory in the presence of pulmonary injury and in any shocked child as the base deficit quantifies the severity of shock and predicts the development of multiple organ failure and continuing haemorrhage. The admission base deficit can be a useful marker and should alert the team to uncompensated shock or potentially lethal injuries. A bedside estimation of the blood glucose should be performed by a nurse and urinalysis performed, once the patient is catheterized or passes urine spontaneously.

Standard radiological investigations in the resuscitation room include x-rays of the cervical spine, chest and pelvis. Imaging of the cervical spine consists of a cross table lateral view, antero-posterior view and an open mouth view. Imaging the high cervical spine can be difficult in the unconscious or intubated patient and the lateral cervical spine x-ray is best performed with traction on the arms. CT imaging of the cervical spine may be required to view C1/C2. However, it is important to remember the higher incidence of ligamentous injury and neurological injury without bone abnormality in children, which may not be apparent on CT. Other modalities such as MRI should be considered if clinical examination suggests the possibility of cord injury despite normal plain radiography. A chest x-ray will identify any significant pneumothorax, haemothorax or pulmonary contusion.

DPL although sensitive for identifying intraperitoneal blood does not provide any information on the type or severity of organ injury, and CT examination of the abdomen and pelvis is the method of choice when further evaluation of the abdomen is required. Children, however, should only be transferred to the CT scanner if they are haemodynamically stable or the same level of ongoing resuscitation and monitoring can be assured. Abdominal ultrasound within the ED may be useful in the hypotensive child considered too unstable to be transferred. In the stable child, ultrasound may have a role in prioritizing imaging studies.

Prognosis

No motor response from the GCS, the Injury Severity Score (ISS) – (International Classification of Disease, Ninth Revision-based Injury Severity Score) and 'unresponsive' from AVPU score have been identified as independent predictors of inpatient mortality in paediatric patients with blunt trauma. In children sustaining severe, multiple traumatic injuries admitted to a Paediatric Intensive Care Unit (PICU) over a 9-year period, a Paediatric Risk of Mortality Score (PRISM) > 35 and a GCS score < 7 represented independent risk factors of death. Children with a head injury had a four-fold greater mortality than those without. Of 957 trauma patients younger than 15 years requiring cardiopulmonary resuscitation (CPR) at the scene or on admission, 225 (24%) survived to discharge, of whom 36% had no functional impairment. A systolic blood pressure below 60 mmHg on admission represented the single greatest predictor of fatality. Those with a GCS < 8 on admission or penetrating trauma were also at greater risk of death.

12.5 Summary

Although trauma is the commonest cause of death in children over the age of one year, it is relatively rare for the ED to be exposed to children with significant injury. It is essential that clinical staff have a systematic approach to the management of an injured child, are aware of how children differ from adults in their response to injury and have a selection of appropriate paediatric equipment readily available.

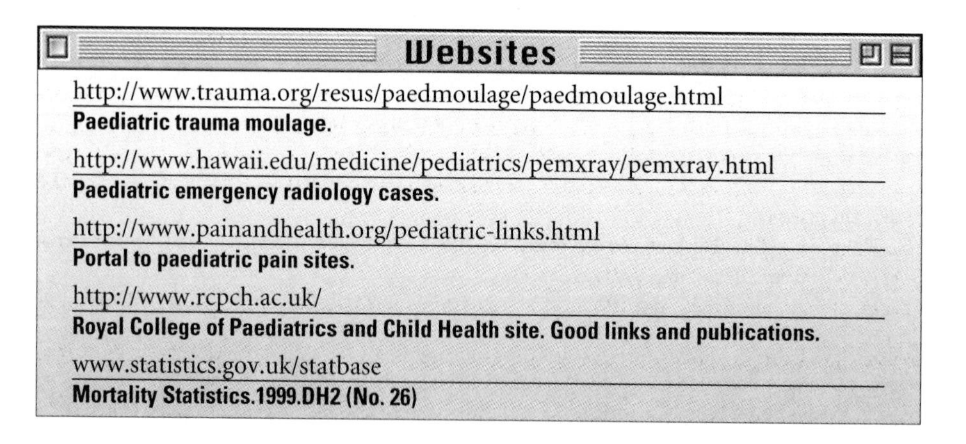
Websites

http://www.trauma.org/resus/paedmoulage/paedmoulage.html
Paediatric trauma moulage.

http://www.hawaii.edu/medicine/pediatrics/pemxray/pemxray.html
Paediatric emergency radiology cases.

http://www.painandhealth.org/pediatric-links.html
Portal to paediatric pain sites.

http://www.rcpch.ac.uk/
Royal College of Paediatrics and Child Health site. Good links and publications.

www.statistics.gov.uk/statbase
Mortality Statistics.1999.DH2 (No. 26)

Further reading

1. **American College of Surgeons Committee on Trauma** (1997) *Advanced Trauma Life Support for Doctors.* American College of Surgeons, Chicago, IL.
2. **Boie ET, Moore GP, Brummett C, *et al.*** (1999) Do parents want to be present during invasive procedures performed on their children in the emergency department? *Ann. Emerg. Med.* 34(1): 70.

3. Bond SJ, Eichelberger MR, Gotschall CS, *et al.* (1996) Non-operative management of blunt hepatic and splenic injury in children. *Ann. Surg.* **223:** 286.
4. Cantais E, Paut O, Giorgi R, *et al.* (2001) Evaluating the prognosis of multiple severely traumatized children in the intensive care unit. *Intens. Care Med.* **27:** 1511.
5. Child Accident Prevention (1989) *Basic Principles of Child Accident Prevention.* Child Accident Prevention Trust, London.
6. Coburn MC, Pfeifer J & DeLuca FG (1995) Non-operative management of blunt hepatic and splenic trauma in the multiply injured pediatric and adolescent patient. *Arch. Surg.* **130:** 332.
7. Di Scala C, Sege R, Li G, *et al.* (2000) Child abuse and unintentional injuries: a 10 year retrospective review. *Arch. Pediatr. Adolesc. Med.* **154**(1): 16.
8. Doyle CJ (1987) Family participation during resuscitation: an option. *Ann. Emerg. Med.* **16:** 107.
9. Gandhi RR, Keller MS, Schwab CW, *et al.* (1999) Pediatric splenic injury: pathway to play. *J. Pediatr. Surg.* **34**(1): 55.
10. Garcia VF, Gotschall CS, Eichelberger MR, *et al.* (1990) Rib fractures in children: a marker for severe trauma. *J. Trauma* **30:** 695.
11. Gross M, Lynch F, Canty T, *et al.* (1999) Management of pediatric liver injuries: a 13 year experience at a pediatric trauma center. *J. Pediatr. Surg.* **34**(5): 811.
12. Hall JR, Reyes HM, Meller JL, *et al.* (1996) The outcome for children with blunt trauma is best at a pediatric trauma center. *J. Pediatr. Surg.* **31**(1): 72.
13. Hannan EL, Farrell LS, Meaker PS, *et al.* (2000) Predicting inpatient mortality for paediatric trauma patients with blunt injuries: a better alternative. *J. Pediatr. Surg.* **35:** 155.
14. Holmes JF, Goodwin HC, Land C, *et al.* (2001). Coagulation testing in pediatric blunt trauma patients. *Pediatr. Emerg. Care* **17**(5): 324.
15. Holmes JF, Brant WE, Bond WF, *et al.* (2001) Emergency department ultrasonography in the evaluation of hypotensive and normotensive children with abdominal blunt trauma. *J. Pediatr. Surg.* **36**(7): 968.
16. Kincaid EH, Chang MC, Letton RW, *et al.* (2001) Admission base deficit in pediatric trauma: a study using the National Trauma Data Bank. *J. Trauma* **51:** 332.
17. Kokska ER, Keller MS, Rallo MC, *et al.* (2001) Characteristics of pediatric cervical spine injuries. *J. Pediatr. Surg.* **36**(1): 100.
18. Li G, Nelson Tang PH, DiScala C, *et al.* (1999) Cardiopulmonary resuscitation in pediatric trauma patients: survival and functional outcome. *J. Trauma* **47:** 1.
19. Mehall JR, Ennis JS, Saltzman DA, *et al.* (2001) Prospective results of a standardised algorithm based on haemodynamic status for managing pediatric solid organ injury. *J. Am. Coll. Surg.* **193**(4): 347.
20. Nakayama DK, Gardner MJ & Rowe MI (1990) Emergency endotracheal intubation in pediatric trauma. *Ann. Surg.* **211**(2): 218.
21. Patel JC, Tepas III JJ, Mollitt DL, *et al.* (2001) Pediatric cervical spine injuries: defining the disease. *J. Pediatr. Surg.* **36**(2): 373.
22. Peclet MH, Newman KD & Eichelberger MR (1990) Patterns of injury in children. *J. Pediatr. Surg.* **25:** 85.
23. Peclet MH, Newman KD, Eichelberger MR, *et al.* (1990) Thoracic trauma in children: an indicator of increased mortality. *J. Pediatr. Surg.* **25**(9): 961.
24. Resuscitation Council (1996) Should Relatives Witness Resuscitation?
Report from Project Team of the (UK).
25. Robinson SM, Mackenzie-Ross S, Campbell-Hewson GL, *et al.* (1998) Psychological effect of witnessed resuscitation on bereaved relatives. *Lancet* **352:** 614.
26. Roux P & Fisher RM (1992) Chest injuries in children: an analysis of 100 cases of blunt chest trauma from motor vehicle accidents. *J. Pediatr. Surg.* **27**(5): 551.
26. Secretaries of State for Health (1992) *The Health of the Nation* 19; 102. HMSO, London.

27. The Advanced Life Support Group (1997) *Advanced Paediatric Life Support – the practical approach.* BMJ Publications, London.
28. The UK Trauma Audit and Research Network. The University of Manchester, data 1994–98
29. Wyatt JP, McLeod L, Beard D, *et al.* (1997) Timing of paediatric deaths after trauma. *BMJ* 314: 868.

13 Trauma in pregnancy

S Fletcher, G Lomas

Objectives

At the end of this chapter the trauma team should understand:

- the anatomy and pathophysiological changes associated with pregnancy;
- the response of the pregnant patient to trauma;
- the assessment and management of the pregnant trauma patient.

13.1 Introduction

The arrival of a pregnant trauma patient in the resuscitation room is a relatively rare but frightening occurrence for all concerned. The trauma team is presented with two patients, mother and fetus. Consequently early obstetric involvement is vital.

Trauma complicates up to 7–8% of all pregnancies and is the leading cause of nonobstetric maternal death. Motor vehicle accidents and falls are the most common causes, while more recently there has been an increasing incidence of assaults.

The pregnant state is associated with changes in anatomy and physiology that alter the pattern of, and response to, trauma. This makes assessment of the severity of injury more complex. Although there are two patients, aggressive resuscitation of the mother is required to save the fetus. Very rarely is delivery of the baby necessary to save the mother.

13.2 The pathophysiology of pregnancy

Pregnancy is associated with many anatomical, physiological and psychological changes. To know what is 'normal' in the pregnant patient requires a basic understanding of these changes.

13.2.1 Airway and ventilation

- Engorgement of the capillaries of the upper airways leads to increased soft tissue bulk of the larynx and narrowing of the airways. This is accompanied by enlargement of the breasts and increased fat deposition in the soft tissues of the face. All these changes lead to an increased incidence of difficult or failed intubation. Smaller endotracheal tubes may be required for intubation.
- Increased vascularity and fragility of the upper airway predisposes the patient to nasopharyngeal bleeding and care must be taken when inserting instrumentation into the airway.

- Minute ventilation is increased mainly due to a 40% increase in tidal volume, respiratory rate is only slightly increased. This 'hyperventilation of pregnancy' results in hypocapnia with a $PaCO_2$ of around 30 mmHg. Normocapnia ($PaCO_2$ ~ 40 mmHg) therefore may be a sign of inadequate ventilation in pregnancy.
- As the uterus enlarges the resulting fall in functional residual capacity diminishes the oxygen reserves. At the same time oxygen consumption is increased. Consequently the pregnant patient's tolerance of hypoxia is reduced.

13.2.2 Circulation

- Heart rate increases gradually throughout pregnancy, reaching 15–20 beats higher than normal by the 3rd trimester. Both systolic and diastolic blood pressures fall by 5–15 mmHg during the 2nd trimester, returning to pre-pregnancy levels by term.
- Cardiac output increases 20–30% (1.0–1.5 l/min) by the end of the 1st trimester due to the increase in blood volume and a decrease in vascular resistance of the uterus and placenta. The uterus eventually receives up to 25% of the cardiac output.
- Blood volume increases steadily by 40–50%, reaching a plateau at 34 weeks. The increase in red cell mass is less than that of plasma resulting in a haematocrit of less than 35%, the 'physiological anaemia of pregnancy'.
- Uterine vessels are incapable of autoregulation – they constrict in the initial response to maternal hypovolaemia severely compromising the fetus with minimal changes in the mother's vital signs.

The pregnant patient may lose up to 1500 ml of blood before any signs of hypovolaemia are seen. Failure to recognize this may lead to underestimation and hence under-treatment of blood loss in the pregnant trauma patient. Once the mother is exhibiting signs of hypovolaemic shock the chance of fetal survival is less than 20%

Cardiac output and blood pressure can both be influenced by maternal position in later pregnancy. In the supine position the weight of the uterus and fetus compress the aorta and vena cava, reducing venous return and cardiac output. This is the basis for the 'supine hypotensive syndrome', where the mother may complain of dizziness, discomfort or nausea whilst lying down. At the same time the fetus may show signs of distress, either bradycardia or tachycardia.

A hypercoagulability state also exists as a result of the elevation in the level of fibrinogen and other clotting factors. Placental abruption may trigger disseminated intravascular coagulation (DIC). This is a life-threatening complication requiring early recognition and treatment.

13.2.3 Gastrointestinal tract

Progesterone has a delaying effect on gastric emptying and also renders the gastro-oesophageal sphincter less competent. This is exacerbated by the uterus displacing the bowel into the upper abdomen. As a result the pregnant patient should always be assumed to have a full stomach and at increased risk of aspiration of gastric contents.

13.2.4 Renal system

- Pregnancy is associated with an increase in both renal blood flow and glomerular filtration rates. Serum levels of creatinine and urea may be only 50% of normal levels.
- Pressure of the uterus on the bladder commonly results in urinary frequency.
- Proteinuria is abnormal, glycosuria is a common finding in normal pregnancy.

13.2.5 Nervous system

Pre-eclampsia, or pregnancy-induced hypertension is a condition requiring urgent treatment. In addition to hypertension, there will be peripheral oedema and proteinuria. The symptoms can be vague and include headache, drowsiness and visual disturbances. Seizures can occur if the pre-eclampsia is not treated and the patient develops full-blown eclampsia. These symptoms can be attributed to a head injury in the pregnant trauma patient and vice versa. Careful assessment of the history and examination of the patient may point to the true cause of the symptoms.

13.2.6 Musculoskeletal system

Pelvic fractures are uncommon as a result of hormonal-induced softening of the joints and relaxation of the sacroiliac joint. The presence of a fractured pelvic in a pregnant trauma patient is therefore an indicator of severe trauma.

13.2.7 Uterus and placenta

- The uterus begins to rise out of the pelvis from the 12th week becoming an intra-abdominal organ. It reaches the umbilicus by 20 weeks and the costal margin at 34–36 weeks.
- The bowel is pushed up into the upper abdomen and the uterus receives the major impact of blunt abdominal trauma. The thick uterine wall initially offers the fetus some protection but this is lost by the 3rd trimester when the muscle becomes stretched and thin.
- Blood flow to the uterus increases throughout pregnancy reaching up to 700 ml/min. Injury to the uterine vessels can result in significant haemorrhage, which may be concealed and therefore difficult to detect.

13.3 Assessment and management

13.3.1 Primary survey and resuscitation

The key to successful management of the pregnant trauma patient is the utilization of a team approach. The team should expand to include an obstetrician, an obstetric nurse and, if there is any likelihood of emergency delivery, a paediatrician. Resuscitating the mother is the best way of resuscitating the fetus. Although obstetrical management is imperative, the ABCs of trauma resuscitation remain the same.

BOX 13.1 Summary of physiological changes of pregnancy

System	Physiological Change
Respiratory	Minute ventilation ↑ (7.5–10.5 l/min)
	Tidal volume ↑ by 40%
	$PaCO_2$ ↓ (40–30 mmHg)
	↓ Functional residual capacity by 20%
	↑ Oxygen consumption by 20%
	↓ Tolerance to hypoxia
	Congested nasal airways
	↑ Incidence difficult intubation
Cardiovascular	↑ Cardiac output (4.5–6.0 l/min)
	↑ Blood volume
	Tolerance of hypovolaemia
	Physiological anaemia
	↓ Peripheral vascular resistance
	↑ Heart rate
	↑ Blood pressure initially
	Aortocaval compression
	↑ White cell count
	Hypercoagulability of blood
Gastrointestinal	Delayed gastric emptying
	Incompetent gastro-oesophageal sphincter
	Full stomach
	Aspiration risk
Renal	↑ Renal blood flow
	↑ Glomerular filtration
	↓ Serum creatinine and urea
Nervous	Pre-eclampsia vs. head injury
Musculoskeletal	Fractured pelvis = major trauma
Uterus/Placenta	↑ Blood flow
	No autoregulation

Resuscitation of the mother is the optimal method of resuscitating the fetus

Airway and cervical spine control

Because of the increased risk of regurgitation and aspiration during pregnancy, early consideration should be given to prevention with a cuffed endotracheal tube. Cricoid pressure should be used in an attempt to minimize the risk of regurgitation. Intubation may be more difficult due to the changes described previously. It is therefore imperative that the airway nurse has a full range of equipment that has been checked, immediately available. If a cervical spine injury is suspected the patient's neck should be immobilized with a semirigid collar and head blocks until the cervical spine has been cleared.

Breathing

High concentrations of oxygen are particularly important in order to ensure fetal oxygenation. If ventilation is required, it is important to remember that 'mild hyperventilation' should be employed ($PaCO_2$ 30 mmHg). The stomach should be decompressed early by gastric tube placement. In late pregnancy, higher inflation pressures will be required as a result of the effects of the uterus on the lungs. Expert help must be sought early, particularly if mechanical ventilation is used, to reduce the risk of barotrauma.

Circulation

Hypovolemia should be suspected before it becomes apparent. Interpretation of maternal pulse and blood pressure readings can be difficult. The fetus may be shocked before the mother develops tachycardia, tachypnoea or hypotension, as blood is shunted away from the uteroplacental circulation to maintain maternal vital signs. If there are team members who are experienced fetal monitoring should be instituted early to help identify significant maternal hypovolaemia.

The increased blood volume and ability to redirect blood from the placental to systemic circulation allows the mother to lose up to one third of her circulating volume before developing the classic signs of shock. Furthermore, the vasodilatation that occurs with pregnancy causes the patient's skin to be warm and pink and dry, even with such a large blood loss.

Vigorous fluid resuscitation should be commenced using warmed crystalloid or a colloid. This should be given through two large bore cannulas (14 g) in the antecubical fossa. Blood for grouping and cross-matching, urea and electrolytes, full blood count should be taken. Prophylactic anti-D must be given to prevent any woman who is Rhesus negative developing Rhesus sensitization.

Meticulous monitoring of the mother's vital signs and her response to the intravenous fluids, along with fetal heart rate if available, will assist with resuscitation. Early consideration should be given to the use of CVP monitoring.

Aortocaval compression may cause or worsen hypotension. To prevent this, patients in the second and third trimester need to be log-rolled onto their left side providing there is no spinal injury. Alternatively, the right hip can be elevated using a sandbag, pillows or a Cardiff wedge, and the uterus manually displaced to the left. If cervical spine injury is suspected, the best method is to have the patient's neck immobilized as above and secured to a long spinal board so that the manoeuvres can be achieved without twisting the vertebral column. Once spinal injury has been excluded, the patient can be nursed in the left lateral position.

Dysfunction

The patient's neurological status is checked in exactly the same way as any trauma patient using AVPU or the GCS. Pre-eclampsia may cause a reduction in level of consciousness and symptoms similar to a head injury. The medical team leader must ensure these are not misinterpreted.

Exposure and environment

This examination should be carried out so that a full assessment of the patient can be made taking care to avoid hypothermia.

The mechanism of injury is also important. As the gravid uterus develops, it becomes an easier target for penetrating trauma. Although the fetus may die following this type of injury, the mother can survive because by the third trimester the uterus acts as a shield for the rest of the abdominal contents. In contrast blunt trauma during this stage of pregnancy may result in uterine rupture with significant haemorrhage. This is associated with a high maternal mortality.

13.3.2 Secondary survey

After the primary assessment has been completed, the secondary survey is carried out systematically with the mother being examined from head to toe and front to back to identify any other injuries. A detailed assessment of the fetus is part of the secondary assessment and should be carried out by an obstetrician.

Assessment of the mother

When examining the abdomen note the fundal height, uterine shape, presence of fetal movement, uterine contractions and any tenderness. A change in shape may indicate uterine rupture or concealed haemorrhage. An irritable uterus can be due to inadequate uterine oxygenation and, if untreated, lead to preterm labour.

Abdominal pain, tenderness or palpation of two abdominal masses suggests uterine injury. This is an obstetric and trauma emergency as maternal shock and fetal death can occur very rapidly. A pelvic fracture may result in damage to dilated uterine veins. The presence of this injury should therefore alert the team to the risk of massive retroperitoneal haemorrhage.

If a vaginal examination is essential, it should be carried out by the obstetric member of the team to allow the uterus, cervical os and the presentation of the fetus to be accurately assessed. Vaginal bleeding or amniotic fluid may be present and some patients may describe having had a sudden gush of fluid. This may be an indication of spontaneous bladder emptying or premature rupture of amniotic fluid. Any fluid lost should be collected to identify amniotic fluid that may have been leaked from the premature rupture of the membranes.

The vaginal opening is inspected for crowning or any abnormal fetal presentation. Prolapse of the umbilical cord is rare but when present must be relieved immediately. If positioning the mother to relieve the pressure on the cord is contraindicated, manual displacement of the presenting part may be needed. Abdominal trauma in late pregnancy can damage the bladder because of crowding of pelvic structures. More commonly, spontaneous voiding occurs because of the increased pressure on the bladder.

Peritoneal lavage can be done if indicated through a supraumbilical minilaparotomy after the patient has a naso-gastric tube and catheter inserted. If the patient requires abdominal surgery this should not be delayed because of the pregnancy.

Assessment of the fetus

Fetal assessment must be carried out by skilled personnel during the secondary assessment, when the mother has been resuscitated.

It is imperative to know the gestational age of the fetus. The most accurate indicator for this will be the last menstrual period. However, in the emergency situation it may not be possible to ascertain this and the fundal height will have to be used instead (*Figure 13.1*). The number of weeks' gestation approximates to the fundal height

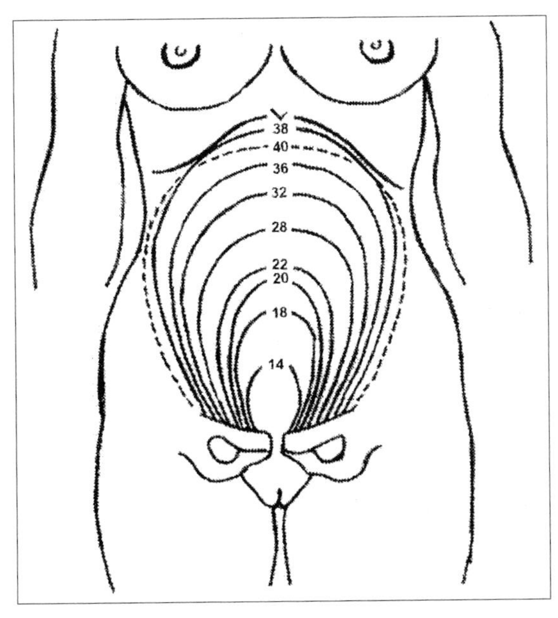

Figure 13.1 Diagram of fundal height

measured in cm from the symphysis pubis. Alternatively, the fundal height reaches the symphysis at 12 weeks, the umbilicus at 20 weeks and the costal margin at 36 weeks.

Fetal evaluation will usually begin by checking the fetal heart tones and rate, and noting fetal movement. The fetal heart tones can be heard by Doppler ultrasonography from 12–14 weeks gestation, and is normally 120–160 beats/min. A fetal heart rate less than 110 is considered a bradycardia. If it is sustained and accompanied with a loss of beat to beat variation then fetal distress is present.

Ultrasound can also be used to assess the placental position, the liquor volume and the presence of intra-amniotic haemorrhage, estimate gestational age, fetal well being, placental laceration and any evidence of separation. Maternal visceral injury by free fluid in the peritoneum may also be detected.

If the patient is over 20 weeks' gestation the fetus can be monitored by a cardiotocograph, to compare uterine contractions with fetal heart rate (*Figure 13.2*). Signs of fetal heart distress include inadequate acceleration of fetal heart rate in response to uterine contractions and late decelerations in response to contractions.

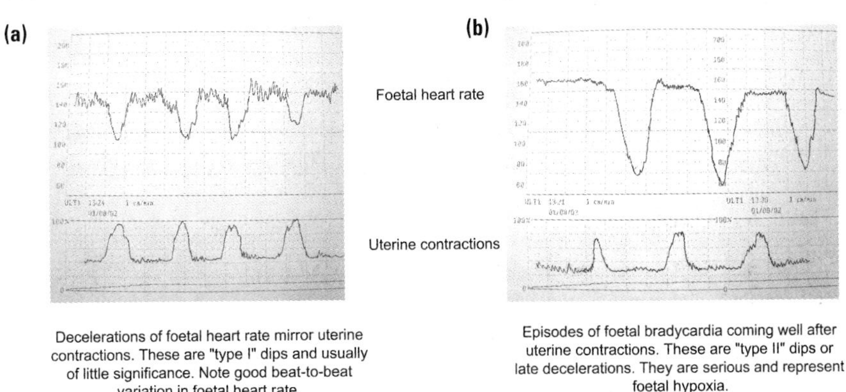

(a) Decelerations of foetal heart rate mirror uterine contractions. These are "type I" dips and usually of little significance. Note good beat-to-beat variation in foetal heart rate.

(b) Episodes of foetal bradycardia coming well after uterine contractions. These are "type II" dips or late decelerations. They are serious and represent foetal hypoxia.

Figure 13.2 Cardiotocograph showing features of foetal distress

AMPLE history

This should have been obtained by the end of the secondary survey. In addition, the trauma team leaders must also take a complete obstetric history. This includes the date of the last menstruation (LMP), the expected date of delivery and any problems or complications of the current or previous pregnancies.

Radiology

Radiography should not be withheld from the pregnant patient; however, unnecessary studies and duplication of films should be avoided. When taking peripheral x-ray films, uterine radiation should be minimized using lead abdominal shields.

13.4 Pregnancy specific injuries

The pregnant trauma patient is at risk of additional obstetric injuries. Premature labour is the most frequent complication seen and whilst placental abruption is not uncommon, uterine rupture is fortunately rare (0.6% of pregnant trauma cases). The following is a brief description of these injuries. These will all require early assessment and management from an obstetric (and paediatric) team.

13.4.1 Premature labour

- Usually noted by the awake patient but may go undetected in an unconscious or intubated patient.
- It may indicate a maternal injury that has yet to be diagnosed.
- The patient may complain of backache or uterine contractions.
- A vaginal discharge, clear or bloody, may be apparent and examination will indicate cervical dilatation or effacement.

13.4.2 Placental abruption

- Apart from maternal death, this is the most common cause of fetal demise especially following motor vehicle accidents.
- It is either total or partial separation of the placenta from the uterine wall and can occur up to 48 hours after trauma.
- Abruption should be suspected if the patient has vaginal bleeding, although this may be absent if the blood loss is concealed retroplacentally.
- Uterine tenderness, premature labour and abdominal cramps along with maternal haemorrhage and hypovolaemic shock may be present.
- Presenting signs can be vague especially in the case of partial separation.
- The only abnormality may be fetal distress, picked up by a change in fetal heart rate.

13.4.3 Uterine rupture

- The signs are numerous and fairly nonspecific: abdominal pain, tender uterus, vaginal bleeding, and maternal shock.
- It is often difficult to assess fundal height and fetal body parts may be palpable.

Uterine rupture usually results in fetal death. It is seen in compression injuries or in those with a history of previous caesarean section. It may be associated with injury to other organs such as bladder or bowel and usually requires hysterectomy.

Perimortem caesarean section

There is little data regarding perimortem caesarean sections. By the time the mother has a hypovolaemic cardiac arrest the fetus will have already suffered severe, prolonged hypoxia. Outcomes of other causes of maternal cardiac arrest may be successful if performed within 5 min of the arrest.

Ongoing thoughts

Recent papers concerning trauma in pregnancy have tried to ascertain which patients can be assessed and then discharged and which need ongoing monitoring. Various maternal and fetal variables have been put forward as predictive factors for poor fetal outcome. These include maternal tachycardia, Injury Severity Score > 9 and abnormalities in the fetal heart rate.

Some centres suggest patients with blunt trauma and no risk factors can be safely discharged home after six, or even four, hours. Others are more cautious, indicating that it is very difficult to predict outcome from these variables and consider a longer monitoring time preferable.

At present there is limited data to support or refute these claims. A prospective multicentre study is necessary to gather sufficient data to clarify the accuracy of these fetal outcome predictors and the role of fetal monitoring.

13.5 Summary

Trauma in pregnancy is a rare occurrence but a significant cause of maternal death and fetal demise. The trauma care providers therefore, understandably, meet it with a certain degree of anxiety. The initial management of the mother is identical to that of the nonpregnant patient following the usual ABCs of resuscitation remembering to consider the pathophysiological changes of pregnancy when assessing the mother. The most effective way of resuscitating the fetus is to adequately resuscitate the mother. The fetus may be in distress even with apparently normal maternal vital signs. The early input of an obstetric team (and paediatrician) to the usual trauma team will provide the best maternal and fetal outcome.

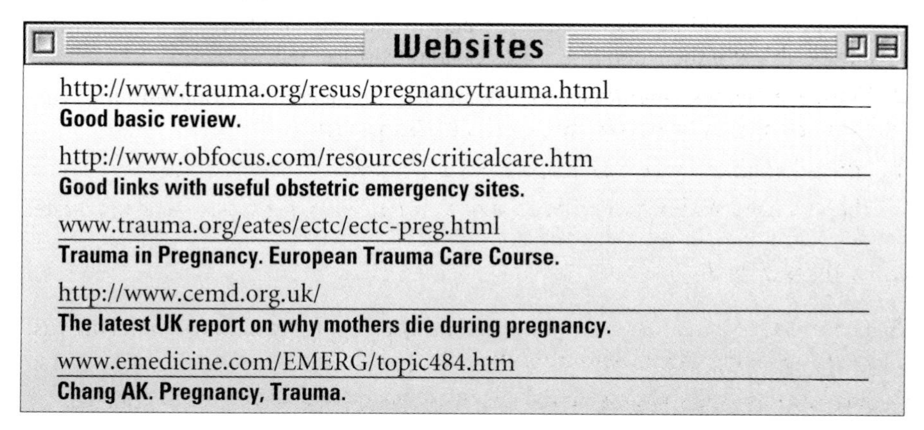

Websites

http://www.trauma.org/resus/pregnancytrauma.html
Good basic review.

http://www.obfocus.com/resources/criticalcare.htm
Good links with useful obstetric emergency sites.

www.trauma.org/eates/ectc/ectc-preg.html
Trauma in Pregnancy. European Trauma Care Course.

http://www.cemd.org.uk/
The latest UK report on why mothers die during pregnancy.

www.emedicine.com/EMERG/topic484.htm
Chang AK. Pregnancy, Trauma.

Further reading

1. **American College of Surgeons Committee on Trauma** (1997) *Advanced Trauma Life Support for Doctors.* American College of Surgeons, Chicago, IL.
2. **Baerga-Varela Y, Zietlow SP, Bannon MP, Harmsen WS & Ilstrup DM** (2000) Trauma in pregnancy. *Mayo Clin. Proc.* 75(12): 1243.
3. **Cardona V & Hurn P (eds)** (1998) *Trauma Nursing from Resuscitation through Rehabilitation*, 2nd edn. W B Saunders Company, Philadelphia.
4. **Colburn V** (1999) Trauma in pregnancy. *J. Perinat. Neonatal Nurs.* 13(3): 21–32.
5. **Curet MJ, Schermer CR, Demarest GB, Bieneik EJ 3rd & Curet LB** (2000) Predictors of outcome in trauma during pregnancy: identification of patients who can be monitored for less than 6 hours. *J. Trauma* **49**(1): 18.
6. **Driscoll P, Skinner D & Earlam R** (2000) *ABC of Major Trauma*, 3rd edn. BMJ Books, London.
7. **Esposito TJ** (1994) Trauma during pregnancy. *Emerg. Med. Clin. North Am.* **12**(1): 167.
8. **Maull KI** (2001) Maternal–fetal trauma. *Semin. Pediatr. Surg.* **10**(1): 32.
9. **Moise KJ & Belfort MA** (1997) Damage control for the obstetric patient. *Surg. Clin. North Am.* 77(4): 835.
10. **Sufrue M & Kolkman KA** (1999) Trauma during pregnancy. *Aust. J. Rural Health* 7(2): 82.
11. **Tillett J & Hanson L** (1999) Midwifery triage and management of trauma and second/third trimester bleeding. *J. Nurse Midwifery* **44**(5): 439.
12. **Trauma Nursing Core Course** (2000) *Course Manual*, 5th edn. Emergency Nurses Association, Chicago, IL.

14 Burn injury

A Kay, R Rickard

Objectives

At the end of this chapter, members of the trauma team will be able to:

- discuss common causes of burn injury and their pathophysiology;
- define the importance of pre-hospital measures in burn injury management;
- define the systematic approach to managing the burned patient;
- carry out burn area assessment and calculate fluid resuscitation requirements;
- list criteria for referral to a specialist burns centre;
- list tasks to be completed in preparation for transfer of the burned patient.

14.1 Introduction

Estimates suggest 175 000 acute burn injuries present each year to Emergency Departments in the UK. Whilst the majority of these injuries are relatively minor, an estimated 16 100 (9%) will require admission and, of these, about 1000 will require intravenous resuscitation. Approximately half of these are children under 16 years of age.

The complexity of the body's response to a burn injury presents a difficult challenge to both nursing and medical staff in the early management of the burn victim. With many advances over recent years, modern burn care is centred on highly skilled, multidisciplinary teams. The *National Burn Care Review* has established a framework to rationalize burn care in the United Kingdom. There is now no place for the occasional burn surgeon in the early and longer-term management of these patients.

The initial emergency management of the burn victim, however, remains within the domain of the ED. Burn victims are trauma victims and accurate assessment, careful initial management and timely transfer to specialist care present the best chance for optimal outcome. Whilst it is important to transfer the severely burn injured patient to a burn centre as quickly as possible (a standard of 4 h from injury being promulgated), adequate resuscitation and careful preparations for transfer are of great importance.

The pre-hospital and emergency management of a burn victim have significant effects on outcome

14.2 Causes of burn injury

- Thermal burns
  - Flame
  - Contact
  - Scalds
- Inhalation injury
  - Airway injury
  - Lung injury
  - Systemic intoxication
- Electrical burns
- Chemical burns
  - Acid
  - Alkali
  - Organic hydrocarbons
- Cold injury
  - Freezing cold injury
  - Nonfreezing cold injury

14.2.1 Thermal burns

Temperature flux

In a thermal burn, tissue destruction depends on the degree of thermal flux, which approximates to the degree of heat encountered multiplied by the duration of exposure.

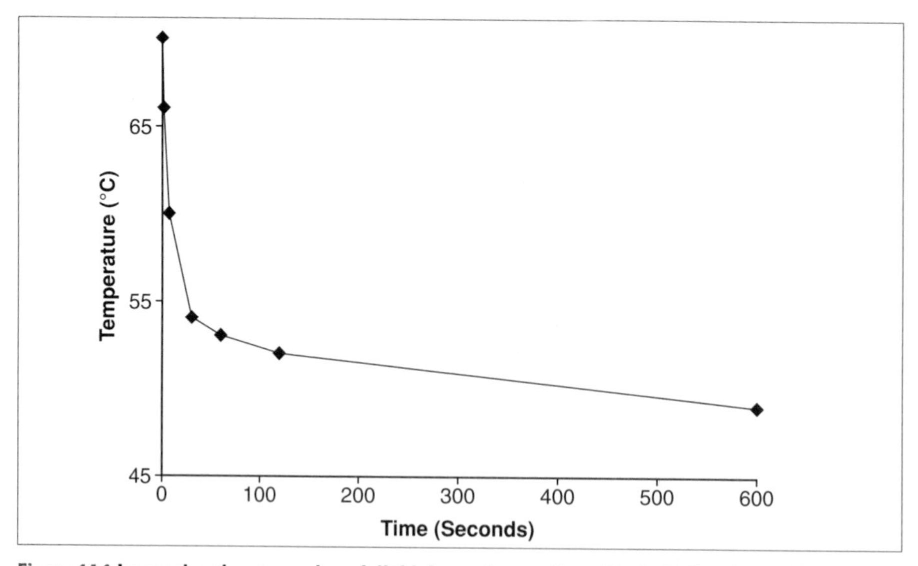

Figure 14.1 Immersion time to produce full thickness burns. From Moritz R, Henriques FC. Studies of thermal injury: The relative importance of time and surface temperature in the causation of cutaneous burns. *Am J Pathol* 23: 695, 1947.

Animal proteins denature above 40°C, and above 45°C cellular repair mechanisms cease. At this temperature, cell death will occur after an hour. In contrast, it takes only one second of immersion in water at 70°C to cause a full thickness burn (*Figure 14.1*).

Hot water splashes and petrol flash burns tend to produce partial thickness burns, as the duration of exposure is short. In contrast, contact burns seen in the elderly who have collapsed against warm plumbing tend to be deep because, although the temperature is relatively low, the duration of contact is often prolonged.

Skin thickness also has a functional relevance. For the same temperature and duration of contact, a functionally deeper burn will be produced in the thinner skin of children and the elderly.

The burn wound

Jackson proposed a burn wound model in 1947 that has remained largely valid (*Figure 14.2*).

Nearest the heat source, where heat cannot be conducted away, the tissues die. This *zone of coagulative necrosis* is surrounded by tissues where the damage is less severe than that required to produce immediate cell death. The burn injury here causes damage to the microcirculation and this zone is known as the *zone of stasis*. Tissues in this zone may progress to necrosis following release of inflammatory cytokines that further embarrass the dermal blood supply over the ensuing few days, with resultant tissue destruction and burn depth progression. Inadequate fluid resuscitation may exacerbate this progression.

Beyond this region is the *zone of hyperaemia*, which represents tissue response to injury with inflammation, cytokine release and increased blood flow. In smaller burns, the tissues of this zone will return to normal after resolution of the hyperdynamic vascular response. In burns over 20%, this zone may include the whole body.

Cooling of the burn immediately following injury has been shown to be beneficial both clinically and experimentally. Inflammatory and microvascular changes are reduced and less necrosis and fibrosis is seen. An increase in epithelial cell growth has also been noted.

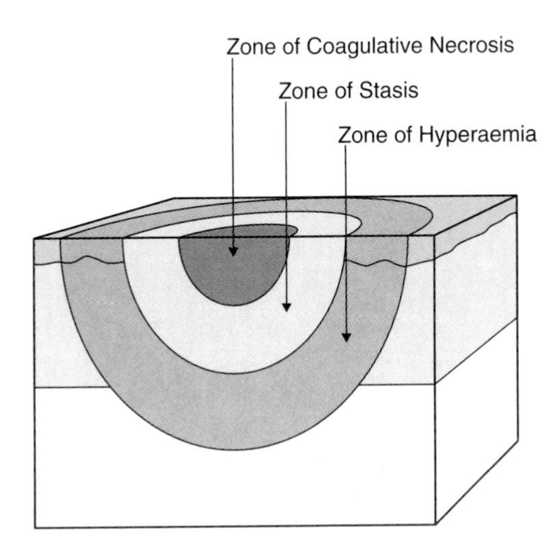

Figure 14.2 Jackson's burn wound model.

Burn depth

As outlined above, the burn wound is dynamic and its appearance can change over the first few days. Furthermore, a burn wound is not a homogeneous wound and a mixed pattern will often be seen. The classification of burn depth used in the UK is purely descriptive, relating to the depth of skin burned. Burns involve either the full thickness or only part of the thickness of the skin. Partial thickness burns are subclassified depending on which parts of the skin are involved – epidermal, superficial dermal or deep dermal.

- Superficial (epidermal) burns: these cause erythema alone, and are most commonly seen as sunburn. They are not included in burn area calculation.
- Superficial dermal burns: superficial dermal burns cause blistering and are wet. The deep dermal vasculature and epidermal appendages remain intact. These burns are associated with erythema, which blanches on pressure, and capillary refill is preserved.
- Deep dermal burns: deep dermal burns damage deeper blood vessels and haemoglobin is sequestered in the tissues. The redness does not blanch on pressure, and is referred to as 'fixed staining'.
- Full thickness burns: The dermis is destroyed and a firm, leathery layer of necrotic tissue known as eschar remains. This necrotic tissue may be waxy white or red. Soot or charred tissue may mask the underlying appearance.

The systemic injury

Lipoprotein toxins released from areas of necrosis drive the systemic inflammatory response. The magnitude of this response is related to the volume of tissue injured, most conveniently expressed as percentage of total body surface area (%TBSA). The most superficial thermal burns cause erythema only, no significant systemic response and in particular no significant capillary leakage. Such areas are therefore not considered part of the burn, and erythema is not included in burn area calculation.

In contrast, in burns of greater than approximately 20% TBSA, inflammatory mediators affect the whole body and patients develop systemic inflammatory response syndrome (SIRS). There is massive loss of fluid from the intravascular space and burn shock develops. Excision of burned tissue reduces the toxin drive behind the response, providing the rationale for early surgery.

A thermal burn of over 20% TBSA is a life-threatening systemic injury

14.2.2 Inhalation injury

Inhalation injury is not a single diagnosis, but consists of three variable components.

Airway injury

The true airway burn is caused by the inhalation of hot gases, flame or steam. The larynx closes quickly and the injury is more frequently limited to the supraglottic airway. Despite the efficient dissipation of heat, the injury is thermal in nature and initially manifest by upper airway swelling. This can cause rapid respiratory obstruction, or this may develop over a period of hours.

Lung injury

The lungs are rarely injured from thermal insult. Rather, products of combustion inhaled beyond the glottis dissolve in the fluid lining the bronchial tree and alveoli, resulting in a chemical injury. Burning building and home decorating materials containing polyvinyl chloride will produce hydrochloric acid and phosgene, whilst polyurethane smoke contains corrosive agents and cyanide gas. Symptoms may be absent initially, but develop with time and rehydration. Inflammation, oedema and decreased surfactant levels cause decreased lung compliance and alveolar diffusion.

Systemic intoxication

Alveolar absorption of combustion products can lead to systemic toxicity. This is usually seen in fires in enclosed spaces, and most commonly involves carbon monoxide and cyanide. Systemic intoxication accounts for the majority of deaths at the scene.

Carbon monoxide (CO) affects the body in two ways. First, it has an affinity for haemoglobin 240 times that of oxygen, and causes tissue hypoxia. Secondly, it has an inhibitory effect on cytochrome oxidase, inhibiting cellular metabolism. Carboxyhaemoglobin levels lower than 10% cause no symptoms and can be found in heavy smokers. Above 20%, higher brain function is impaired, with progressive loss of neurological function to 60%, where death occurs.

Like carbon monoxide, cyanide causes inhibition of cellular metabolism through its effects on the cytochrome oxidase system. At very low concentrations, the patient will complain of headaches and dizziness. Usually, however, the inhaled concentration of cyanide is such that the victim becomes dyspnoeic and rapidly loses consciousness.

Inhalation injury is not a single entity

14.2.3 Electrical burns

Resistance to conduction of electricity through the body produces heat that can cause burns. The degree of damage caused is a function of the resistance of the tissue, the duration of contact and the square of the current. Bone provides most resistance, followed by skin, fat, nerve, muscle and body fluids. Burns of the skin may be seen which do not reflect the severity of underlying tissue destruction. Furthermore, many electrocutions result in falls, and there is therefore a high risk of associated injury. Cardiac arrhythmias may occur following discharge of current across the thorax.

Electrical injuries are divided into three groups: low voltage, high voltage and lightning strike.

Low voltage

Electrical burns are classified as low voltage below 1000 V. These include domestic mains supply at 240 V, single-phase alternating current and industrial power supply at 415 V, three-phase current. The common car battery is capable of producing a direct current of sufficient amperage at only 12 V to cause a significant thermal burn when short-circuiting through jewellery. Low voltage electrical burns most commonly involve local tissue destruction, with charring of the skin and necrosis of tissues immediately beneath. Duration of contact may be prolonged due to muscle tetany caused by domestic alternating current at 50 Hz.

High voltage

High voltage electrical burns occur over 1000 V, although often these reach 11 000 to 33 000 V, as encountered in high tension transmission cables. Even higher voltages occur in power stations and substations.

High voltage injuries occur through either flash burns or current transmission. Relatively small entry and exit wounds may be associated with massive underlying damage of muscle and bone and entire compartments may be destroyed. Multiple entry and exit wounds may be seen, especially if the current has arced across joints on its passage to earth. Secondary damage through compartment syndrome may occur.

The superficial wound of an electrical burn may hide the serious nature of underlying tissue destruction

Lightning strike

Although uncommon in the UK, lightning injuries result from ultra high tension, high amperage short duration electrical discharge of direct current. A direct strike, where the discharge occurs directly through the victim, is almost invariably fatal and thankfully rare. More commonly, a 'side strike' or 'splash' occurs, when lightning strikes an object of resistance, such as a tree and is then deflected through the victim. Typically the current flows over the surface of the victim causing partial thickness burns, although there may be significant burns of the feet. Wounds may have an unusual arborescent or splashed-on appearance known as Lichtenberg flowers. Though deep organ damage is not often seen, respiratory arrest may occur through the reversible effects of discharge on the medulla. Prolonged efforts at resuscitation are justified.

14.2.4 Chemical burns

Two-thirds of those who suffer chemical burns are male. The hands are most commonly affected, followed by the lower limbs. The Control of Substances Hazardous to Health (COSHH) regulations were introduced in the UK under Health and Safety legislation in 1988 and have reduced the number of chemical burns in industry through the introduction of safer working practices. The majority of work-related chemical burns seen are due to cement (*Figure 14.3*). More than 50% of chemical burns are now due to domestic products, often oven and drain cleaning compounds. Less than 5% of all such injuries require admission.

COSHH regulations stipulate that Safety Data Sheets should be available for all industrial processes

With two notable exceptions, chemical burns can largely be divided into those caused by acids, those caused by bases or alkalis and those caused by organic hydrocarbons. Acids produce coagulative necrosis similar to a thermal burn and as such prevent deep penetration of the burning agent through formation of an eschar. Alkalis, in contrast, cause injury through liquefactive necrosis and saponification of fats, and penetrate deeper into tissues. Organic hydrocarbon compounds, such as petrol, can cause a chemical burn without ignition by liquefaction of lipids.

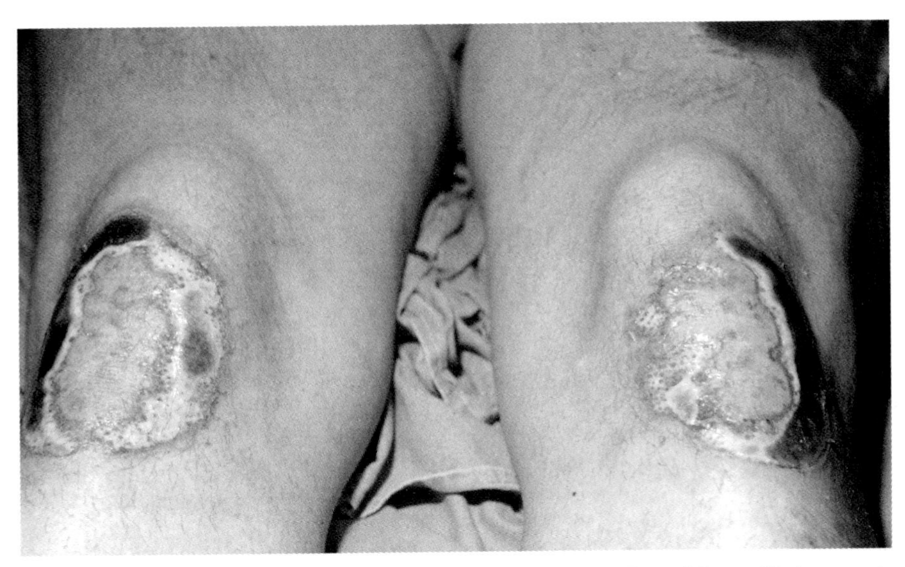

Figure 14.3 Cement burns. The patient had been kneeling in cement. The calcium oxide in cement reacts with water to produce calcium hydroxide. It is the calcium hydroxide which causes the burn. This photograph demonstrates beautifully that the area of maximum pressure, from which water and cement were expelled, has been spared.

Hydrofluoric acid is used in glass etching, fluorocarbon manufacture, PTFE and high-octane fuel manufacture. In burns caused by hydrofluoric acid, the fluoride ion is absorbed and chelates calcium and magnesium ions, causing bone demineralization, cell death and potassium release. The fall in serum calcium and rise in serum potassium can be very rapid and lead to arrhythmias, refractive VF and death. Of note, hydrofluoric acid burns can be fatal at less than 2.5% TBSA.

White phosphorus burns are largely seen in the military, where the compound is used as an igniter in ordnance and in tracer rounds. Phosphorus ignites on contact with air. It is extremely fat soluble and produces yellow blisters with a characteristic garlic smell. If absorbed, hepatorenal toxicity may occur and death has been recorded with as low a dose as 1 mg/kg. Management of these burns involves removal of particles under water or following irrigation with copper sulphate, brushing particles away or picking them off directly with forceps. Identification of the remaining particles is helped by irrigating the wound with copper sulphate. The resulting reaction causes the phosphate particles to blacken as well as reducing their burning. Beware though that copper sulphate is toxic in its own right and needs to be subsequently removed from the wound by irrigation.

14.2.5 Cold injury

In the United Kingdom, cold injuries are most commonly associated with social deprivation and neglect. Those patients injured through mountaineering or on Arctic expeditions are seldom seen in the acute phase, and most present late on return from another country. A number of conditions are described and nomenclature can be confusing. The following definitions are used by the Royal Navy in the treatment of injured Royal Marines commandos.

Freezing cold injury (FCI)

FCI or frostbite is a cold injury where the tissues freeze. FCI which, within 30 min of starting rewarming, recovers fully leaving no residual symptoms or signs is known as *frostnip*. Also described is freeze-thaw-refreeze injury (FTRI). As its name suggests, this is FCI where freezing occurs more than once, with thawing of tissues in between. FTRI can be particularly destructive.

Nonfreezing cold injury (NFCI)

NFCI is a cold injury in which tissues are subjected to prolonged cooling insufficient to cause freezing of the tissues. The diagnosis consists of a group of conditions with similar symptoms, signs and sequelae, and includes trench foot, immersion foot and shelter limb. Prolonged exposure of one or more limbs results in reduced blood flow, followed by a period of reperfusion which is accompanied by an acute syndrome of hyperaemia, swelling and pain which may itself be followed by a chronic disorder.

14.3 Pre-hospital approach to burn patient management

Good first aid management of a burn injury can significantly improve outcome

14.3.1 First aid measures

- Always use a SAFE approach:
  - shout/call for help;
  - assess the scene;
  - free from danger;
  - evaluate the casualty.
- Remove the burning source and stop the burning process.
  - Thermal burns. Remove all soaked or burnt / burning clothing and all jewellery, which can act as reservoirs of heat. Bring bagged clothing to hospital for examination.
  - Chemical burns. Beware injuring oneself, or the patient further. Wear thick rubber gloves, and cut off clothing contaminated with the chemical agent, rather than removing it over the victim's head, for example. Dust off any chemical powders. Retrieve the container or Safety Data Sheet and bring it to hospital.
  - Electrical burns. Isolate the power source. If this is not possible, use an electrically insulated tool to pull the victim from the current source.

Beware of other injuries

- First aid.
  - Assess ABCs. Beware of other injuries. Give oxygen by high flow (15 l/min), nonrebreathing mask. Cannulate for analgesia as necessary, but limit to two

attempts and do not allow cannulation to prolong on scene time. If successful, fluid replacement with crystalloid (normal saline or Hartmann's solution) can be started. If possible, fluids should be warmed.

- Cool the burn and warm the patient. Irrigate with flowing, cold tap water applied as soon as possible after burning, and for *at least* 10 min, and perhaps for up to an hour. Immediate cooling of the burn wound modifies local inflammation and reduces progressive cell necrosis.[4] The water should not be ice cold. Proprietary wet gel preparations (e.g. Burnshield®) may have a role in this regard, but their clinical efficacy has yet to be proven. With chemical burns, irrigation must be continued for much longer – at least 30 min. Beware of inducing hypothermia particularly when dealing with children, small adults and large burns.

Cool the burn, warm the patient

- Assess the burn severity. The type of burn is more important than %TBSA. Methods of %TBSA *estimation* include Wallace's 'Rule of Nines' (*Figure 14.4*) and Burn Serial Halving (*Figure 14.5*). The latter has been proven to be an accurate method of estimation and may be easier to remember. Small burns may be assessed remembering that the *patient's* hand (including fingers) represents approximately 1% TBSA.
- Dress the wounds. Dress thermal and electrical burns loosely with clingfilm. If possible, continue to irrigate chemical burns.

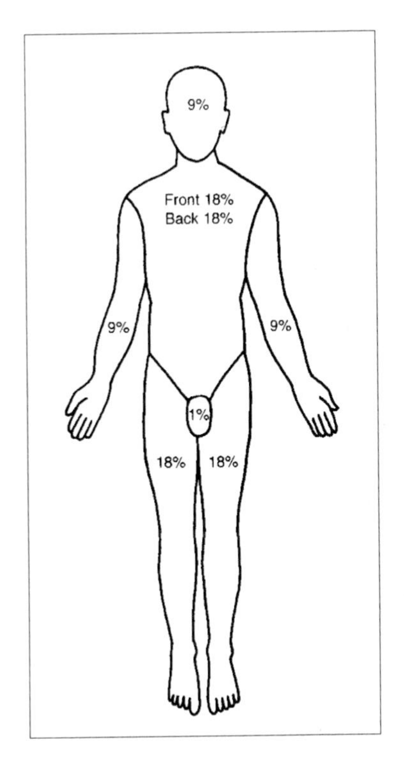

Figure 14.4 Wallace's rule of nines.

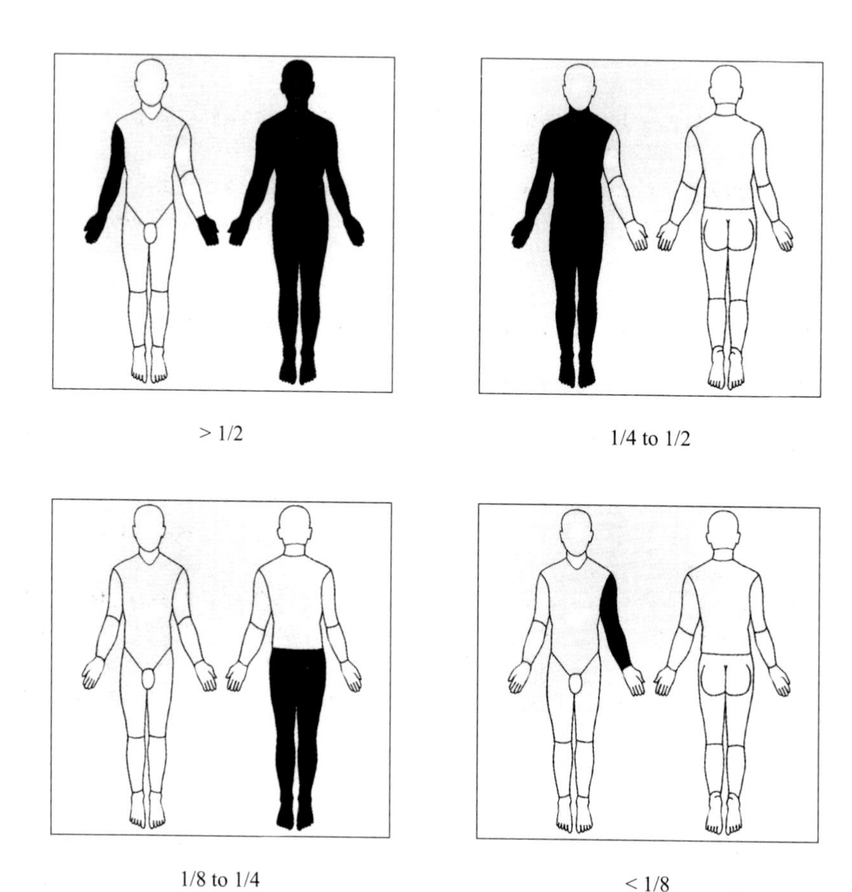

Figure 14.5 Serial halving. Figure marked >1/2 – more than half of the skin is burnt. 1/4 to 1/2 – less than half, but more than a quarter of the skin is burnt. 1/8 to 1/4 – more than one eighth, but less than a quarter of the skin is burnt. < 1/8 – less than one eighth is burnt.

- Analgesia. Intravenous opiate with antiemetic should be titrated to effect in adults. Intranasal diamorphine may be useful in children. Entonox has varying efficacy and reduces oxygen delivery.

14.3.2 Communication

Information should be passed back to the ED as per the national standard:

- Age, gender, incident, ABC problems, relevant treatment carried out, ETA. Be alert for:
  - > 25% TBSA;
  - airway concern;
  - high voltage electrocution;
  - carbon monoxide poisoning;
  - associated serious injuries.

14.3.3 Transport

- All treatment should be carried out with the aim of reducing on-scene times and delivering the patient to the appropriate treatment centre.

Transport should not hinder continuing cooling of the burn wound.

The patient should be transported to the nearest ED for assessment and stabilization. Local protocols may allow for direct transfer to a burns facility.

14.4 Emergency Department management of the burn patient

14.4.1 Introduction

Major burn victims are trauma victims and their initial assessment is the same as for any other seriously injured patient. Furthermore, those patients with a major burn may have injuries other than the burn and these must be excluded or treated. Burn of greater than 10% TBSA and all high voltage electrical injuries should be assessed and treated in a resuscitation bay.

Although normally carried out before arrival, ensure that the burning process has been stopped. Continue to cool the burn. Benefit from cooling may still be seen even if cooling has not been started within 30 min from the time of burning. Beware hypothermia, however, and a decision to stop cooling needs to be based on patient core temperature.

14.4.2 Primary survey

A full primary survey needs to be carried out using (see Section 1.6.1). The full manifestations of the burn injury will evolve over several hours, and the primary survey is to identify any injuries that may compromise survival while a more thorough assessment of the burn is undertaken.

Airway and breathing

In the initial assessment of the airway and breathing the most important aspect is to diagnose any degree of inhalation injury. Potential complications can therefore be anticipated and appropriate interventions instigated.

The development of signs and symptoms from airway oedema and pulmonary injury occurs progressively over several hours. The key to diagnosis is therefore a high index of suspicion with the frequent re-evaluation of those considered to be at risk.

A high index of suspicion is the key to diagnosing inhalation injury

The presence of any of the following indicate the possibility of an inhalation injury:

- a history of exposure to fire and/or smoke in an enclosed space such as a building or vehicle;
- exposure to a blast;
- collapse, confusion or restlessness at any time;
- hoarseness or any change in voice;

- harsh cough;
- stridor;
- burns to the face;
- singed nasal hairs;
- soot in saliva or sputum;
- an inflamed oropharynx;
- raised carboxyhaemoglobin levels;
- deteriorating pulmonary function.

In all cases administer a high concentration of oxygen, preferably humidified.

If any degree of upper airway obstruction is present, endotracheal intubation is mandatory. In severe cases this may require the use of a surgical airway. The presence of stridor indicates a degree of obstruction already exists. If there is a strong suspicion of inhalation injury but obstruction is not evident, an experienced anaesthetist should be called urgently to assess the patient. Swelling will increase over the first few hours. If in doubt, intubate.

If inhalation injury is suspected, experienced anaesthetic expertise is required promptly. If in doubt, intubate

Circulation

It should be noted that hypovolaemic shock secondary to a burn takes some time to produce measurable physical signs. If the burn victim is shocked early, other causes should be excluded. A history of a blast, vehicle collision or a fall whilst escaping the fire should raise suspicion of other injuries.

If the patient has hypovolaemic shock, this should be treated as outlined elsewhere in this manual independent of the severity of burn.

Early hypovolaemic shock is rarely due to the burn

Establish intravenous access with two large bore cannulae. It is possible to cannulate through burnt skin but this should be avoided if possible. If necessary use cut-downs, intraosseous or, as a last resort, central routes. Send blood for laboratory baseline investigations including carboxyhaemoglobin levels if an inhalation injury is suspected.

Disability

Reduced level of consciousness, confusion and restlessness normally indicate intoxication and/or hypoxia secondary to an inhalation injury. Do not, however, overlook the possibility of alcohol or drug ingestion and the presence of other injuries.

Exposure

Remove all clothing, including underwear, jewellery, watches and any other restricting items. The risk of hypothermia is often overlooked. The removal of clothing and liberal use of cold water at the scene, during transfer and in the emergency department leads to the not uncommon event of the burns centre receiving a hypothermic patient.

Judicious local cooling of the burn should be accompanied by covering uninvolved areas and aiming to get the ambient room temperature to 30°C.

Hypothermia is a significant risk during the management of burns

Before progressing to the specific management of the burn and a full secondary survey, reassess the patient's ABCs.

14.4.3 Management of the thermal burn

Inhalation injury

There is little else that can be done in the emergency department beyond intubation and ventilation. Any patient with a suspected inhalation injury should be closely observed in an area equipped for intubation. If there is an inhalation injury the patient needs to be managed by an experienced anaesthetist until arrival at the receiving burns centre.

Remember to interpret pulse oximetry readings with caution, especially in the presence of carboxyhaemoglobinaemia. Obtain arterial blood gas analysis and a chest x-ray. These may be normal initially.

There is no evidence that administration of steroids is beneficial (although pre-injury users should continue their medications).

There should be an extremely low threshold for elective intubation if the patient is going to be transferred to another hospital.

Cutaneous burn

Whatever the cause of the burn, the severity of the injury is proportional to the volume of tissue damage. In terms of survival, the percentage of the total body surface area (%TBSA) involved is the most important factor. *Functional* outcome is more often dependent on depth and site of the burn.

Calculating %TBSA burn

Use of the 'rule of nines' or serial halving is sufficient only for a rapid guess of %TBSA in the pre-hospital setting. This method is not accurate enough for calculating fluid requirements. A more detailed assessment should be made using a Lund and Browder burns chart (*Figure 14.6*).

When using this chart it is important to be precise. Very carefully and accurately draw the burnt areas onto the chart and then sit down and calculate the %TBSA. Ignore simple erythema. In very large burns it can be easier to calculate the size of area not burnt. Differentiating between full and partial thickness burns is not essential.

Ignore simple erythema

The palmar surface of the patient's hand including the fingers equates to 1% TBSA and can be used to estimate small areas of burn.

Calculate the %TBSA accurately. Do not guess

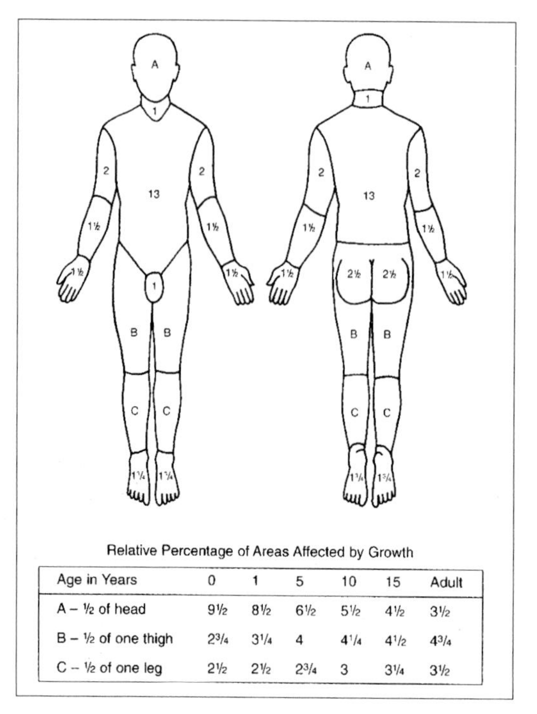

Relative Percentage of Areas Affected by Growth

Age in Years	0	1	5	10	15	Adult
A – ½ of head	9½	8½	6½	5½	4½	3½
B – ½ of one thigh	2¾	3¼	4	4¼	4½	4¾
C – ½ of one leg	2½	2½	2¾	3	3¼	3½

Figure 14.6 Lund and Browder chart.

Preventing burns shock

Any burn greater than 10% TBSA in a child and 15% TBSA in an adult is going to require intravenous fluids to prevent the development of burn shock.

Intravenous fluid resuscitation is required for all burns greater than:

15% TBSA in adults

10% TBSA in children

The volume required is given by the Parkland formula:

2–4 ml Hartmann's solution × %TBSA burn × kg body weight

Use the higher value of 4 ml initially. Weigh the patient or ask their weight. Guessing is notoriously inaccurate. A child's weight can be obtained by using a recognized formula or a Broselow tape.

The formula gives a volume of fluid. Half this volume is administered in the first 8 h and the second half over the next 16 h. The requirement of fluid starts at the time of injury. The rate of administration therefore needs to allow for any catch-up.

Monitoring

The Parkland formula provides an estimate of the fluids required. It does not allow for other losses, or for maintenance needs. It is therefore essential to monitor the adequacy of the fluid resuscitation. This is best achieved in the emergency department by measuring urinary output and a urinary catheter must therefore be inserted.

Aim for urine outputs of:

- 1 ml/kg/h in adults.
- 2 ml/kg/h in children.

14.4.4 Management of the thermal burn wound

The aim of burn wound management is to maximize the functional and cosmetic outcome. Apart from small superficial burns, wound management needs to be supervised by a burns centre. Beyond stopping the burning process and cooling the burn as described above, there is rarely any indication for the emergency department team to interfere with the burn wound.

Initial treatment

If there is to be no undue delay in transfer to a burns centre the only need for most burns is to reduce heat and water loss and to make the wound less painful. This can be achieved by loosely covering the burn with clingfilm. Hands can be placed in plastic bags. The patient should then be kept warm with dry blankets. Accurate assessment of the wound will take place at the burns centre and there should be as little interference with it as possible. There is no indication for applying any form of topical antiseptic solution or cream and indeed these will make it more difficult for the burns team to assess the wound.

Do not use ointments or creams

Escharotomy

A circumferential full thickness burn can act like a tourniquet and compromise circulation. Division of the constriction is known as escharotomy. This is not a straightforward undertaking and should be performed in an operating theatre by skilled persons. There is rarely a need to perform an escharotomy within the first few hours. The exception is a full thickness burn of the entire trunk that is preventing respiration. In this situation pre-transfer escharotomy should be discussed with the burns centre.

14.4.5 Other initial interventions

Ensure immunity against tetanus. In the absence of any specific indications such as associated contaminated wounds, there is no requirement for antibiotic prophylaxis. Insertion of a nasogastric tube and urinary catheter will be required.

Antibiotics are not indicated in the early management of burns

Burns are painful and the patients are often terrified. Furthermore, pain will lead to further adrenaline (epinephrine) release and may potentiate burn depth progression. Adequate intravenous opiates should be administered early.

Adequate intravenous opiates should be administered early

14.4.6 Management of the chemical burn wound

Apart from a very few exceptions (see below), specific antidotes to chemical injury are not indicated, as exothermic reactions may worsen the burn wound. The mainstay of treatment is copious and continued irrigation with water. Irrigation should be carried out for at least 30 min in the case of an acid burn, and for at least an hour for an alkali. Hypothermia should be avoided and the water used to irrigate need not be cold. It is important that the diluted chemical is not allowed to pool around the body, as further injury may occur. Indicator paper can be placed intermittently on the skin to see if pH is returning to normal. Chemical burns of the eye require prolonged irrigation and early consultation with the local ophthalmic service.

Chemical burns require prolonged irrigation with water

Specific antidotes are required for the following agents:

- hydrofluoric acid: 1% Ca gluconate;
- white phosphorus: 1% $CuSO_4$.

Once the chemical has positively been removed and the wound is clean, treatment is as for a thermal burn.

14.4.7 Management of the electrical burn

Associated injury

High voltage electrical injury carries a high risk of fatality at the site of electrocution. Victims who have arrested at the site, but who have made it alive to the ED will require continued and prolonged cardiopulmonary resuscitation. Electrical workers may have been thrown from a height and suffered additional serious injury. Primary and secondary survey of all high voltage electrical injuries must therefore be carried out in a resuscitation bay.

Dysrhythmias

In all cases of electrocution, a 12-lead ECG should be performed. If abnormal, continuing cardiac monitoring should be employed and a cardiac opinion should be sought. In the absence of ECG abnormality or cardiac history, continued cardiac monitoring is of no proven benefit.

Fluid resuscitation

As previously mentioned, the cutaneous burn from electrical contact can belie the seriousness of underlying injury. Reliance on the Parkland formula may therefore underestimate fluid requirements and careful monitoring of urine output is essential.

In patients with deep damage, haemochromogenuria may occur and deposition of haemochromogens in the proximal tubules may cause acute renal failure. Resuscitation fluids should be increased to maintain a urine output of 2 ml/kg/h. Haemochromogen excretion may also be promoted using a forced alkaline diuresis. This should only be undertaken after advice from the local burns intensivists.

Reliance on standard formulae in electrical burns may underestimate fluid requirements

Limb injury

Hourly assessment of peripheral circulation in injured limbs must be carried out. Assessment includes:

- skin colour;
- oedema;
- capillary refill;
- peripheral pulses;
- skin sensation.

The primary symptom of compartment syndrome is increasing pain that is not relieved by opiates and appears out of proportion to the cutaneous injury. Signs include altered sensation in the distal limb and pain on passive stretching of the ischaemic muscles. A pale pulseless hand or foot is a very late sign and usually signifies the need for amputation. If in doubt, or there is likely to be delay before transfer to definitive burn care, a local plastic surgery or orthopaedic opinion must be sought and fasciotomies carried out as necessary.

14.4.8 Management of cold injury

Freezing cold injury (FCI)

Immediate aid to the victim of FCI is centred upon the decision as to whether or not to attempt to rewarm and thaw affected tissues. This, in turn, is determined by the ability to sustain warmth and to protect the thawed tissues from further freezing or trauma. If there is any risk of the affected parts becoming frozen again, then the threat of massive tissue destruction by FTRI militates against any rewarming. Once the decision to thaw has been taken, then ideally the whole affected extremity should be immersed in thermostatically controlled stirred water at between 38 and 42°C, and kept there until tissue temperatures are uniformly in excess of 30°C. If the ability to monitor deep tissue temperature is lacking, the extremity should be immersed for 30 min beyond the point where normal consistency returns. Deeply frozen tissues may require prophylactic decompression prior to thawing to prevent compartment syndrome. The process of rewarming may be extremely painful and opiate analgesia should be administered.

Non-freezing cold injury (NFCI)

If it is established that the extremity has not become frozen, and is therefore presumed to be NFCI, evidence is that rapid rewarming should be avoided. Slow rewarming of the affected extremity, whilst the rest of the patient is rewarmed from hypothermia may be employed. Following rewarming, some patients may require analgesics.

The subsequent management of the affected parts requires specialist care and referral should be made to a burns centre or plastic surgery unit. Avoidance of secondary infection is important but antibiotics should be reserved for treatment rather than prophylaxis.

14.5 Transfer to definitive care

In all cases, early contact with a burn centre should be made. Advice on initial management and transfer will be given.

14.5.1 National Burn Injury Referral Guidelines

The British Burn Association guidelines for referral take into account not only the size of the skin injury, but other less succinct predeterminants of complexity. All complex burns should be sent to the local burn centre or burn unit.

Complex burn injuries

A burn may be deemed complex if one or more of the following criteria are met:

- age
  - under 5 years or over 60 years;
- area
  - burns over 10% TBSA in adults;
  - burns over 5% TBSA in children;
- site
  - burns involving face, hands, perineum or feet;
  - any flexure, particularly the neck or axilla;
  - any circumferential dermal or full thickness burn of the limbs, torso or neck;
- inhalation injury
  - any significant inhalation injury, excluding pure CO poisoning;
- mechanism of injury
  - high pressure steam injury;
  - high voltage electrical injury;
  - chemical injury >5% TBSA;
  - hydrofluoric acid injury (>1% TBSA);
  - suspicion of nonaccidental injury; adult or paediatric;
- existing conditions
  - cardiac limitation and/or MI within 5 years;
  - respiratory limitation of exercise;
  - diabetes mellitus;
  - pregnancy;
  - immunosuppression for any reason;
  - hepatic impairment; cirrhosis;
- associated injuries
  - crush injuries;
  - major long bone fractures;
  - head injury;
  - penetrating injuries.

Associated injuries may, in some circumstances, delay referral of the burn. In such instances advice about burns management should always be sought.

Complex nonburns

Complex nonburns should also be referred:

- inhalation injury alone
  - any significant inhalation injury with no cutaneous burn, excluding pure CO poisoning;
- vesicobullous disorders over 5% TBSA
  - epidermolysis bullosa;
  - staphylococcal scalded skin syndrome;
  - Stevens–Johnson syndrome;
  - toxic epidermal necrolysis.

14.5.2 Preparations for transfer

Once the decision to transfer a patient is reached, in consultation with the nearest burn unit, safe transit of the patient must be ensured. A member of staff should be designated to find the nearest available burn bed. This may not be in the nearest burn centre, and its location will have implications for the mode of transfer. Even with greater centralization of burn expertise, there are few reasons why patients in the majority of the UK cannot reach definitive care promptly. With some longer distance transfers, rotary or even fixed wing aircraft may be required.

Before transfer it is important to carry out the following:

- a thorough secondary survey has been performed and any injuries identified be appropriately managed;
- maximum feasible inspired oxygen is being administered;
- if there is any suspicion of an inhalation injury, the patient has been assessed by an experienced anaesthetist and intubated if necessary;
- adequate intravenous access is secured and appropriate fluid resuscitation has started;
- the burn wound is covered with Clingfilm and the patient is being kept warm;
- adequate analgesia;
- urinary catheter in place;
- free draining nasogastric tube in place;
- all findings and interventions, including fluid balance, are clearly and accurately documented.

All patients should be transferred with an appropriately trained escort.

If it is likely that a delay in transfer will exceed 6 hours then the situation needs to be discussed further with the burn centre. In this circumstance it may be deemed necessary for:

- escharotomies to be performed;
- the burn wound to be cleaned and a specific dressing applied;
- the commencement of maintenance intravenous fluids and/or nasogastric feeding.

Websites

http://www.nlm.nih.gov/medlineplus/burns.html
Good starting point for burns websites.

http://www.burnsurgery.org/
Excellent peer reviewed website.

http://www.baps.co.uk/documents/nbcr.pdf
UK national burn care review.

http://www.safety.odpm.gov.uk/fire/
UK government site with fire statistics and recommendations.

Further reading

1. **Department of Trade and Industry** (2001) Home and Leisure Accident Research, Consumer Safety Unit. Department of Trade and Industry.
2. **National Burn Care Review Committee** (2001) Standards and Strategy for Burn Care. A review of Burn Care in the British Isles. National Burn Care Review Committee Report.
3. **Jandera V, Hudson DA, deWet PM, Innes PM & Rode H** (2000) Cooling the burn wound: evaluation of different modalities. *Burns* **26**: 265–270.
4. **Arturson G** (1985) The pathophysiology of severe thermal injury. *J Burn Care Rehab* **6**: 129–146.
5. **Sheridan RL, Ryan CM, Quinby Jr WC, Blair J & Tompkins RG** (1995) Emergency management of major hydrofluoric acid exposures. *Burns* **21**: 62–64.
6. **Oakley EHN** (2000) A review of the treatment of cold injury. Institute of Naval Medicine Report No. 2000.026.
7. **Smith JJ, Scerri GV, Malyon AD & Burge TS** (2002) Comparison of serial halving and rule of nines as a pre-hospital assessment tool. *J Emerg Med* **19**(suppl.): A66.

15 Hypothermia and drowning

J Soar, C Johnson

Hypothermia

Objectives

The objectives of this section are that members of the trauma team should understand:

- how to define hypothermia;
- the pathophysiology of hypothermia;
- how to diagnose hypothermia;
- initial management of the hypothermic patient;
- rewarming techniques;
- difficulties in diagnosing death in the hypothermic patient.

15.1 Definition

Hypothermia is defined as a core body temperature less than 35°C. When considering signs, symptoms and treatment it is useful to classify it as mild (35–32°C), moderate (32–30°C), or severe (less than 30°C). These temperature ranges are arbitrary and other classifications are available.

15.2 Pathophysiology

Humans regulate their body temperature very accurately and even minor variations in the temperature of vital organs can lead to psychological and physiological disturbance. Under normal circumstances, the temperature of the environment is sensed by specialized nerve endings in the skin and the body temperature by nerves in the great vessels and viscera. This information reaches the hypothalamus via the spinothalamic tracts in the spinal cord. By balancing heat loss and production, the hypothalamus controls the body temperature.

The commonest cause of hypothermia is heat loss. This occurs as a result of:

- conduction: the direct transfer of heat between a warm object to a cooler one, for example when lying on a cold floor;

- convection: heat is transferred to surrounding air or water which moves away taking the heat with it;
- radiation: the loss of heat by the emission of infrared radiation from a warm body to a cooler one. Normally, this is the main method of heat loss accounting for up to 60%;
- evaporation: liquid water on the surface of the skin or a wound turns to water vapour, lowering the temperature of the liquid remaining. This then absorbs heat energy from the body, which then cools.

With their larger surface area to volume ratio, children have a greater rate of heat loss by all these mechanisms, while vasodilatation from any cause increase heat loss by conduction, convection and radiation.

Those with normal thermoregulation are at high risk of hypothermia when exposed to cold environments, after immersion in cold water (see Section 15.8), or exposed to wet and windy conditions. Body heat is lost rapidly in these situations via the mechanisms described above. Still air is a good insulator and, consequently, when blown away by the wind, this insulating layer is lost and body temperature falls.

The combination of temperature and wind is called the wind chill factor

Water has an even greater thermal conductivity than air and wet clothes and damp conditions increase the speed of heat loss.

Heat production can also be reduced, usually as a result of a decrease in metabolism, for example, unconsciousness, hypothyroidism, hypopituitarism, while the elderly have a reduced capacity to increase heat production. Reduced heat production alone is not a common cause of hypothermia, it is more often a contributing factor to increased heat loss.

The main method of reducing heat loss is by vasoconstriction. This, however, can be blocked by drugs, particularly alcohol. The process is usually supplemented by behavioural responses, such as putting on extra clothing, avoiding the cold and reducing surface area by curling up. Heat production is increased by shivering which increases the metabolic rate and generates heat. Unfortunately, this mechanism is lost as the core temperature falls below 32–30°C.

Several studies have shown that trauma victims have lower core temperatures than expected, particularly in cases of severe injury. The cause of this is probably multifactorial and includes environmental conditions, metabolic changes, blood loss or the injury itself. Whatever the cause, trauma patients with a low core temperature have a worse prognosis and therefore every effort must be made to prevent further falls in temperature after arrival in the Emergency Department.

15.3 Diagnosis

Hypothermia should be suspected from the clinical history and a brief external examination. The symptoms are often nonspecific (Box 15.1).

As the core temperature falls below 32°C, the anatomical and physiological dead space increase which, along with a left-shift of the oxyhaemoglobin dissociation curve, significantly impairs tissue oxygenation. A sinus bradycardia, resistant to atropine,

BOX 15.1 Signs and symptoms of hypothermia

Mild: 35–32°C

- Pale and cold
- Shivering
- Increased:
  - respiratory rate
  - pulse rate
  - blood pressure
- Conscious

Moderate: 32–30°C

- Pale and cold
- Minimal shivering
- Reduced:
  - respiratory rate
  - pulse rate
  - blood pressure
- ECG changes
- Confused, slurred speech, lethargic

Severe: below 30°C

- Pale and cold
- No shivering
- Hypoventilation
- Severe bradycardia or arrhythmia
- Hypotension
- Coma, areflexia
- Dilated pupils

develops that eventually progresses to atrial fibrillation with a slow ventricular response (*Figure 15.1*), nodal rhythm, ventricular fibrillation and finally asystole (see Box 15.2). Below 28°C, the myocardium becomes very sensitive and even the slightest stimulus such as moving the patient may trigger ventricular fibrillation. This is usually

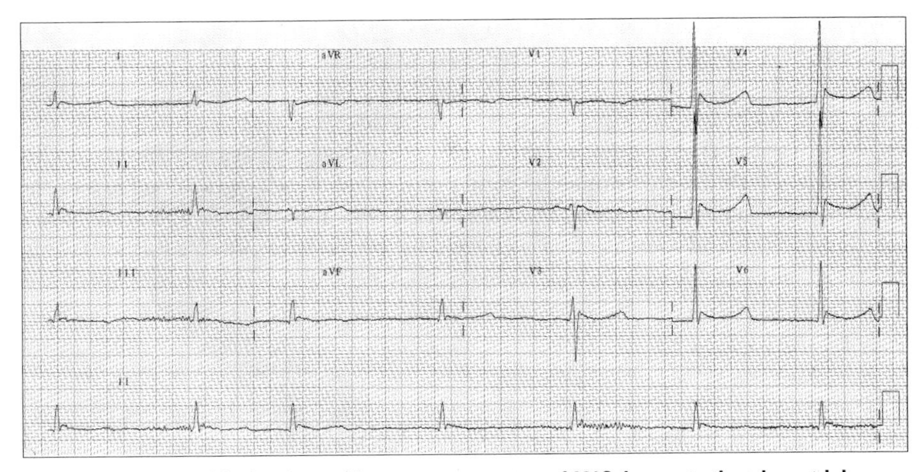

Figure 15.1 12-lead ECG of patient with a core temperature of 23°C demonstrating slow atrial fibrillation and J waves (characteristic humps at the end of the QRS complex) (courtesy Dr J. Nolan).

BOX 15.2 ECG changes associated with decreasing temperature

- Shivering
- J waves
- Sinus bradycardia
- Atrial fibrillation
- Ventricular fibrillation
- Asystole

resistant to defibrillation until core temperature is over 30°C. Renal concentrating ability is reduced leading to a 'cold diuresis' which, in addition to a shift of plasma into the extravascular space, results in hypovolaemia. Cerebral metabolism is reduced by the fall in temperature, evident as a reduction in the level of consciousness, and loss of gag and cough reflexes, placing the victim at increased risk of aspiration. Prolonged immobility may cause rhabdomyolysis, hyperkalaemia and acute renal failure.

15.4 Initial management of the hypothermic patient

The same principles as described throughout this book for primary survey and initial management apply equally to the hypothermic patient.

15.4.1 Primary survey and resuscitation

Open, clear, and maintain a patent airway and administer oxygen. If there is inadequate or no spontaneous respiratory effort, commence ventilation with a high concentration of oxygen. If tracheal intubation is indicated, it must be performed as carefully as possible, particularly in the presence of severe hypothermia, to avoid the risk of inducing VF. The cervical spine must be immobilized appropriately, with great care being taken if the patient is hypothermic after immersion in water. Oxygen should be preferably warmed (40–46°C) and humidified. In severe hypothermia it may be difficult to identify the presence of a pulse, and therefore a major artery must be palpated for up to a minute whilst looking for signs of life before concluding that there is no cardiac output. A Doppler ultrasound probe may also be useful in these circumstances. Peripheral venous access may be difficult and early consideration should be given to alternative techniques. All fluid must be warmed and care taken with the rate of administration as the cold myocardium is intolerant of an excessive fluid load.

If the patient requires CPR the tidal volumes and rates for chest compression are the same as for a normothermic patient, although chest wall stiffness may make this difficult to achieve. Arrhythmias tend to revert spontaneously with warming and usually do not require immediate treatment. Bradycardia may be physiological in severe hypothermia, and cardiac pacing is not indicated unless it persists after rewarming. Defibrillation may not be effective if the core temperature is less than 30°C. If the patient does not respond to three initial defibrillation attempts, subsequent defibrillation attempts should be delayed until the patient is warmed to above 30°C.

Central vascular access is preferable for the administration of drugs as they may pool when given peripherally due to venous stasis. Drug metabolism is reduced and accumulation can occur to toxic levels in the peripheral circulation if drugs are administered repeatedly via this route in the severely hypothermic victim. The efficacy of drugs at their site of action is also reduced and the use of inotropes and anti-arrhythmic drugs is unlikely to be helpful in severe hypothermia until rewarming has been established. These patients need urgent transfer to a critical care setting where full invasive haemodynamic monitoring can be established. The effects of inotropic drugs and anti-arrhythmic drugs can then be carefully titrated during the warming process.

The patient's neurological state will be affected by the degree of hypothermia and as a result, may lead to an underestimation of their level of consciousness. Alternatively a reduced level of consciousness due to head injury may be wrongly attributed to the patient's temperature. Clearly as the patient rewarms, their conscious level should improve. Any failure to do so should raise the suspicion of a co-existing head injury.

During the primary survey, the diagnosis of hypothermia must be confirmed by measuring core temperature using a low reading thermometer. No single site is ideal for temperature measurement but the easiest sites are rectal, tympanic or oesophageal. If rectal temperature is measured there is often a significant lag between changes in core temperature and the measured temperature. Tympanic temperatures are slightly better, but are dependent on a clear view of the drum and there may be differences between the two tympanic membranes. An oesophageal temperature probe is probably the best method for continuously monitoring core temperature during rewarming in the intubated patient. The accuracy of thermometers also varies, so it is important to be consistent with the site of monitoring when tracking temperature changes and to take repeated readings.

15.4.2 Secondary survey

As with all victims of trauma, a thorough head-to-toe examination must now be performed to identify any life-threatening injuries. It is also at this point that concerted efforts will be made to start rewarming the patient.

Rewarming

If advanced warning is given of the arrival of a hypothermic patient, every effort should be made to receive them into a warm environment. The temperature of the resuscitation room should therefore be raised and all drafts prevented. The team need also to ensure an adequate supply of warm fluids, blankets and access to warming devices.

Rapid rewarming may cause an increase in cardiovascular instability due to fluid and electrolyte shifts. Some believe that victims should be rewarmed at a rate that corresponds with the rate of onset of hypothermia. This is difficult to gauge in practice, however, and rewarming a patient too slowly may increase the time that the patient is vulnerable to the harmful effects of hypothermia.

Rewarming may be passive external, active external, or active internal (core rewarming)

Passive warming can be achieved with blankets, hot drinks and a warm room. It is suitable for conscious victims with mild hypothermia. Only supervised victims with mild hypothermia who are otherwise well should lay in a warm bath. A hot shower whilst standing may cause fainting due to rapid vasodilatation. In moderate hypothermia rewarming needs to be more active. The use of warm air blankets together with warm intravenous fluids is usually all that is required. These patients should also receive warm humidified oxygen.

In severe hypothermia or cardiac arrest active warming measures are required. A number of techniques have been described although there are no clinical trials of outcome to determine the best method. Techniques include the use of warm humidified gases and gastric, peritoneal and pleural lavage with warm fluids at 40°C. Ideally the preferred method in these patients is active internal rewarming using extracorporeal devices such as cardiopulmonary bypass because it also provides a circulation, oxygenation and ventilation while the core body temperature is gradually rewarmed.

In practice, facilities for cardiopulmonary bypass are not always available and a combination of methods may have to be employed. Alternative extracorporeal warming may be performed using continuous veno-venous haemofiltration. The extracorporeal circuit should be warmed and replacement fluids heated to 40°C. This is only possible in those with a circulation.

During rewarming, patients are likely to require large amounts of fluids as their vascular space expands due to vasodilatation. All intravenous fluids should be warmed prior to administration. Careful haemodynamic monitoring (continuous arterial blood pressure and central venous pressure) is important and these patients are best managed in a critical care environment.

Investigations

Investigations must include regular measurements of arterial blood gases and electrolytes, particularly potassium, as rapid changes (hyperkalaemia) can occur during the rewarming period. Blood gas analysers measure patient blood gas values at 37°C, and if corrected for the patient's temperature, tend to be lower as gases are more soluble in blood at lower temperatures. To interpret corrected values, results would have to be compared with the normal value for that particular patient temperature. It is, therefore, easier to interpret uncorrected arterial blood gas measurements, as it is then only necessary to compare them with the well-known normal values for 37°C. This also simplifies comparison of results from serial blood gas samples during rewarming.

Hyperglycaemia is often associated with hypothermia as a result of the reduced metabolic ability of the cold tissues. Insulin must not be administered as this will exacerbate the normal fall during rewarming and render the patient dangerously hypoglycaemic. Repeated estimations are therefore required and intravenous glucose may be required in patients whose condition is due to enforced immobility and exhaustion. Blood cultures, thyroid function tests, alcohol levels and a toxicology screen should also be performed.

15.4.3 Prognosis

A full recovery without neurological deficit is possible after prolonged hypothermia even when associated with cardiac arrest, as hypothermia confers a degree of protection to the brain. However, an extremely low core temperature and significant co-morbidity are both predictors of a poor outcome.

15.5 Death and hypothermia

Hypothermia may mimic death so beware of pronouncing death in the hypothermic patient. Outside hospital, if practical, treatment and resuscitation should commence to allow transfer to hospital. Death should only be confirmed if the victim has obvious lethal injuries or if the body is frozen making resuscitation attempts impossible. Severe hypothermia may protect the brain and vital organs from the effects of hypoxia by slowing metabolism. Warming may also reverse arrhythmias associated with hypothermia. Fixed dilated pupils and stiffness can be due to hypothermia. In a patient with cardiac arrest found in a cold environment hypothermia may be the primary cause but it is difficult to distinguish from secondary hypothermia after cardiac arrest due to myocardial infarction or other causes. Ideally death should not be confirmed until the patient has been rewarmed or attempts at rewarming have failed to raise core temperature. This may require prolonged resuscitation. In the hospital setting the clinical judgement of senior team members should determine when resuscitation can stop in the hypothermic arrest victim.

There is not a prescriptive temperature below which death should not be diagnosed

Drowning

Objectives

The objectives of this section are that members of the trauma team should understand:

- the definitions associated with drowning;
- the aetiology of drowning;
- the pathophysiology of immersion and submersion in water;
- the initial resuscitation and specific therapies;
- factors that effect outcome after submersion in water.

15.6 Definitions

Immerged victims have their head above water and problems are usually due to hypothermia and cardiovascular instability (*Immersion* injuries). Submerged victims (head below water) develop problems secondary to asphyxiation and hypoxia (*Submersion* injuries). Victims of both immersion and submersion may aspirate fluids into their lungs. *Near drowning* refers to survival, at least temporarily, after immersion or submersion with aspiration of fluids in the lungs. *Drowning* refers to submersion events where the patient is pronounced dead within 24 hours of the event. Death occurring after this period is termed 'drowning-related death'.

15.7 Aetiology

Worldwide half a million people die each year due to drowning. It is a leading cause of death in children. There were 104 drownings in children aged 0–14 years in the UK in 1998 (see Box 15.3) and the incidence is rising possibly as a result of the increased number of garden pools and ponds. Alcohol use is involved in about 25–50% of adolescent and adult deaths associated with water recreation.

BOX 15.3 Location of drownings in children aged 0–14 years in the UK, 1998

Location	Number
River, canal, lake	31
Bath	25
Garden pond	21
Pools	11
Sea	10
Other	6

Modified from Sibert *et al. BMJ* 2002; **324:** 1070–1071

15.8 Pathophysiology of immersion and submersion

Immersion (head above water) in thermoneutral water (temperature greater than 25°C) causes hydrostatic pressure on the body resulting in an increase in venous return, cardiac output and work of breathing. The increase in cardiac output and volume shifts result in a diuresis. The latter is enhanced by peripheral vasoconstriction due to cold when the water temperature is less than 25°C (as found in most inland and offshore waters in the UK). This causes a further increase in urine output that is most severe at water temperatures below 5°C. The heart rate and cardiac output increase, causing a raise in myocardial oxygen demand that can cause ischaemia, arrhythmias and cardiac arrest. Respiratory drive is initially enhanced producing large gasps followed by hyperventilation and difficulty in breath holding. These initial effects of immersion in cold water make swimming very difficult and account for the large number of deaths in apparently 'good swimmers' close to safety. Muscle function diminishes further increasing the difficulty in swimming.

Survival rates improve by wearing:

- insulative clothing;
- a life-jacket that keeps the head out of the water;
- face-protection to prevent cold water from splashing onto the face.

Submersion (head below water) results in the victim trying to breath-hold for as long as possible. Ultimately there is swallowing and aspiration of water. The amount of water aspirated may initially be limited by laryngospasm. Hypoxaemia occurring after submersion results in secondary cardiac arrest. It is important to remember that primary cardiac arrest may occur prior to submersion such as due to myocardial ischaemia and ventricular fibrillation whilst swimming.

Hypothermia may develop after immersion or submersion. In icy water (less than 5°C) hypothermia develops rapidly. Brain cooling prior to the onset of severe hypoxaemia and secondary cardiac arrest may confer a degree of protection from neurological damage. Successful resuscitation with full neurological recovery has occurred in victims of prolonged submersion in extremely cold water. For example, survival in a 2-year-old child has been reported after submersion for 66 minutes in water at 5°C. The pathophysiological effects of hypothermia have been described earlier in this chapter.

15.9 Rescue

Rescuers must take care of their personal safety and keep risks to a minimum in attempting to reach or recover the victim. They should try and use a boat, raft, surfboard or flotation device to reach the victim.

If the victim has clinical signs of serious injuries, a history of diving, motorized vehicle crash, or fall from a height, especially if associated with water sports activity, protection of the cervical spine should be considered. Victims who have been in water for prolonged periods must be treated with care as they are relatively hypovolaemic due to the hydrostatic squeeze on their body. Removal from the water can result in cardiovascular collapse and many cases of postimmersion sudden death have been reported. It is, however, vital to remove the victim from the water as soon as possible. This may be achieved by floating the victim supine onto a spinal board before removing the victim from the water. Try to avoid constricting the chest with any harness and if possible keep the casualty horizontal. Once rescued keep the victim still, and protect them from further heat loss.

15.10 Assessment and management

15.10.1 Primary survey and resuscitation

The same principles as described throughout this book for primary survey and initial management apply. The management is the same whether the submersion incident occurred in salt or fresh water.

Open the airway with a jaw thrust rather than head tilt and chin lift if spinal cord injury is suspected. The patient's spine should be immobilized with a cervical collar and spinal board (see Section 1.6.1).

Special training and skills are needed to perform resuscitation in the water and should therefore not be routinely attempted by rescuers as it will delay removal from the water. Rescue breaths are almost impossible to perform unsupported in deep water. However, rescue breathing may be attempted once the rescuer can stand in the water or the victim is out of the water.

Debris should be removed manually or with suction if available once dry land is reached. There is no need to remove water from the airway. Some victims aspirate no water because of breath holding or laryngospasm on submersion. At most, there is only a small amount of water aspirated into the lungs and this is rapidly absorbed into the central circulation. Tipping the patient head down will not help to drain water or secretions from the lungs and may precipitate vomiting. Abdominal thrusts to remove water from the stomach and lungs should not be performed for the same reasons.

Vomiting is common after submersion. If it occurs, turn the victim's head to the side and remove vomitus manually or with suction. Patients should be tilted on a spine board or log-rolled if spinal injury is suspected. Early tracheal intubation and controlled ventilation is essential in the unconscious victim. Severe hypoxaemia is likely so as high a concentration of oxygen as possible should be given.

Hypothermia often accompanies submersion injury, so more time (up to a minute) may be needed to assess the circulation. The same principles apply for the hypothermic submersion patient as described in the section on hypothermia. Submersion produces a multisystem insult. These patients need to be managed in a critical care setting. They are at high risk of developing an acute lung injury, which may progress to acute respiratory distress syndrome (ARDS). Respiratory support with continuous positive airway pressure (CPAP) and assisted ventilation may be required to protect the lungs. During prolonged immersion the hydrostatic pressure of the water exerts a 'squeeze' effect that reduces the circulatory volume. On removal from the water, loss of this hydrostatic 'squeeze' can result in circulatory collapse due to hypovolaemia. Intravenous fluids should be administered with care and guided by clinical judgement and haemodynamic monitoring to prevent precipitating pulmonary and cerebral oedema.

15.10.2 Secondary survey

It is important that those who have drowned undergo a secondary survey, head-to-toe examination (Box 15.4). Many of these patients will be transferred early to the intensive care unit and, if this is the case, it is important on hand-over to establish that the secondary survey has not yet been completed.

Pneumonia is common in those victims requiring ventilation. Antibiotic therapy should only be started if there are signs of infection and after appropriate culture specimens have been taken. Broncho-alveolar lavage (BAL) may be useful to detect lung organisms in the ventilated patient. There is no good evidence that prophylactic antibiotics or steroids improve outcome. A nasogastric tube should be inserted to decompress and empty the stomach once resuscitation is underway.

BOX 15.4 Suggested investigations for near-drowning patients

- Arterial blood gases
- Electrolytes
- Glucose
- Urea and creatinine
- Creatine kinase
- Full blood count
- Coagulation screen
- Blood cultures
- Sputum or broncho-alveolar lavage (BAL)
- Chest x-ray
- ECG
- Toxicology screen

Further management and prognosis

Patients who have a spontaneous circulation and breathing when they reach hospital usually have the best outcome. A very small number of patients have survived after prolonged CPR. It is difficult to set any limits for duration of submersion after which withdrawal of CPR should be considered. However, the chances of survival are limited in both adults and children after submersion for more than 25 min in water with a temperature greater than 5°C. Children do not seem to have a better outcome than adults. Rapid cooling prior to cardiac arrest and brain hypoxaemia seems to be protective. Up to a third of near-drowning victims have moderate to severe brain damage. Death is often due to hypoxic brain injury in those who have survived initial resuscitation attempts.

In some areas attendances to the emergency department are common after immersion and submersion incidents. Discharge should only be considered if there is no evidence of aspiration and after a period of observation (at least 6 h) if:

- the patient is clinically normal, with no fever, cough, or respiratory symptoms. Pulmonary oedema is common with aspiration and may occur several hours after the event;
- the arterial oxygen tension and saturation is normal when the patient is breathing room air;
- chest examination is normal and the chest radiograph is clear;
- there are no other worrying symptoms.

Patients with evidence of aspiration need longer observation. On discharge patients and their carers should be given instructions to return if respiratory symptoms develop.

15.11 Summary

The same principles as described throughout this book for primary survey and initial management apply to victims of hypothermia and drowning. Passive or active external methods of warming are needed for victims of mild or moderate hypothermia. In severe hypothermia and cardiac arrest active internal methods such as cardio-pulmonary bypass may be needed. Death should be diagnosed with care in victims of hypothermia. Cooling in cold water prior to cardiac arrest confers a degree of protection from neurological damage.

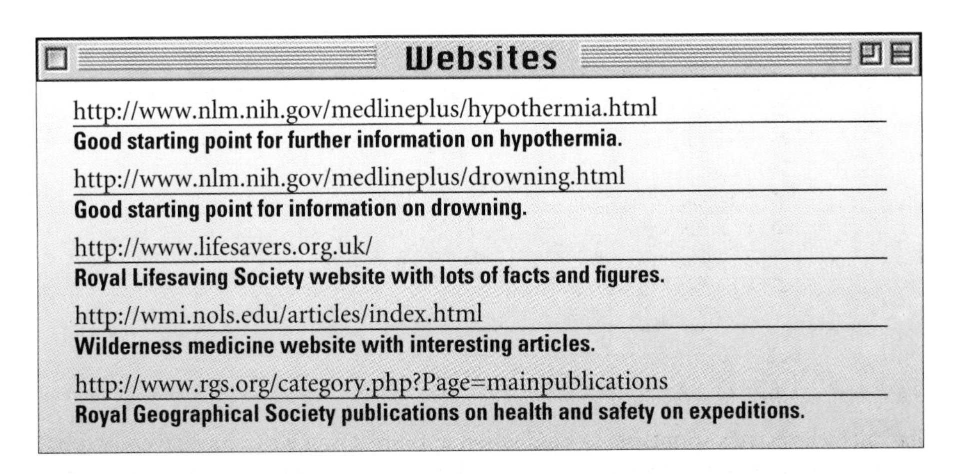

Websites

http://www.nlm.nih.gov/medlineplus/hypothermia.html
Good starting point for further information on hypothermia.

http://www.nlm.nih.gov/medlineplus/drowning.html
Good starting point for information on drowning.

http://www.lifesavers.org.uk/
Royal Lifesaving Society website with lots of facts and figures.

http://wmi.nols.edu/articles/index.html
Wilderness medicine website with interesting articles.

http://www.rgs.org/category.php?Page=mainpublications
Royal Geographical Society publications on health and safety on expeditions.

Further reading

1. **Auerbach PS (ed.)** (2001) *Wilderness Medicine. Management of Wilderness and Environmental Emergencies*, 4th edn. Mosby.
2. **Bolte RG, Black PG, Bowers RS, *et al.*** (1998) The use of extracorporeal rewarming in a child submerged for 66 minutes. *JAMA* **260:** 377.
3. **Gilbert M, Busund R, Skagseth A, *et al.*** (2000) Resuscitation from accidental hypothermia of 13.7 degrees C with circulatory arrest. *Lancet* **355:** 375.
4. **Golden F St C, Tipton MJ & Scott RC** (1997) Immersion, near drowning and drowning. *Br J Anaesth* **79:** 214.
5. **Koller R, Schnider TW & Neidhart P** (1997) Deep accidental hypothermia and cardiac arrest – rewarming with forced air. *Acta Anaesth Scand* **41:** 1359.

6. Simcock T (1999) Immediate care of drowning victims. *Resuscitation* **41:** 91.
7. Suominem P, Baillie C, Korpela R, *et al.* (2002) Impact of age, submersion time and water temperature on outcome in near drowning. *Resuscitation* **52:** 247.
8. Walpoth BH, Walpoth-Alsan BN, Mattle HP, *et al.* (1997) Outcome of survivors of accidental deep hypothermia and circulatory arrest treated with extracorporeal blood warming. *NEJM* **337:** 1500.
9. Watson RS, Cummings P, Quan L, *et al.* (2001) Cervical spine injuries among submersion victims. *J Trauma* **51**(4): 658.

16 Pain relief after trauma

T Johnson, J Windle

Objectives

The aims of this chapter are to help the trauma team to:

- understand the physiology of pain;
- appreciate the variability in patients' response to pain;
- manage trauma patients' pain more effectively;
- understand the progression to chronic pain states.

16.1 Introduction

Pain is a common human experience that functions as a protective mechanism to both external and internal stimuli, raising the body's awareness of physical or emotional damage. The perception of pain involves sensations, feelings and emotions that are unique and specific to an individual and is the most common reason for a patient to seek medical care. This individual response presents trauma team members with a complex phenomenon that may be difficult to understand, it is not easily quantifiable like the recording of a blood pressure or pulse. Pain is both personal and private; the experience cannot easily be articulated or interpreted by another person, increasing the likelihood of subjectivity.

Patients with severe and complex injuries represent a challenge to the trauma team; their pain is often derived from multiple sources, it may be very severe and can often evoke the strongest of physiological and emotional responses that may exist for a significant length of time. A clear understanding of the physiology of pain will assist all the team members in assessing the patient's pain and allow them to make informed choices regarding appropriate and effective modes of treatment. Recognition of innovative and challenging methods of pain control, as alternatives, will ultimately increase the priority of pain relief for trauma patients.

16.2 Physiology of the experience of pain

The perception of pain can be affected by many external stimuli such as anticipation, comprehension, anxiety, fatigue or a sense of danger. These stimuli have the potential to increase or decrease an individual's pain response. In contrast to patients undergoing planned surgery or procedures the trauma patient is unprepared for the events surrounding the injury. As a result the noxious stimuli are interlinked with emotional and sensory responses. The body's physiological reaction to a noxious stimulus is termed nociception and pain is the associated unpleasant experience. The manifestation of pain from injury is the result of a complex chain of communication between the body and brain.

The nervous system is the sensing, thinking and controlling system of the body. Sensory information is collected from many sources, such as the skin, internal tissues, through sight and sound, and eventually transmitted to the brain for cognitive processing and interpretation. The peripheral and central nervous systems are the main components involved in the transmission and interpretation of pain.

16.2.1 Peripheral nervous system

Pain receptors or nociceptors are located in the skin, periosteum, joint surfaces, arterial walls, subcutaneous tissues, muscles, viscera and fascia. These are all common sites of trauma-related injury. The majority of deep tissues have relatively few pain receptors, resulting in a less specific location of the pain stimulus. In the skin, the perception of pain begins in nerve fibres the density of which varies; large quantities are found in highly sensitive areas, for example, the thumbs, fingers or lips while smaller quantities are found in areas such as the back and internal organs. Each nerve ending has a receptor that responds to mechanical, thermal and chemical stimuli resulting in appreciation of heat, touch, pressure, joint position and pain sensations.

Tissue damage

Tissue damage causes the release of powerful inflammatory mediators such as serotonin, histamine and bradykinin, resulting in stimulation and sensitization of the chemoreceptors. The cell membrane becomes destabilized, further sensitizing the pain receptor to other stimuli. The chemical effect on the receptors is thought to produce the pain of inflammation, particularly in those tissues surrounding the actual area of damage. These chemicals decrease the threshold of all receptors in the body, converting them functionally to nociceptors (pain receptors). In effect those chemicals, released as a consequence of pain due to injury, now increase the intensity of that response.

Once an injury has occurred the stimulated nociceptors convey their pain message along A-delta or C peripheral afferent nerve fibres. A-delta fibres are fine, myelinated fibres that conduct rapidly (5–30 m/s). This is the first pain sensation sensed, usually sharp, pricking and well localized. C fibres are smaller, unmyelinated and are stimulated by mechanical, thermal and chemical sources producing dull, aching, and burning sensations. C fibres are widely distributed in both the skin and deep tissues and mediate 'slow pain' sensations. The conduction velocity of C fibres is one tenth that of A-delta fibres and this results in sensations less easily defined as to their intensity or point of origin. For example, the source of pain from a crush injury to a digit is easily localized without seeing it, but an abdominal injury usually results in generalizing the location of their pain.

Nociceptors are usually silent, but after stimulation by tissue damage, they become more sensitive to further damage and also respond to what is usually a nonpainful stimulus, for example, warmth becomes hot or burning while touch becomes tenderness. This is called allodynia and is an example of primary (local) hyperalgesia. Spinal mechanisms result in areas surrounding the injury also developing allodynia (secondary hyperalgesia). This results in the injured part and a surrounding zone being protected, by withdrawal from normal use. In most circumstances this promotes resolution of the pain and healing.

Chemical changes within the dorsal horn of the spinal cord affect the synapsing between peripheral and secondary neurons and their interneurons. This has been described as a 'pain gate'. The sensitivity depends on pre-existing sensitivity and current input. Neuroregulators are either excitatory (neurotransmitters) or regulatory (neuromodulators), and are responsible for further defining the pain message when transmitting the impulse across a synaptic cleft. An important neurotransmitter of pain impulses is an excitatory peptide called Substance P. The delayed action of Substance P explains why pain can be prolonged after the source or cause has been removed. Other transmitters and neuromodulators include glutamate, serotonin, norepinephrine, dopamine and the endogenous opioid peptides.

16.2.2 Central nervous system

Nociceptive messages entering the spinal cord are relayed on to the thalamus and then to the cerebral cortex via the spinothalamic tracts (*Figure 16.1*). The exact mechanisms and pathways of central pain processing are poorly understood – there is no discrete area of the brain responsible for pain, rather pain perception, emotion, autonomic function, memory and motor responses are linked in a complex matrix.

Pain modulation

The nervous system adapts to pain stimuli. Peripheral mechanisms usually result in enhancement of sensitivity whilst central mechanisms can exaggerate response (fear,

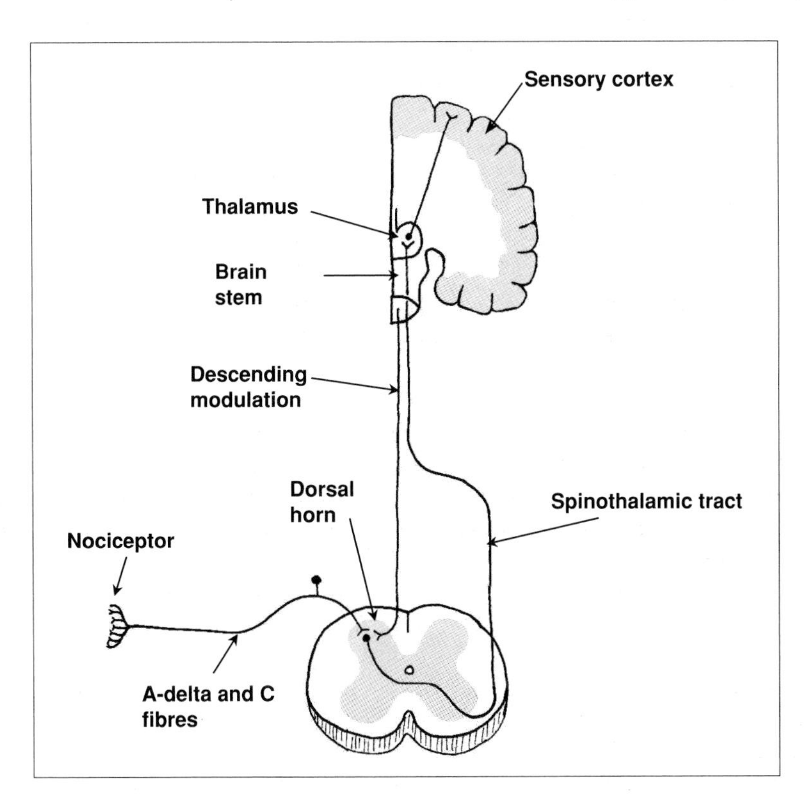

Figure 16.1 Spinal cord pathways of pain transmission

anxiety) or dampen response (bravado, hypnosis). Changes in serotonin and the endogenous opioid peptides are involved in both.

Spinal reflexes may increase pain following trauma. The stimulation of motor reflexes results in the muscle spasms often seen in trauma. Muscle spasm heightens the pain response possibly by inducing local metabolic changes. This often accounts for the dramatic improvement in pain control achieved after immobilization of a fracture.

16.3 Clinical management of pain

It requires a team approach to address the psychological, pharmacological and physical needs of patients in order successfully to control their pain: the 'Three Ps of Pain Management'.

16.3.1 Psychological

There is clear evidence that as anxiety increases the pain threshold lowers, exacerbating the pain response, in contrast, feelings of confidence and control have an inhibitory effect. This effect can and should be utilized by the trauma team members to limit anxiety and inhibit pain by ensuring a calm environment, providing frequent reassurance, and demonstrating effective teamwork. Furthermore, the individual response is also related to the acute experience and the events surrounding the injury. Pain associated with major injury in a dangerous and highly charged situation, such as escaping from a burning building, may be ignored or overlooked. Pain associated with relatively minor injuries sustained during civil disturbance, where an innocent onlooker becomes a victim, may appear excessive.

Previous painful experiences modify the neural systems creating a memory of past events and enhancing behaviour. Repeated exposure to noxious stimuli lowers the patients' threshold and increases their sensitivity. For example, a chronic back pain sufferer who sustains an acute injury may well experience an increased response to the pain stimulus. Once nociceptors have been sensitized, only slight stimuli are needed to produce a significant pain response or hyperalgesia. Early assessment and appropriate control of pain can prevent the development of hyperalgesia and reduce the overall long-term pain response.

An individual's response to illness or injury is also influenced by their cultural background, where behaviours are taught or learned. This influence can be manifested by a stoic acceptance seen particularly in the elderly population who often under-report pain or conversely an open display of pain often seen in the very young. Whilst there is no evidence that tolerance is different in various ethnic or cultural groups, outward expression of pain varies enormously. This influence of culture and beliefs also extends to trauma team members who may impose their own values and personal influence when evaluating the pain. To avoid personal bias in pain assessment, the multi-dimensional nature of pain, including physical, emotional, social and environmental components must be considered. The patient's contribution should be valued and included whenever possible.

Paediatric patients

A variety of behavioural responses are seen in children, some of which are cultural, including irritability, grimacing, guarding, pushing away, withdrawal, crying and over-reacting to minimal stimuli. Although these may simply be a response to pain, they may also indicate fear and anxiety as a result of previous unpleasant experiences with hospitals. Children who are fearful or mistrust health care workers are more anxious, which ultimately leads to an increased pain response. Trauma team members must be aware of child development in relation to chronological age in order to understand the expected behaviour and language skills, thereby improving communication with a distressed child, gaining their trust and cooperation.

Elderly patients

This group of patients often present with pre-morbid conditions that complicate, and compound, the acute trauma phase. Many elderly patients live with a degree of pain daily and accept this discomfort as part of the ageing process. Again the observation for pain behaviours is important and discussing their options for pain relief, which may be pharmacological but could also include appropriate comfort measures such as appropriately positioning and supporting the patient.

The trauma team

The way in which the trauma team work has an important effect on the patient's pain. Confidence is essential and explanation and justification at each stage in an appropriate and sensitive manner is as effective as pharmacological anxiolytics. Even in the worst circumstances, trauma patients may be very worried about the effects of what has happened to others, for instance their relatives. Understanding and reassurance will go a long way in playing a part in helping contribute to relief of anxiety and its effects on pain.

Assessment of pain

Due to the highly subjective nature of pain and the influences described above, only the patient can be truly aware of their pain. The relationship between the trauma nurse and patient affords the ideal opportunity to assess the patient's pain, plan their care and intervene with appropriate and timely analgesia. An accurate assessment will also increase the effectiveness of treatment.

The picture of pain may include:

- mechanism of injury;
- patient behaviour (e.g. facial expression, mobility);
- physiological response (e.g. tachycardia, sweating);
- patient report of pain (assessment tool).

Assessment tools

Pain assessment tools have been used in the treatment of chronic pain for some time, but acute care settings have been slow to appreciate the proven advantages. In the ED, any tool needs to be quick, accurate and flexible for varying situations and ages.

Verbal descriptor scales using groups of words that either describe pain, for example, burning, aching or stabbing or its severity, for example, mild, moderate, severe, are common, as they are quick and adaptable. These can be enhanced if used in conjunction with a visual analogue scale. The simplest and quickest consists of a line with a scale ranging from zero to 10, where zero represents 'no pain' and 10 the 'worst possible pain'. The scale may also indicate the parameters associated with mild, moderate and severe pain and patients participate by marking their level of pain on the scale. A horizontal line is preferred as vertical lines indicate a rapid increase and may reduce the sensitivity of the tool.

Adequate pain assessment in the child poses a challenge, especially in the very young. Words used to describe the levels can be altered to suit the age group but are of little use to the pre-verbal child. Sensory, visual pain scales have proven to be effective in children over the age of 3 years (and in patients with learning difficulties). A modification of the scale, using a range of happy, smiling faces, to sad, crying faces serves as a quick reference and useful mode of assessment. In addition, it is also useful to observe a child over time and note any refusal to play or move normally. Acute pain relief in children is possible with accurate assessment, timely analgesia and will calm parents and carers.

Behaviour scales have been introduced into emergency care to offset the subjectivity of the assessment and provide practitioners with a more objective means of establishing pain levels. The Manchester Triage System (MTS) (1997), used in over 80% of emergency departments in the UK, combines three assessment tools into one 'Pain Ruler' (*Figure 16.2*).

There is no direct relationship between the strength of a stimulus and the perception of pain. Because of the variation and complexity of the mechanisms described, the correlation between the degree of pain and classification of injury is unreliable and should never replace the individual assessment of the patient's unique pain experience.

The following illustrate this process.

- Patient 1 walks into the emergency department, limping but unaided, following an inversion injury to the ankle. When shown the pain ruler he points to five on the scale indicating moderate pain.

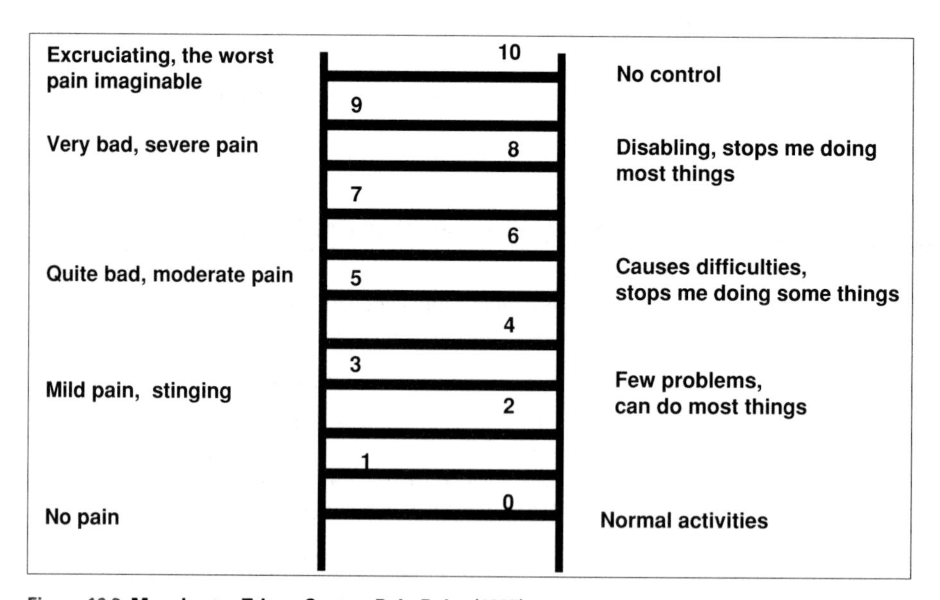

Figure 16.2 Manchester Triage System Pain Ruler (1997)

- Patient 2 having sustained a similar injury, hops into the department, stops frequently to rest and his face is red with the effort. He is sweating and grimaces on each movement, relieved to sit down in triage. On assessment with the pain ruler he points to 6 on the scale, again moderate pain.

This demonstrates how the objective pain score can be a vital part of the decision-making process. The use of a quick assessment tool is beneficial to both the patient and staff. Whether an established format is chosen or a unit specific tool is developed, a pain assessment tool increases awareness of the patient's pain, improves assessment skills and ultimately guides pain management decisions.

The accurate assessment of pain by the trauma team nurse must be coupled with the ability to offer adequate analgesia; there is little point in documenting and agreeing a mild to moderate pain score when a patient will have to wait for some considerable time before receiving analgesia. The introduction of Patient Group Directions for the administration of simple analgesia at triage ensures timely and appropriate pain management resulting in reduced pain, stress and anxiety for the patient and a feeling of empowerment for the practitioner.

16.3.2 Pharmacological

Drugs are the mainstay of providing pain relief after trauma and a wide variety of agents can be used. The following concentrates on those most commonly used in the UK.

Opioids

These provide effective analgesia for most trauma patients. Side effects include the following.

- Nausea: this is often exacerbated by the delay in gastric emptying as a result of trauma. Provided vomiting does not compromise the patient, it may bring relief.
- Respiratory depression: respiratory rate may fall towards normal levels with effective analgesia – clinical trends are more helpful than specific values. A low respiratory rate after opioid analgesia enough to reduce pain suggests other pathology. Where there is doubt about the effects of opioids on central respiratory drive, analysis of arterial blood gases may help (see Box 16.1).

BOX 16.1 Typical changes in $PaCO_2$ seen after the administration of opioids

$PaCO_2$	Comment
Low	In the conscious patient, consistent with pain and/or anxiety. If in pain, it is likely to be safe to proceed with opioid titration
Normal	Commonest situation – proceed or continue with analgesia
High	Indicates that ventilation is inadequate and need to distinguish between: Mechanical cause of inadequate ventilation e.g. pneumothorax or flail segment – repeat primary survey Pain from chest trauma – administer effective analgesia Central respiratory depression, e.g. opioids, head injury – repeat primary survey

- Pruritus and urinary retention (usually with higher doses).
- Sedation: this is usually minimal with judicious titration of opioids. In patients with a head injury, a reduction in level of consciousness beyond a calming and analgesic effect will be detected by an appropriately performed assessment of the patient's Glasgow coma score.

Concerns over use of opioids

- The potential to mask pathology. This is now known to be unfounded and relief of severe pain allows more effective clinical examination in a less distressed patient.
- Miosis (small pupils). This is a result of a central effect on the brainstem. It does not mask the development of pupillary abnormalities associated with intracranial pathology. A unilateral fixed dilated pupil will be more obvious as a result of the miosis in the unaffected pupil.
- Hypotension. Under normal circumstances the effect is minimal. In the trauma patient, pain may mask the presence of hypovolaemia as a result of cardiovascular stimulation increasing the pulse and helping maintain blood pressure. Care is therefore needed in the trauma patient with pain, a tachycardia but normal or low blood pressure is indicative of hypovolaemia and fluid resuscitation should precede the use of opioids.

Overcaution regarding the side effects of opioids is one of the major obstacles to analgesia being achieved

Occasionally, the effect of opioids may need to be reversed for diagnostic or therapeutic purposes. This may be achieved with small doses of naloxone – 400 μg diluted in 10 ml saline and given initially in 1 ml increments. Severe pain must be anticipated in some cases and alternative methods of analgesia, for example, nerve blocks, considered.

Morphine

This is considered the 'gold standard' analgesic and, with appropriate use, most patients will get rapid and effective analgesia. It is available for administration by a number of routes but it must be remembered that in patients with renal failure a metabolite, morphine-6-glucuronide, is more potent than morphine and will accumulate.

Intravenous titration of morphine

- The usual dose required ranges from less than 4 mg in the frail elderly patient to 100 mg in younger opioid tolerant patients.
- The safest method of administration is by diluting an ampoule (usually 10 mg) to 1 mg/ml using normal saline.
- Incremental doses of 2 mg or 3 mg are appropriate in an adult.
- In the frail, shocked, elderly or children the dose must be reduced (0.02–0.05 mg/kg in children).
- Intravenous opioids work quickly and subsequent doses can be given after 3–5 min, (longer in the elderly with slower circulation).

- It is important that observation of conscious level, respiratory rate, pulse and blood pressure are performed at 5-min intervals and continued for at least 15 min after the last dose.

Patient controlled analgesia (PCA)
This is best thought of as a method of maintaining analgesia rather than attaining it. Having achieved an agreed level of analgesia using the technique described above, the PCA patient device can allow the patient to self-medicate as the initial doses wear off.

Terminology for PCA

- Loading dose – quantity of drug to establish analgesia (as above).
- Bolus dose – incremental dose of drug by patient demand to maintain analgesia.
- Lockout interval – duration of time after a successful bolus dose during which the device will not respond to further requests.

Typical settings for an adult are:

- bolus dose of 1 mg;
- lockout interval of 5 min;
- opioid requirements are very variable between patients and therefore the maximum dose (for example, amount permissible in 4 h) is an unnecessary restriction;
- opioid tolerant patients may need high bolus doses, for example 4 mg, but usually the lockout interval remains constant.

Many elderly patients will not or are unable to use PCA effectively, even after a seemingly good explanation, and other routes must be used. Other opioids, for example fentanyl, may be used by the PCA route according to local protocols. For PCA purposes 20 μg fentanyl is equivalent to 1 mg morphine.

Intramuscular analgesia
This has a slower onset of action than intravenous titration and in the trauma patient poor peripheral blood flow will further reduce absorption making it difficult to achieve initial adequate pain control. However, when opioid requirements have been established it may be the preferred method of maintaining analgesia, particularly in elderly patients unable to understand and use PCA.

Intravenous infusion

- Require reliable intravenous access.
- Patients must be under close supervision to enable effective rate adjustment without the risk of overdosage.
- Usually restricted to patients in a HDU or ICU.

Oral route

- An ideal way for continuing analgesia.
- Patients must be able to tolerate an oral intake.
- Severe pain may need high oral doses of opioids.
- Can be continued after discharge from hospital.

- May avoid the need for admission to hospital after some injuries despite severe pain.
- Must be balanced against the potential for misuse in some populations.

Other opioids

Fentanyl

- An alternative morphine for instance when there is allergy.
- An initial dose of 0.1 mg is equivalent to approximately 10 mg of morphine.
- Has a short duration of action.
- As with all opioids, careful titration and observation is required.

Pethidine

- Short duration of action.
- Relatively impotent against severe pain.
- Associated with severe nausea and vomiting.
- Metabolites are proconvulsant.

Codeine (methyl morphine)

- Metabolized to morphine to become active.
- 10% of the population are unable to metabolize codeine to morphine (i.e. no analgesic effect).
- Conversion is unreliable, therefore providing variable analgesia.
- Can only be given orally or intramuscularly, intravenously associated with severe hypotension.
- Traditionally used for analgesia in patients with head injury, increasingly replaced with morphine.

Tramadol, buprenorphine and nubaine

- Little clinical benefit in most emergency situations compared with morphine.
- Less potent than morphine.
- Side effects similar to morphine.
- The use of this group of drugs may compromise the efficacy of morphine at a later stage, making control of severe pain difficult to achieve.
- Much more expensive than morphine.

Oxycodone and hydromorphone

- Relatively new opioid antagonists.
- Do not have significant active metabolites.
- May be an advantage for patients in renal failure.

Nonopioid drugs

Nonsteroidal anti-inflammatory drugs (NSAIDs)

- This group of drugs work by inhibiting an enzyme called cyclo-oxygenase (COX) the inhibition of which results in a reduction of prostaglandin formation.

- There are two types of COX:
  - COX-1, which is involved in production of prostaglandins responsible for gastric mucosal protection and platelet aggregation.
  - COX-2, involved in the production of prostaglandins in injured tissues and involved in inflammation and pain.
- Older, nonspecific NSAIDs inhibit both forms of COX, recently COX-2 specific NSAIDs have been introduced which have less adverse effects.
- The analgesic effect is similar across all agents and there is a ceiling effect because other mechanisms of pain generation are not affected.

A summary of preparations and their potential for side effects is shown in Box 16.2.

BOX 16.2 NSAID preparations and their potential side effects

	Nonspecific NSAIDs	COX-2 NSAIDs
Oral preparations	Ibrufen 200 mg qds Diclofenac 50 mg tds	Rofecoxib 50 mg daily
Intravenous preparation	Ketoralac 10–30 mg	Paracoxib 20–40 mg
Asthma	Both are avoided in aspirin sensitivity and asthma associated with recurrent nasal polyps. Safe if history of uneventful NSAID usage	
Upper GI ulceration	Avoid if significant recent history	Reduced risk of ulceration
Renal failure	Both are avoided in critical illness, hypovolaemia or established poor renal function	
Haemorrhage	May potentiate bleeding by inhibiting platelet aggregration	Little or no effect on platelet function
Bone healing	Both may inhibit bone healing (animal model evidence only)	

Although NSAIDs are very useful in the management of trauma pain, their anticoagulant and renal effects make them unsuitable for the initial management of patients with major trauma. They should therefore be reserved for use in those patients who have been fully resuscitated.

Paracetamol

- Effective in many forms of acute pain.
- It is inexpensive by either the oral or rectal route.
- It is probably under used particularly in patients who are unable to have non-steroidal anti-inflammatory NSAID treatment.
- An intravenous preparation is available but is currently unlicensed for use in the UK (propacetamol 2 g iv 6 hourly – equivalent to 1 g oral paracetamol 6 hourly).
- Very effective when used in combination with opioids ('morphine sparing effect').

All patients with severe pain will benefit from having a combination of an opioid and either a NSAID or paracetamol

Entonox

This is a mixture of 50% oxygen and 50% nitrous oxide. It is administered to spontaneously breathing patients via a demand valve using a facemask or mouthpiece. There is probably both analgesia and euphoric effect. It should not be used in patients with possible pneumothorax or pneumocranium because of the risk of expansion of gas within enclosed spaces.

Ketamine

This is an intravenous anaesthetic agent, very useful in extreme situations such as emergency amputation or removal of large embedded object. The airway and circulation are relatively well maintained compared with the use of other intravenous anaesthetic agents but this should not be used as an excuse for complacency. It has been used safely in circumstances where access to the patient is difficult. A dose of 1 mg/kg intravenously will produce anaesthesia for several minutes although movement and vocalization may still occur. Reduced doses will provide profound anaesthesia but the maximal effect may take several minutes to onset. Many fit young adults will experience profound hallucinogenic effects that can be reduced by the concurrent administration of a benzodiazepine for example diazepam 2–5 mg, iv.

In extreme circumstances, ketamine can be administered intramuscularly, but the effects are very unpredictable, particularly in circumstances where peripheral perfusion may be impaired. An individual with appropriate anaesthetic training should supervise the use of ketamine.

Local anaesthetic techniques

These can be extremely useful in the trauma patient and range from simple local infiltration analgesia to nerve blocks. Whatever technique is used, it is important that an appropriate concentration of local anaesthetic agents to avoid the risk of toxicity (CNS and cardiac excitation and or depression) and for each patient calculate the maximum safe dose and ensure that this is not exceeded.

Recommended maximum doses

- Lignocaine plain – 3 mg/kg.
- Lignocaine with adrenaline (epinephrine) – 5 mg/kg.
- Bupivacaine ± adrenaline (epinephrine) – 2 mg/kg.

The relationship between the amount of drug, concentration and volume is given by the formula:

$$\text{Volume (ml)} \times \text{concentration (\%)} \times 10 = \text{dose of drug (mg)}$$

For example: 20 ml of 2% lignocaine

$$20\ \text{(ml)} \times 2\ \text{(\%)} \times 10 = 400\ \text{mg}$$

Toxicity is also increased using more concentrated solutions therefore always use the lowest effective concentration, for example, 0.5% lignocaine is adequate for infiltration analgesia.

Although there are a large number of nerve blocks that can be usefully applied in the trauma patient, the authors feel that there are two that all trauma team leaders should be familiar with: intercostal and femoral nerve blocks. These have a 'high benefit:low risk' ratio. Those interested in other blocks should refer to one of the many excellent texts available.

Intercostal nerve block

Useful for rib fractures to aid coughing and deep breathing. The intercostal nerve runs in the subcostal groove along the inner, inferior border of the rib, accompanied by the intercostals vessels. The nerves associated with the lower seven ribs are most accessible and blocked at the angle of the ribs. There is a small risk of pneumothorax so patients need to remain under close supervision after they have been attempted.

- The patient is best placed in the lateral position, affected side uppermost. The upper arm is then placed above their head to remove the scapula from over the ribs.
- The site of injection is approximately a hands breadth from the spine.
- The site is cleansed with antiseptic and the area draped.
- The lower border of the rib is identified by the operator's nondominant hand.
- The skin over the rib is then 'pushed' upwards (cranially).
- The syringe containing local anaesthetic solution, with needle attached, is held like a dart and the needle introduced perpendicularly through the skin to make contact with the rib.
- The tension in the skin is then released allowing the needle to be 'walked' down the rib until it just slips off the inferior border.
- The needle is then angled at 45° and advanced a further 0.5 cm to place the tip in the groove beneath the rib.
- The syringe is then aspirated looking for blood or air to ensure that the tip of the needle is not in the vessels or within the lung respectively.
- Local anaesthetic, usually 3–4 ml of 0.5% bupivacaine, is then injected and the needle withdrawn.
- The procedure is then repeated at the next rib.

Femoral nerve block

This supplies most of the periosteum of the femur and block allows fractures to be reduced or traction applied effectively with minimal discomfort avoiding the need for opioid analgesia. It is important to use an appropriate technique and regional anaesthesia needle to minimize risk of damage to the nerve.

- The inguinal ligament is identified, running from the anterior superior iliac spine to the pubic tubercle.
- The femoral artery is identified at the midpoint, just below the ligament and the area cleansed.
- A finger is placed on the pulsation of the femoral artery.
- A 21 g, short bevel needle, attached to a syringe containing local anaesthetic, is inserted 1 cm laterally to the artery, at 45° and advanced to a depth of 3–4 cm.
- In the conscious patient, if paraesthesia is elicited, withdraw the needle slightly
- Aspirate to ensure that the needle tip is not within a blood vessel.
- Inject local anaesthetic, usually 20 ml of 0.5% bupivacaine.

- If paraesthesia is not obtained or the patient is unconscious, inject the local anaesthetic in a fanwise manner from adjacent to the artery, moving laterally, 3–4 cm.

16.3.3 Physical treatments

Immobilizing an injured limb not only reduces pain but will also reduce blood loss, the risk of neurovascular damage and fat emboli from underlying fractures. This can be achieved using box splints, gutter splints, air or vacuum splints. Traction splints for the lower limb (see Section 9.5.7) are designed to provide immobilization and maintain reduction of a fracture. There is a wide range of modern devices, all of which are based upon the original design by Hugh Owen Thomas.

Surface cooling of an injured limb, particularly around joints, will help to reduce oedema and pain. This is best achieved using commercially available ice packs, which are stored at 5°C and reusable. Ice should never be applied directly to the skin.

Superficial burns are very painful and hypersensitive to touch, including exposure to air currents. Covering the burned area with a sterile dressing will reduce pain and help protect from contamination. A variety of propriety dressings are available in an emergency, however, PVC is cheap, sterile and nonadherent.

Finally, avoiding long waits on spinal boards or trolleys will all be helpful.

16.4 Analgesia for difficult conditions

Use of analgesic or anaesthetic medications intravenously, alone or in combination with sedatives, to produce suitable operating conditions is widely practised and often provide a means of rapidly reducing fractures or dislocations. The main risks are of airway obstruction and aspiration of regurgitated gastric contents.

The administration of intravenous benzodiazepines to the point of inducing a state resembling general anaesthesia is not appropriate. Where there is any doubt, an experienced anaesthetist should supervise with protection of the airway.

16.4.1 Cancer pain patients (e.g. pathological fractures)

Patients may already be on large doses of opioids and will be tolerant to the effects such that very large doses may be required. Opioids are usually effective but very much increased doses are necessary. Early involvement of the acute pain team is strongly recommended.

16.4.2 Drug abusers or patients on methadone maintenance programmes

As always a careful assessment of pain and analgesia is required. These patients suffer pain from injury just like any others and are often fearful that requests for analgesia will be ignored and this may increase their demanding behaviour. A traumatic episode is unlikely to be a good time to institute a drug withdrawal programme – remember that they already have a substance abuse problem and withholding adequate analgesia for obvious injury is unlikely to be helpful. Opioids will be relatively ineffective but if used this must be at an appropriately high dose. Other forms of analgesia, such as NSAIDS and local blocks, will usually be very welcome. Opioid maintenance will need to be continued. Liaison with the local drugs team may provide future support.

16.4.3 Recurrent trauma (e.g. fractures of brittle bones or recurrent osteoporotic fractures)

It may be helpful to draw up a plan for analgesia if admission is regular. On occasions an effective analgesia plan may avoid admission, for example, initial doses of intravenous morphine, whilst diagnosis is made followed by discharge on strong oral opioids with planned reduction as pain resolves.

16.5 Progression to chronic pain

A large proportion of chronic pain is initiated by a traumatic episode. Injury produces pain and hypersensitivity. Tenderness of injured tissue can be described as:

- allodynia – innocuous stimuli such as touch on the painful area being sensed as pain;
- hyperpathia – an accentuation of what would otherwise be a painful stimulus.

This protective hypersensitivity normally limits movement and function until healing can occur.

Hypersensitivity normally resolves but in a small number of patients this does not occur and an exaggerated and prolonged pain syndrome may develop. The resulting pain is usually out of proportion to the inciting event and diagnostic delay and confusion, with perhaps inappropriate reassurance that all will resolve, often adds to the patient's difficulties.

16.5.1 Examples of chronic pain syndromes

Complex Regional Pain Syndrome (CRPS) type 1

Previously known as Reflex Sympathectomy Dystrophy (RSD), this is most commonly seen after minor peripheral limb trauma, either soft tissue injury or fracture. An early warning sign is high pain levels despite immobilization. This often leads to further and prolonged immobilization. The limb becomes swollen, sensitive, discoloured and there may be circulatory or growth changes in the skin, nails and hair. Both peripheral and central neuronal mechanisms are involved explaining why traditional attempts at treatment blocking the sympathetic chain or systemic anti-adrenergic agents are disappointing. Early mobilization with aggressive analgesia (systemic or local anaesthetic) appears to offer the best chance of a good outcome.

Immobilization of injuries beyond the first few hours unless an absolute necessity is contraindicated as a form of analgesia

CRPS Type 2 (previously known as causalgia)

A similar syndrome that results from a specific injury to a peripheral nerve, for example, following gunshot wounds or lacerations. Treatment uses the same principles as described above.

Examples of these would be low back pain or cervical whiplash injury. Road traffic accidents result in many injuries, usually dealt with by clinical examination, x-ray, radiography, advice and discharge. Back and neck pain are in any case common complaints in a normal community. Typically the pain of acute neck or back sprain increases over the first few hours and days. It may result in a re-referral or visits to the GP. Appropriate advice at an early stage is vital – inappropriate rest or fear of further damage may result in a chain of events leading to substantial disability (see Figure 16.3).

Careful reassurance that there is no evidence of significant mechanical disruption must include the possibility that pain and stiffness may increase before resolving. Obviously patients will need to be advised to return if there are specific symptoms such as numbness or weakness associated with spinal injury but proper reassurance may avoid attendance for reassurance about pain which has not resolved or which has increased.

Anticipation of increasing pain after whiplash type injury may be reassuring provided it is combined with advice to return for specific problems

Further *early* aggressive diagnostic tests, for example scans, may be very useful in encouraging normal activity in the presence of persisting pain symptoms, thus preventing months of diagnostic uncertainty for the patient with the risk of permanent disability.

16.6 Summary

The vast majority of patients attending the emergency department do so with minor, single system injuries, commonly to limbs. This group of patients often report mild to moderate pain, the sensation is usually short-lived, and relief is either spontaneous or requires only simple analgesia. In contrast, patients with severe and complex injuries represent a challenge to the trauma team as their pain is often derived from multiple sources. Severe pain, as experienced by the trauma victim, can often evoke the strongest of physiological and emotional responses that may exist for a significant length of time. By understanding the psychological, pharmacological and physical needs of the trauma patient their pain will be managed more appropriately and reduce the risk of progression to a chronic pain state.

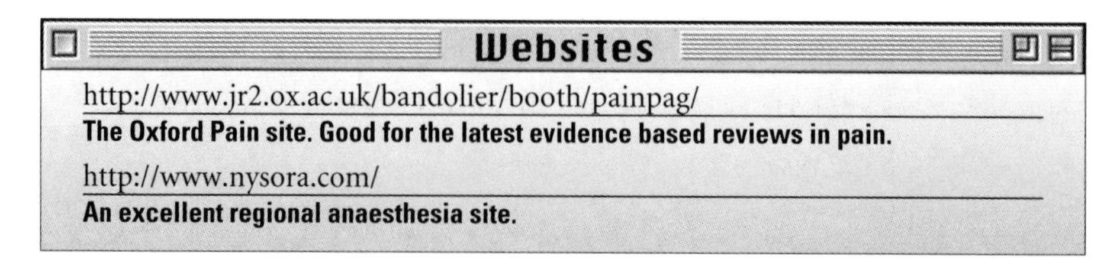

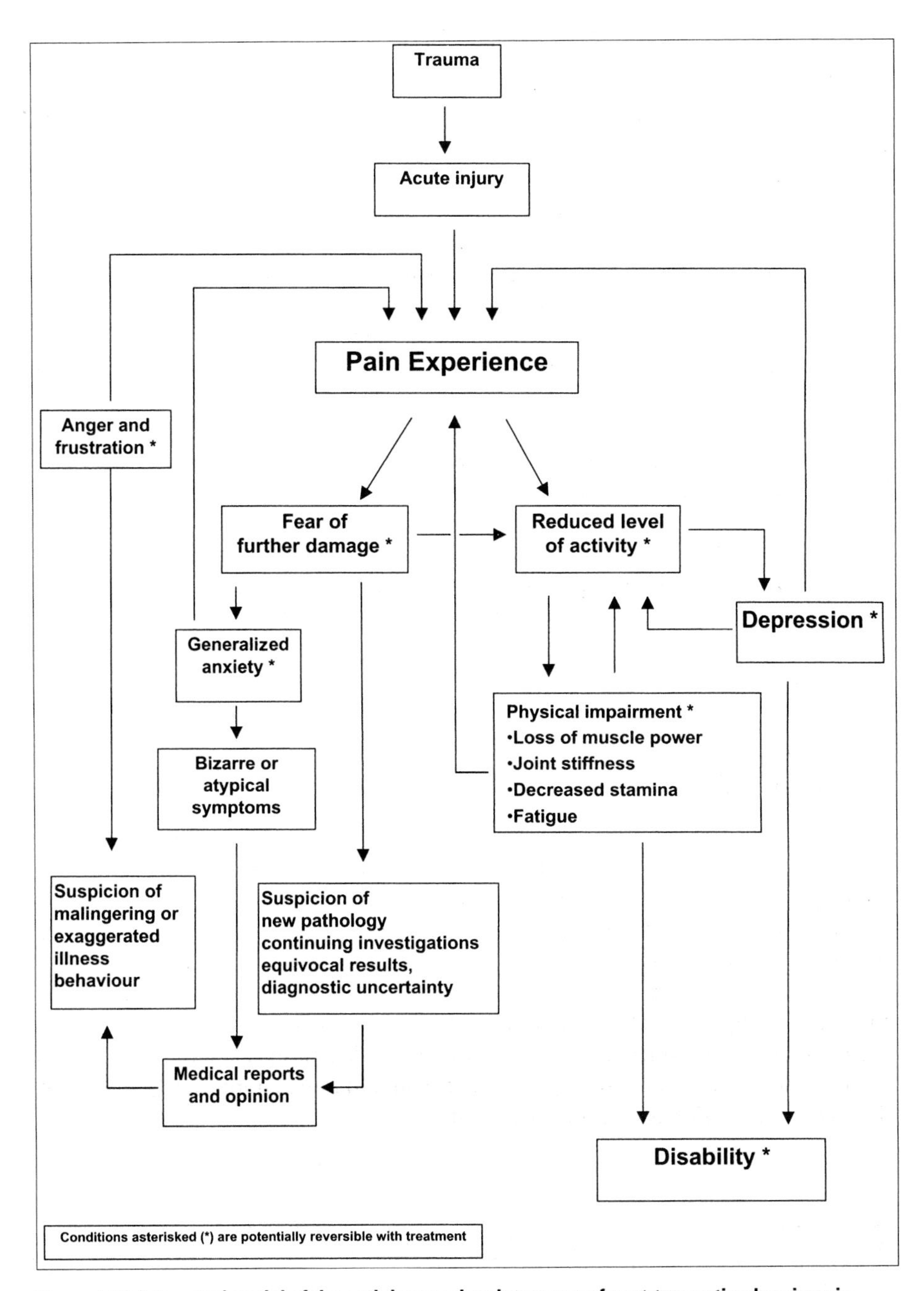

Figure 16.3 Integrated model of the aetiology and maintenance of post-traumatic chronic pain

Further reading

Mackway-Jones K (ed) (1997) *Emergency Triage.* BMJ Publishing Group, London.

17 Inter- and intra-hospital transfer of the trauma patient

K Lennon, S Davies, P Oakley

Objectives

At the end of this chapter, members of the trauma team responsible for transferring a patient should understand:

- the indications for secondary transfer;
- the composition of the transfer team;
- the equipment and drugs required;
- the phases of transfer.

17.1 Introduction

Each year in the United Kingdom, thousands of critically ill patients are transferred between hospitals. A significant proportion of these transfers involved trauma patients undergoing secondary transfer from district general hospitals to specialist units. Inter-hospital transfer of critically injured patients is a much more serious and potentially complicated process than many people realize and the occurrence of adverse incidents are well recognized.

17.2 Indications for secondary transfer

Major trauma patients require secondary transfer for a variety of reasons, both clinical and nonclinical including a lack of:

- surgical expertise (e.g. no neurosurgical service);
- specialist intensive care support (e.g. no neuro/trauma intensive care facility);
- equipment for specialist investigation (e.g. 24-h computerized tomography);
- intensive care beds, due to inadequate staffing or absolute overflow.

Repatriation is a less common nonclinical indication for humanitarian or economic reasons.

Specific clinical indications for secondary transfer usually relate to the anatomical injury and the associated specialist service (see Box 17.1). Single specialty hospitals (e.g. stand alone neurosurgical and cardiothoracic centres) pose a particular risk to the blunt trauma patient, as major blunt trauma rarely affects isolated body regions. The indications for transfer vary in their urgency depending on whether the transfer is an emergency for life-saving surgery, urgent for life-threatening states requiring specialist

BOX 17.1 Indications for secondary interhospital transfer

1. Severe head injury
   - Requiring a neurosurgical operation
   - Requiring neurosurgical assessment or intensive neurological monitoring
2. Suspected mediastinal injury
   - Aortic tear
   - Tracheobronchial rupture
   - Ruptured oesophagus
3. Burns
   - Extent (surface area and depth)
   - Particular site (e.g. airway and flexures)
4. Spinal injuries
   - Unstable fracture
   - Spinal cord injury
5. Limb and pelvic injuries
   - Pelvic (including acetabular) reconstruction
   - Vascular injuries
   - Open tibial fractures with extensive soft tissue injuries
   - Severe hand injuries
6. Severe faciomaxillary injuries
7. Liver injuries
8. Severely injured children
   - Requiring specialist paediatric surgery
   - Requiring intensive care
9. Severely injured patients
   - With multiple injuries, according to regional trauma system guidelines, where it has been agreed to centralize major trauma in a trauma centre
   - Requiring regional or supraregional intensive care techniques
   - Requiring rehabilitation
   - Requiring repatriation or treatment in their home area

intensive care but no surgery, or elective for reconstruction, rehabilitation or repatriation.

17.3 Transfer team composition

Inter-hospital transfer is a multidisciplinary specialty and a team approach is required. Due to the isolated working environment and the often complex nature of the patient's medical condition, team members should be of sufficient seniority and have appropriate skills. All trainees should undergo a formal training programme and be directly supervised until deemed competent. Attendance on courses specific to training in inter-hospital transfer, such as the Safe Transfer and Retrieval (STaR) Course (Advanced Life Support Group 2002), should become a mandatory requirement. It is recommended that anaesthetists accompany head-injured patients. Other medical specialists (e.g. emergency physicians and nonanaesthetist intensivists) can perform this role, provided that they have proven competency in resuscitation, airway care, ventilation, other organ support and intensive care monitoring techniques in addition to acute trauma management.

Component roles from four different disciplines provide the necessary elements for the transfer team (see Box 17.2).

BOX 17.2 Component roles for a transfer team

1. Medical (anaesthetist, intensivist, emergency physician, or other doctor with appropriate training for clinical assessment and intervention)
2. Nursing (emergency department or intensive care nurses to provide holistic care and communicate with team members, the patient, and the patient's family)
3. Technical (operating department practitioner or intensive care technician to operate and troubleshoot problems with machinery such as monitors and ventilators)
4. Transport (ambulance paramedics or technicians to handle and secure the patient together with being responsible for the mobile environment.

Multidisciplinary training allows for members from each of these backgrounds to learn to perform complementary skills. The exact number of accompanying personnel will then depend on the clinical circumstances in each case. A complex, unstable case will require a team that includes all four specialists. Overlapping skills will allow a smaller team to manage safely less complex cases.

Retrieval teams are routinely used in the secondary transfer of paediatric patients to specialist paediatric centres. When using such teams for major trauma, one has to be wary of the time-limited situation, as mobilization of the team and travel to the primary hospital can be very time-consuming. This may occasionally necessitate a child being transferred by nonspecialists in paediatric transfer. Alternatively, the transfer team could consider bringing the specialist surgeon to the patient in extreme situations. While this may offer an advantage for the individual patient, it depletes resources at the specialist centre.

17.4 Equipment and drugs

A critically injured patient must be transferred in a 'portable intensive care' environment. All equipment must be robust, durable and lightweight. Everything should be serviced regularly and checked both daily and before transfer. The team must be familiar with the equipment (see Box 17.3) and drugs (see Box 17.4) in the transfer kit and with that available in the transfer vehicle itself.

Electrical equipment needs to be able to run reliably on batteries and spares, with a much longer life than the maximum possible journey time. Nickel-cadmium type batteries should generally be avoided. Modern ambulances are equipped with electrical power capabilities and equipment such as syringe pumps can often be connected directly into the ambulance power supply.

A monitored oxygen supply is required with enough reserve to cover a doubling of the expected journey time in case of breakdown or other delay. Portable mechanical

BOX 17.3 Essential equipment for transfer

- Portable monitor with ECG, NIBP, SaO_2, $EtCO_2$, three invasive pressures, and temperature
- Portable sucker (which does not depend on electricity or gas)
- Self-inflating bag-valve-mask and intubation equipment, including back-up cricothyroidotomy
- Portable ventilator with disconnection and high pressure alarms, and variable settings (V_T, rate, FiO_2, PEEP, I:E ratio)
- Extension hose with Schraeder probe (as extension to ventilator oxygen hose to reach distant supply)
- Rucksack transport kit with respiratory and cardiovascular equipment rolls (including venous access equipment) and a drug pack
- Chest drain equipment
- Battery powered syringe drivers
- Battery powered IV volumetric pumps
- Defibrillator
- Urinary catheters
- Warming blanket
- Spare batteries
- Head light
- Protective clothing (high visibility clothing and protective helmet)
- Communication aids
- Scissors and tape

BOX 17.4 Essential drugs for inter-hospital transfer

- Hypnotics/sedatives, e.g. midazolam, propofol, etomidate, ketamine
- Muscle relaxants, e.g. suxamethonium (for intubation or re-intubation), atracurium, cisatracurium, vecuronium
- Local anaesthetics, e.g. lidocaine (lignocaine), bupivacaine
- Analgesics, e.g. fentanyl, morphine
- Anticonvulsants e.g. diazepam, thiopental
- Mannitol
- Inotropes, e.g. adrenaline, norepinephrine (noradrenaline)
- Resuscitation drugs according to Resuscitation Council guidelines

ventilators must have disconnection and high-pressure alarms. Variable inspiratory/expiratory (I/E) ratio is invaluable in severe lung injury or ARDS. The ability to provide pressure controlled ventilation, pressure support and continuous positive airway pressure (CPAP) are desirable.

Multichannel, portable monitors with a clear illuminated display and resistance to motion artefact is essential. Alarms need to be visible, as well as audible, in view of the noisy environment.

Syringe drivers and infusion pumps should be used in preference to gravity-dependent drips, which are inaccurate and unreliable in moving vehicles. Pumps should be mounted below the level of the patient and infusion sets fitted with anti-siphon valves.

A well-designed, dedicated transfer trolley can simplify the whole transfer process. This should be chosen in full consultation with the local ambulance service and must be compatible with local ambulance specifications to fit in place in the vehicle.

A mobile phone (despite the risk of interfering with electronic equipment), essential contact telephone numbers and cash/credit cards should be available for use in an emergency.

17.5 The five phases of inter-hospital transfer

Inter-hospital transfer can be considered in five phases as outlined in Box 17.5.

BOX 17.5 The five phases of inter-hospital transfer

1. Initial assessment: identification of injuries with resuscitation and stabilization of physiological systems
2. Consultation and referral: decision to transfer and communication with the receiving centre and transport agency
3. Preparation for transfer
4. Transportation: handling the patient and the environment
5. Handover and return

17.5.1 Phase one: initial assessment

Assessment, resuscitation and stabilization should follow the recommendations as laid out in Section 1.5. Trauma care is time-limited. Failure to identify injuries and thoroughly resuscitate and stabilize the patient prior to transfer may lead to serious, life-threatening complications in transit. A patient persistently hypotensive despite resuscitation must not be transported until all possible causes of the hypotension have been identified. Correctable causes of major haemorrhage (e.g. splenic injury) should be dealt with prior to transfer. A fundamental requirement before transfer is to ensure satisfactory and stable organ perfusion and tissue oxygen delivery. Following severe head injury it is essential to avoid hypoxia and hypotension to reduce the risk of secondary brain injury.

The transfer team should liase with the ambulance service to confirm the availability of an appropriate transfer vehicle. All equipment and drugs must be fully checked prior to setting off. Oxygen requirements should be calculated and then doubled to account for unexpected delay. Originals or copies of case notes, investigation results and x-rays must be collected together, along with a referral letter and any blood or blood products that must accompany the patient on the transfer. A pre-transfer checklist is advisable to minimize the risk of forgetting anything. A sample transfer checklist for neurosurgical patients is shown in Box 17.6. The receiving hospital should be contacted and given an estimated time of arrival.

It is not necessary to wait until the entire set of initial investigations is complete before considering transfer, or indeed contacting the receiving unit. However, the referring clinician must possess sufficient knowledge about the patient's overall condition in order to present a sufficiently accurate account for which to base the consultation.

17.5.2 Phase two: consultation and referral

The need to transfer a patient to another unit may be obvious from the outset. For example, a patient with a severe head injury, or may be more complex and linked to

BOX 17.6 Transfer checklist for neurosurgical patients

System	Checklist
Respiration	$PaO_2 > 13$ kPa, $PaCO_2 < 4.5$ kPa Airway clear and protected adequately Intubation and ventilation required OG tube in situ (if intubated)
Circulation	MABP > 90 mmHg (SBP > 90 mmHg with potential trunk bleeding) Pulse < 100/min Peripheral perfusion 2 reliable large iv cannula *in situ* Estimated blood loss already replaced
Head injury	GCS, GCS trend (improving/deteriorating) Focal signs Skull fracture
Other injuries	Cervical spine injury, chest injury, fractured ribs, pneumothorax Intrathoracic, intra-abdominal bleed Pelvic, long bone fracture Extracranial injuries toileted and splinted
Escort	Doctor, nurse, ODP, ambulance crew adequately experienced Instructed about THIS case Adequate equipment and drugs Adequate oxygen Can use equipment and drugs Case notes, investigation results, radiology films and reports, and referral letter Contacted the receiving unit and know exactly where to go to Telephone numbers programmed into portable phone Portable phone battery fully charged Name and bleep number of receiving doctor Cash/credit cards in case of emergency Family aware of details

other factors, such as lack of intensive care beds. Either way any decision to transfer a patient to another hospital must be made at consultant level and must involve the on-call intensive care consultant and all other specialist consultants involved in the patient's care. The consultant coordinating the transfer must ensure that the transfer team, once assembled, are fully aware of all details relevant to the patient and the transfer plan. Communication within the team is also essential. They must be fully aware of each other's roles and responsibilities.

Once the decision has been made that a transfer is necessary, one of these consultants, ideally a designated on-call consultant with responsibility for coordinating inter-hospital transfers, must communicate the need for transfer with the on-call intensive care consultant and all other relevant specialist consultants at the receiving hospital. Information should be exchanged in concise and unambiguous terms.

It is essential for a plan of transfer to be agreed between the referring and receiving consultants. This will include:

- any further investigations or interventions prior to transfer;
- the mode of transfer (e.g. land or air ambulance);
- the timing of transfer;
- the exact location to which the patient should be transferred.

As soon as a decision has been made to transfer, ambulance control must be contacted. They need to be involved in deciding on the mode of transfer and will need time to mobilize sufficiently experienced crews. Any delay in communicating with the ambulance service will lead to unnecessary delays in setting off.

Sensitive communication with the patient (if awake and competent) and the family must never be forgotten. They need to be made fully aware of the clinical situation and the reasons for transfer. The relatives require accurate directions to the receiving hospital, together with contact telephone numbers. These could be pre-printed for the hospitals used as regular referring units from the transferring hospital. On no account should relatives attempt to keep pace with the transferring ambulance. Ideally they should follow on some 10 or 15 min after the patient and transfer team have left for the receiving hospital.

Good communication is a cornerstone of a successful and uneventful transfer. This is never more important than at the time of referral and when the patient is handed over at the end of the transfer.

17.5.3 Phase three: preparation for transfer

Preparation for transfer begins with proactive investment and training. Checklists prior to transfer are invaluable and will ensure that no aspect of the transfer process is omitted, thereby reducing the potential of adverse incidents.

In any particular situation, there may be important preparations prior to transfer, in response to the discussions with the receiving unit. Treatment may be added or modified, for example, adjusting intravenous fluids in a major burn. The transferring team must still retain responsibility, so that adjustment to such changes, for example, are made according to the urine output and the overall clinical picture.

Some preparations are generic, such as securing lines and tubes, keeping the patient well wrapped and warm. The patient should have been log-rolled off the spinal board during the secondary survey. A vacuum mattress is to be preferred to reapplying a hard spinal board in a patient with a known or an uncleared spine. If no alternative is available, a spinal board may be re-used for short transfers, though it is probably best avoided. Pressure sores rapidly develop (*Figure 17.1*).

A key consideration at this stage (as in all stages) is airway management.

When in doubt intubate prior to transfer

Intubating a complex trauma patient, with an uncleared spine, is difficult enough in the resuscitation room, let alone in the confined space of an ambulance. The indications for intubation after head injury are shown in Box 17.7. Once intubated, the patient must be kept adequately paralysed and sedated. Sedative, analgesic and muscle

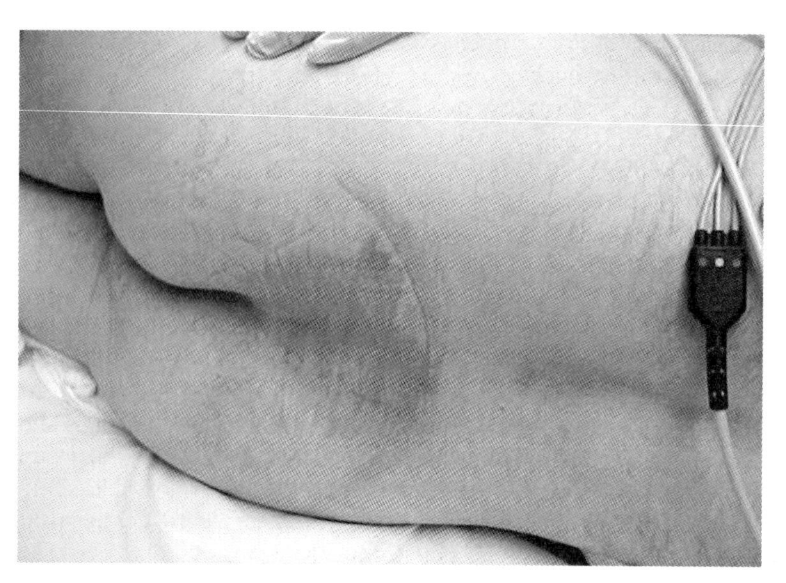

Figure 17.1 **Pressure sore formation**

relaxant drugs are best delivered by infusion. Fifteen minutes after connection to the portable ventilator, blood gases must be analysed. This will allow adequate time for any adjustment that is necessary to ensure adequate oxygenation and ventilation. Intubated head-injured patients must be transferred with a PaO_2 greater than 13 kPa and a $PaCO_2$ of 4.0–4.5 kPa. In the presence of a pneumothorax or significant fractured ribs, a chest drain should be inserted prior to transfer. A large bore gastric tube must be passed in an intubated patient.

BOX 17.7 Indications for intubation and ventilation after head injury

Immediately

- Coma – not obeying commands, not speaking, not eye opening, i.e. GCS < 9
- Loss of protective laryngeal reflexes
- Ventilatory insufficiency as judged by blood gases
  - Hypoxaemia (PaO_2 < 9 kPa on air or < 13 kPa on oxygen)
  - Hypercarbia ($PaCO_2$ > 6 kPa)
- Spontaneous hyperventilation causing $PaCO_2$ < 3.5 kPa
- Respiratory arrhythmia

Before the start of the journey

- Significantly deteriorating conscious level, even if not in coma
- Bilateral fractured mandible
- Copious bleeding into mouth (e.g. from skull base fracture)
- Seizures

Hypovolaemic patients tolerate transfer poorly and intravenous volume loading may need to be undertaken prior to transfer. Even after surgery, do not underestimate ongoing losses from other sources, such as fracture haemorrhage and third space losses. A central venous catheter can be used to optimize filling and administer drugs and fluids during transfer. In the head-injured patient without an intracranial pressure monitor the mean arterial blood pressure should be kept above 90 mmHg to optimize cerebral perfusion pressure. In patients with potential trunk bleeding, who cannot be operated on at the referring hospital (e.g. in a tear of the thoracic aorta being referred to a cardiothoracic centre), the systolic blood pressure should be kept at a maximum of 90 mmHg. This may necessitate the use of vasodilators. On the rare occasion where both injuries co-exist, the risk of haemorrhage is greater than the risk of secondary brain injury. A systolic pressure of 90 mmHg is acceptable under these circumstances.

Dislocations and significantly displaced fractures should be reduced and immobilized prior to transfer. Open wounds should be irrigated with sterile saline if contaminated and then covered to reduce the risk of infection. Open fractures should be inspected once and a photograph taken to allow others to visualize the wound. The wounds should be covered with an antiseptic dressing. If iodine is used it should not be used in excess. Depending on the urgency of transfer, formal debridement in an operating theatre may be necessary before commencing the transfer.

17.5.4 Phase four: transportation

Provided the patient has been meticulously investigated, stabilized and packaged (*Figure 17.2*) prior to setting off, transportation should be relatively straightforward, requiring few, if any, interventions en route. If there is any doubt about the patient's stability then the transfer should be delayed. Monitoring must be continuous throughout the transfer.

Sedation and paralysis should be optimized before departing, this will ensure that sudden movement, such as moving the trolley out of the vehicle or transferring the patient from trolley to bed, does not cause coughing or other movements, which may compromise the patient.

Most transfers in Great Britain take place using land ambulances. The environment is one of restricted movement in a confined space in a moving vehicle with limited access to the patient and temporary isolation from help, drugs and equipment. Vibration, noise and poor lighting affect practical procedures and interfere with the reliability of monitoring devices. An emergency vehicle travelling at high speed puts both the patient and staff at risk of death or serious injury. If there are significant problems during transfer the vehicle should be stopped and if staff have to get out, high visibility clothing and protective helmets must be worn. On any issue of safety the paramedic crew must be obeyed.

The senior medical attendant present should dictate the speed of travel, the aim is a smooth and steady ride, rather than fast and stop start – safety, not speed is paramount. The ambulance should be driven speedily on straight stretches of road, but slower around bends. The use of police escorts will be dictated by local policy and, if appropriate, these will be coordinated by the ambulance service control.

Staff should remain seated at all times and wear their seatbelts. If a member of staff has to undo their seatbelt to attend to the patient then they should inform the crew and kneel in the 'tripod position' rather than stand and sway. Vehicles should therefore be designed and equipped to provide an optimal transport environment and maximize the comfort and safety of both patients and staff.

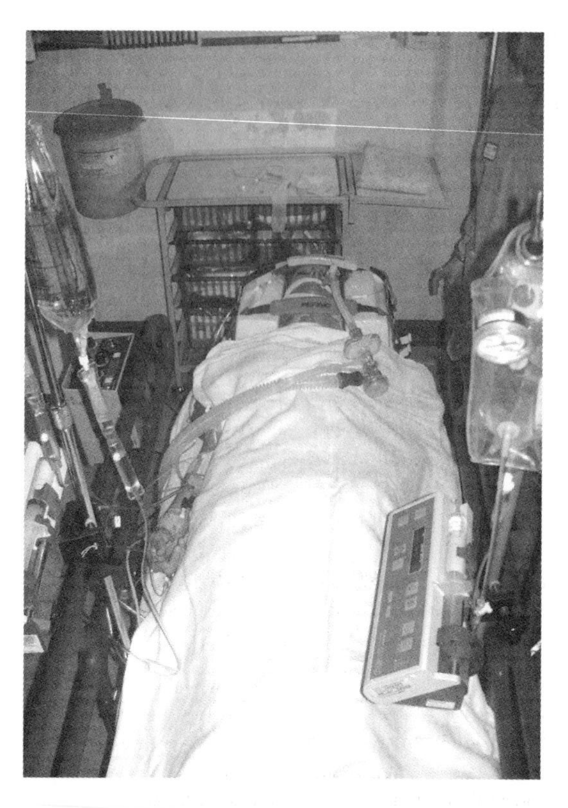

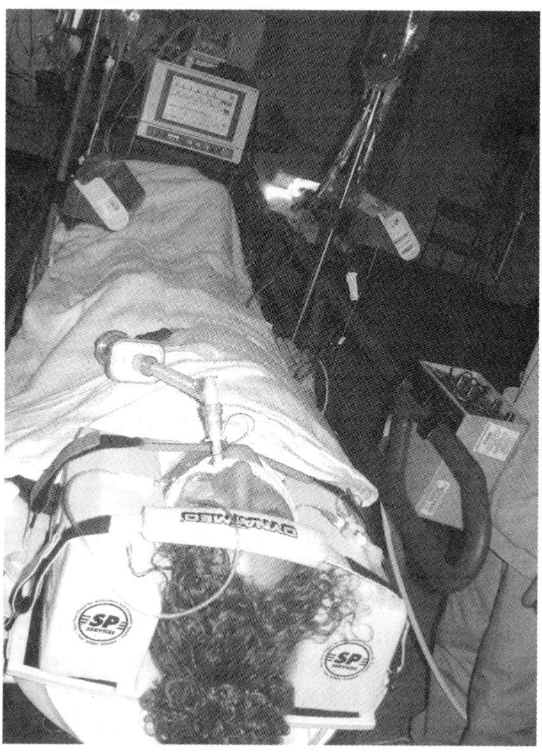

Figure 17.2 Packaging a patient for transfer

A continuous written record must be kept during the transfer, with particular reference to critical incidents.

The design considerations for intensive care land ambulances shown below in Box 17.8 are taken from the latest Intensive Care Society Guidelines for the transport of the critically ill adult.

BOX 17.8 Design considerations for intensive care land ambulances

Vehicle

- Driven by suitably trained personnel
- Able to carry up to four members of hospital staff in addition to ambulance crew
- Seats for staff should ideally be rear facing or forward facing (not side facing)
- Seats to be fitted with head restraints and three-point inertia reel seat belts
- Hydraulic ramp, winch or trolley system designed to enable single operator loading
- Patient trolley central mounted allowing all round patient access
- Stable comfortable ride with minimal noise and vibration levels
- Regular service and maintenance contracts

Services

- Standard 12-volt DC supply. In addition:
  240 V 50 Hz AC power supply from an inverter or generator (recommended minimum output 750 watts. This is generally sufficient to power a portable ventilator, monitor, and infusion pumps)
  Minimum of two standard 3 pin 13 amp outlet sockets in the cabin
- Minimum of two F size oxygen cylinders in secure housings
  Manifold system with automatic cylinder change over, and audible oxygen supply failure alarm
  Minimum of two wall mounted outlet valves for oxygen
  (Oxygen concentrators may be an alternative)
- Medical air supply is also desirable but the space required by additional cylinders or compressors may be a limiting factor
- Adequate lighting, heating, air conditioning, and humidity control

Equipment

- Mobile telephone to enable communication with referring/receiving hospital
- Defibrillator and suction equipment
- Adequate storage and stowage for ancillary equipment

An increasing number of secondary inter-hospital transfers are being carried out using helicopters. In some remote areas of Great Britain, for example, the Orkney Islands fixed wing aircraft are used. The transferring staff must understand how to approach and leave a helicopter safely. As a general rule, movements around the aircraft should not be undertaken when the rotors are still running. Staff should only approach a helicopter after receiving express permission to do so by the aircraft crew. They must at all times follow any instructions the aircrew may issue. A request for the use of a helicopter (civilian or military) should be made through ambulance control as it is the ambulance service who have the statutory responsibility to undertake the transfer.

17.5.5 Phase five: handover and return

Responsibility for the patient remains with the transfer team until an agreed time during handover at the receiving hospital. The handover should include a clear, concise verbal and written account of the patient's history, vital signs, therapeutic interventions and significant clinical events both prior to and during transfer. A template for a structured handover at the receiving hospital is recommended in Box 17.9.

BOX 17.9 Handover template

Immediate information

- Personnel: introduce yourselves
- Patient: introduce your patient
- Priority: indicate any major problem that needs immediate attention

Case presentation

- Presentation: mechanism and time of injury
- Problems: simple list of injuries and other major problems
- Procedures: simple list of major interventions and investigations
- Progress: system review
  - Respiratory (e.g. oxygenation and ventilator settings)
  - Circulatory (e.g. haemodynamic status and blood transfused
  - Nervous system (e.g. conscious level and sedation/paralysis)
  - Metabolic (e.g. urine output and glucose level)
  - Host defence (e.g. temperature, antibiotics and steroids)

After handing over, the transfer team may need a brief period of refreshment before returning back to their hospital. A debriefing session should be considered after complicated transfers. All transfers should be audited and a system for reporting critical incidents should be in place.

Do not forget to return with ALL the equipment you took with you!

17.6 Summary

With the increasing centralization of hospital services in the United Kingdom, the number of secondary transfers for victims of major trauma is likely to rise, unless there is a government mandate to introduce a network of regional trauma systems. If such a network were to be established, injured patients would be taken directly to a hospital specializing in their reception and ongoing care and the number of secondary transfers would then be significantly reduced. Until such time arises, the trauma team must ensure that any patient who requires transfer, for whatever reason, receives the optimal care using the system described above.

Websites

http://www.trauma.org/prehospital/index.html

This prehospital link covers a number of transfer related issues.

http://www.gov.ns.ca/health/ehs/air_ambulance.htm

There are numerous websites about air ambulance services. This is one of the better ones.

A number of professional associations such as the Intensive Care Society (http://www.ics.ac.uk/ICS.html) have transfer guidelines available on the web. The best require membership and passwords to view.

Further reading

1. **Advanced Life Support Group.** (2002) Safe Transfer and Retrieval. The Practical Approach. BMJ Publications, London.

Index